YOUR

POWER UP YOUR HEALTH

MIGHTY

IGNITE YOUR TRANSFORMATION

INNER

RECLAIM YOUR SELF

HEALER

———

NATY HOWARD

FOREWORD BY DON OSCAR MIRO-QUESADA

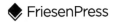
FriesenPress

Suite 300 - 990 Fort St
Victoria, BC, V8V 3K2
Canada

www.friesenpress.com

Email: info@natyhoward.com
Website: https://www.natyhoward.com
Editorial: Janet Matthews; www.janetmatthews.ca janet@janetmatthews.ca
Cover Design: Michele Davison

Disclaimer:
The contents of this book and all contents found at www.natyhoward.com website are for educational purposes only. You should consult your doctor prior to undertaking any dietary changes including juice fasting, cleansing or doing a detox. Naty Howard, Yoga Spirit Medicine, The Realign Ranch. and its contributors cannot be held liable for any damages that result from following any of the ideas presented on this book and on this website. As well, we will not assume any responsibility for any information or opinions posted on this website by any third party poster.

Attention:
Quantity discounts are available to your company, educational institution or writing organization for reselling, educational purposes, subscription incentives, gifts or fundraiser campaigns.
For bulk purchasing information please contact info@natyhoward.com.

FB— Yoga Spirit Medicine
IG— naty_howard
#YourMightyInnerHealer

ISBN
978-1-5255-5698-2 (Hardcover)
978-1-5255-5699-9 (Paperback)
978-1-5255-5700-2 (eBook)

1. HEALTH & FITNESS, HEALING

Distributed to the trade by The Ingram Book Company

ARE YOU READY

TO

UNLEASH

YOUR

MIGHTINESS?

"A powerful and unique book. Naty has drawn from ancient and modern sources and blended this knowledge with her own rich experience and personal wisdom to create a marvellous and inspirational journey back to wholeness. This book supports the reader to integrate powerful practices with the regenerative powers of Ayurvedic principles as they are applied in the use of high vitality foods and wild nutritional medicines. Written as a masterpiece and designed to take us deeply into the shamanic energetics of the plant world and nature to support the shift in consciousness."

— Shantree Kacera, R.H., D.N., Ph.D., Author of Ayurvedic Tongue Diagnosis and Founder and co-director of The Living Centre

---

"Coming from her own single-pointed journey towards healing, Naty creatively presents a multi-dimensional approach to becoming all that we are. Her passionate and honest voice reminds us of the profound link between physical healing and spiritual awakening, and she generously gives us an abundance of practical tools to bring it into our lives."

— Caroline Marie Dupont, M. Sc., Soul Coach & Holistic Nutritionist

---

"If you don't understand the absolute need to detox your body, increase your nutritional intake and develop a more integrated way of living in better balance within yourself as well as with the Earth, this book will set you on the right path of healing and wholeness. Enjoy and empower yourself to thriving and living raw and juicy!"

— Ingrid Cryns, Registered Psychotherapist and Eco Architect

"Naty's absolute intention to be a clear vessel in this world on all levels has allowed her to transform her difficult journey into a mastery that will assist you in your transformation through her gentle words in her amazing book-Your Mighty Inner Healer. Her story is one of hope, courage, remembrance, and transformation that will uplift your heart and encourage your soul."

— Cindy Mahealani Sellers-Founder Angel Farms Cleanse,
Author-You Don't Have to Hurt Anymore.
Speaker, recording artist, Nutritionist, Iridologist, Spiritual Healer

---

"Your Mighty Inner Healer brilliantly illumines how pivotal a plant based self-care approach to human spiritual evolution is and furthermore clearly discloses Naty's own courageous process of healing and Self-transformation. This book is a sacred gift to all who read it, a steadfast altruistic dedication to the Great Work, to the seven generations and a roadmap helping humankind re-Member its essential purpose for Being, which is to serve the entire web of life through teaching Love in the way we live."

— don Oscar Miro-Quesada, respected kamasqa curandero and altomisayoq adept from Peru, founder of The Heart of the Healer (THOTH), originator of Pachakuti Mesa Tradition cross-cultural shamanism.

"Naty Howard's book reads like a manifesto of her personal triumph over heavy metal toxicity and her journey towards balance and spiritual well being. By unpacking the healing modalities she encountered, she coaches and encourages you to find yours. Through the voice of her Mighty Inner Healer and the wisdom found in her personal process, she inspires you to take the risk to heal yourself."

— (Rev.) Andrew Blake, RP, Buddhist Chaplain & Psychotherapist

TABLE OF CONTENTS

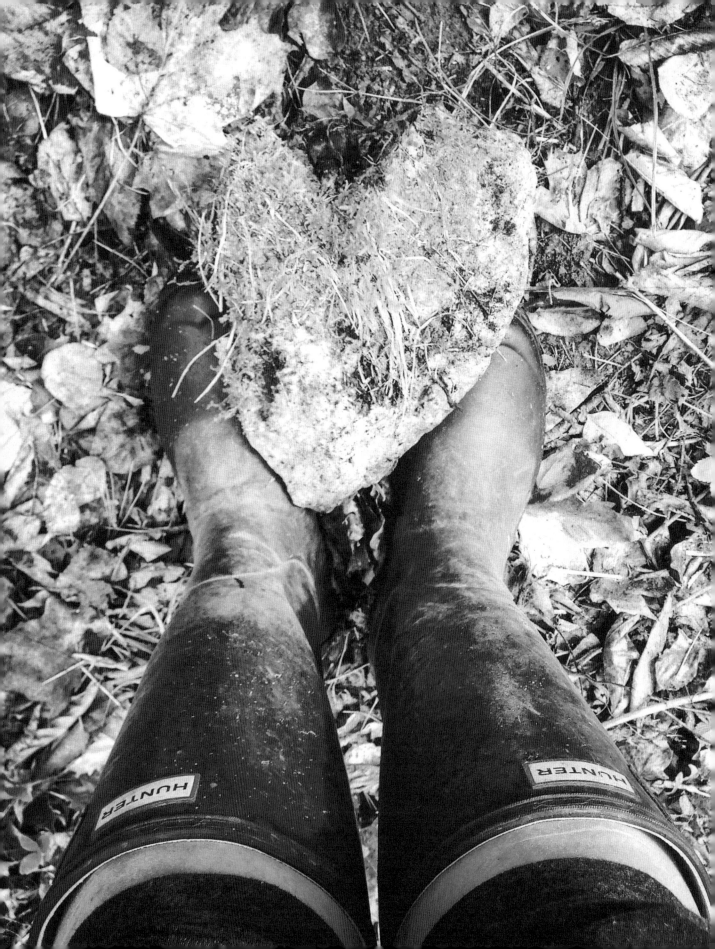

To the greatest challenge of my life, that brought me to my knees and became my greatest teacher, as it gifted me with the greatest deep healing journey of all:

The reclaiming of my self.
The awakening to my truth.
The anchoring deep into the earth, in service to you.

To the beautiful life that has blossomed by going in and through,
To the magic and the medicine that awakened me.

To you, for your courage to step into your own revolution as you reclaim not only your health, but your sense of belonging and your mightiness to be your best self going forward.

It's your road, and yours alone.
Others may walk it with you, but no one can
walk it for you.

— Rumi

FOREWORD

It is undeniable that increasing levels of toxicity on a global scale are insidiously impacting our inner and outer health. Our relationship to the ever evolving interdependent sacred web of life stands in delicate balance. The question is: How do we begin to clean up the current toxic mess contaminating our bodies, minds and planet? Finding an answer to this question may appear rather daunting except to those already engaged in the purifying and health restorative virtue of conscious breathing, of eating organic food, of daily juicing and weekly fasting, of gracefully lived synergy with the natural world, of flowing movement, dance, drumming, song, of embodied reverence and of gratitude empowered living as a whole.

Today, more than ever, we need courageous heart awakened and trusted consciousness expanding guides to help usher in a beneficent co-creative healing partnership between humankind and our natural world. My dear friend and shamanic soul ally Naty Howard is one of these luminous guides, a true shining light in the world. In her highly comprehensive and wisely practical book, *Your Mighty Inner Healer*, Naty has given poignant expression to how the health of our planet is inextricably connected to our personal and interpersonal lives—from the dietary choices we make to the human and non-human relationships we nurture and sustain.

The first time I met Naty I was struck by the peaceful fullness of her presence, the powerful stillness of her posture, the widely loving openness of her service disposition. All these personal attributes shine brightly throughout the pages of Your Mighty Inner Healer, in which she brilliantly discloses how pivotal a plant based self-care approach is to physical, emotional, mental and spiritual wellbeing. With the wisdom and dedication akin to an alchemist of old, Naty begins this ground breaking book with her own story of progressive liberation from the bodily ravages of environmental toxins we all now face in our daily living. She then offers her readers a meticulously user-friendly delectable banquet of self-care insights, mind-body practices and time proven natural remedies guaranteed to restore healthful wholeness in our lives.

In essence, this book is a genuine sacred gift to the world, a much needed dose of altruistic service to the Great Work, as well as a seven generation road map for our re-Membering as a spiritually awake human species born of Creation's dreaming. I thus pray this humble contribution of worded recognition and deserving praise for *Your Mighty Inner Healer* serves to wildly disseminate the adoption of its inherent wisdom beauty throughout our Four Directions—so mote it be!

don Oscar Miro-Quesada,
Originator of Pachakuti Mesa Tradition cross-cultural shamanism; Founder, The Heart of the Healer (THOTH)
www.heartofthehealer.org

DEAR WELLNESS WARRIOR:

The work works only when you work it. So, work it well. You are powerful beyond measure, and the depth of the healing you seek is equally seeking you, for life always wants to live and thrive.

This mighty book was born out of my own challenges when I discovered I was suffering from elevated heavy metal toxicity, causing numbing pain on the right side of my body. It is my gift to you, because I too have travelled my own pathway of deep healing into the inner space of source and sacredness. The teachings I found there are now a part of my everyday life, and are the teachings I share with you here, and through my own service into the world.

Amid your struggles and search, take a moment and be still. Now, in that place of stillness, imagine living your life radiantly healthy, in great harmony and balance. Breathe into that image of yourself and allow it to expand through every fibre of your body. This book is your pathway to manifesting that vision—to living as your most radiant, glowing, healthy, Mighty self. You are the hero of your own journey. It is up to you to rise above your challenges, in and through your conflicts, and reclaim yourself "alive" along the way.

I believe in your power to make it happen and, because I do, I have created this book to give you tools and practices for deep healing. They will assist you on your journey through your obstacles to your inner space of home, of wellness, and to connecting deeply with the source within. Throughout these pages, you will find inspiration and practical wisdom you can use today on topics that include:

- Foundations for health
- 13 tools, tips, and tricks for healthy gene expression
- 3 root causes of disease

- Multiple tools and practices to engage deep healing
- Wisdom on how to let your inner shine glow using liquid nutrition
- 108 liquid nutrition recipes to power up your health
- The ritual of detox including a one day guided Mighty detox
- The art of mindfulness, plus 13 practices
- The alchemy of inner questing, includes four self-inquiry exercises
- How to be your own revolution
- 18 tools to unleash your mightiness

As you begin to work your magic, you will be the recipient of the greatest of all medicines: a) an awakened heart, b) a glowing, radiant, healthy body in alignment with the nature of the cosmos, and c) the ability to anchor deeply into the Earth, as you engage through sacred action into the world.

This is a gift for you, so own it. Gift yourself with this opportunity to detoxify, repair, rebuild, rejuvenate, and regenerate. Begin to walk, breathe, move, and act in a way that is congruent with the emergence of your truest desires. Gift yourself with the possibility of healing deeply, beyond what may seem possible to you now, beyond what others may be claiming to be true for your state. Gift yourself with a radiant vision of you—already vibrantly healthy, already whole. And though healing is non-linear journey, take massive, imperfect, sustainable action towards your own wellness. I promise you the universe will conspire to assist you.

I *invite you to get a journal* that will serve you for your own process through this book. I invite you to take this opportunity to empower yourself as you heal deeply.

As you continue reading, I want you to really sink into this process; go slowly and take it one step at a time. I also want you to direct your attention inward. Take time to pause … and to reconnect with what's really in your heart. This will help you to realign with what matters most, and to find your *true north* once more.

It is my hope that you find a place of deep healing and refuge in this book. I hope that some of the tools and practices I share on these pages become tools and practices that allow you to power up your health, ignite your transformation, and spark your own revolution towards new vitality and radiant health. The ultimate goal of mighty is to allow you to manifest and project your best possible self into the world.

FORWARD OR, RATHER, INWARD

The journey of deep healing towards radiant health and ultimately personal revolution, can take many roads. The opportunity to rise up can present itself in the form of a challenge or health crisis that ultimately forces us to look into our hearts; for the answers lie within, and the wisdom we seek requires only an awakening. The seeds of our own potential destiny already reside in the space within our hearts, but most of us are too busy looking elsewhere for the love, compassion, and grace that we already are.

My own path to radiant health, or rather my path to reclaiming the fragmented pieces of my sacred self, arrived with the birth of our third son. Along with the joyous occasion of his arrival came the shock of an unexpected truth. I had become a toxic, ticking time bomb that was getting close to its last tick.

I didn't know it at the time, of course. I only knew that over those first couple of weeks, (always primal in its essence) where time seemed to stop and the boundaries of space seemed to merge in between worlds, after a new life had emerged from the depths of my being … the right side of my body had started to go painfully numb.

A long list of tests came and went. Tears and desperation came and stayed, along with a bundle of medications I refused to take. There was no apparent answer for what was happening. All the tests came back normal, for which I am to this day thankful. But the pain and numbness persisted, along with the bottles of pain medication that stared at me from across my kitchen counter. I was never one to take meds; my system is so sensitive that a simple Tylenol does a number on me. So I began to seek, to read, and to try to understand. As I attempted to find the wisdom within, my body started to speak. As it did, I began to slowly put the pieces of my broken map back together, and quite quickly realized they were leading me into my heart, into my own personal revolution, and the deepening of life as I knew it.

I started paying close attention to when this painful numbness was strongest. I was vegan already, but soon realized that when I ate anything cooked, especially oils, the pain was strongest. When I ate raw foods, it seemed the pain was not as strong. Once I had this realization, it was not hard to make the choice to eat only raw foods. At this point I became 100% raw vegan, and the numbness started to shift. After six months of eating this way, the numbness was gone entirely, and then everything changed: I discovered my brave new world. First I discovered the world and the power of *living nutrition*, but soon I was deeply humbled by the power of *liquid nutrition*.

I already had a habit of juicing. Throughout my pregnancy I had juiced daily. Raw juice was what I craved, every single day and sometimes night. But as I moved more and more into my brave new world, I began discovering the world of green smoothies, of wheatgrass juice, and elixirs. I discovered the world of building my immunity, and better assisting my body in the task of detoxification through regular juice fasts that would last between one and seven days. Then, in 2012, I heard the call to dive deeper: I did a forty-day juice fast alongside a deepening of my yoga and meditation practices. *Everything changed again*: alchemy found its way into my heart.

I have always believed our bodies have the ability to heal themselves. We just have to understand the language of their expression. And so I did, and came to decipher the code of my dis-ease, of my dis-harmony. At the time, I was living in the countryside just outside of Toronto, Canada. We had moved to the country in search of fresh air, forests, and a life in greater resonance with nature. What we didn't realize was that life in this particular place was not as picture-perfect as we had dreamt. Environmental toxicity is a bitch, and the consequences of our global total disregard for the environment caught up with me, just as they have caught up with many of you. On our country road were two sod farms that were endlessly spraying herbicides. We were there for seven years, and during that time five other sod farms opened up shop on our same long country road. By the time we left, the creek that crossed our backyard had begun turning fluorescent neon green with the chemical runoff.

I was angry at what was happening to me. I felt my body breaking down during that time, and as I read and read, I became more aware about the effects of chemical toxicity, both from the environment "out there," and from what we expose ourselves to personally in our home and work environments. I became angrier when I began to realize that my own toxic journey had indeed started long ago. Long before I had kids or moved to the country I had been a photojournalist. For fourteen years, I had worked in a darkroom using loads of chemicals, and even though we wore gloves and masks, the toxic impact of those chemicals still found its way into my bloodstream. Unbeknownst to me, my toxic body had become a ticking time bomb.

As an alchemist at heart, it was easy for me to realize how the perfect synergy between the photo chemicals, the environmental toxic exposure from the sod farms, and the anesthesia from a third C-section had sent my body into toxic overload, and caused this ticking time bomb to explode. The outer evidence was the painful numbness of the right side of my body.

My healing journey has been another process of great alchemy, this time a positive one. As such, it led me into a process of falling in love with life all over again, a process of remembrance, of awakening to the inner sacred space of the heart and its expression in the form of right action in sacred reciprocity to the world.

My journey has also been a process of necessarily turning my anger into a source of empowerment so I could move forward into the brave new world I had discovered. It was as if a vortex had opened, and with it came many a long night. Yet when I awoke, it was to greater clarity and a greater awareness about the nature of my path.

The power of living and liquid nutrition began to remove the veils of separation between my body, my physical life, and my greater body: Mother Earth. I began to study Ayurveda and, as I did, the universal laws of interrelationship and interconnectedness became clear. The toxicity that was running through me is at present running through all rivers on this planet, and is in the process of destroying all life on Earth. This opportunity allowed me to deepen my wisdom of permaculture[1] and forest gardening and tap into the magic, the medicine, and the mysticism of shamanic, yogic, and Vedic traditions. In so doing, they have expanded my heart and my life, and fuelled the emergence of my own becoming.

This is a journey forward, or rather, inward—very much like a spiral. My challenge has become both my greatest teacher and the spark that ignited my personal revolution. The cracks in our hearts show us the path of involution, for the fragmented pieces of our sacred self must reunite deep within the inner space of the heart, in order for us to access the cognitive memory where all lives. Where the actions and non-actions of our ancestors reside, awaiting our remembering, enabling us to move beyond the stories that have shaped us, to a place where we can consciously create our own stories. This sacred reciprocity is a gift to the seven generations that will come after us, and beyond us.

As the saying goes, there is no magical pill, but there is a magical process.

---

1   Permaculture: "an agricultural system or method that seeks to integrate human activity with natural surroundings so as to create highly efficient self-sustaining ecosystems." Merriam-Webster Dictionary.

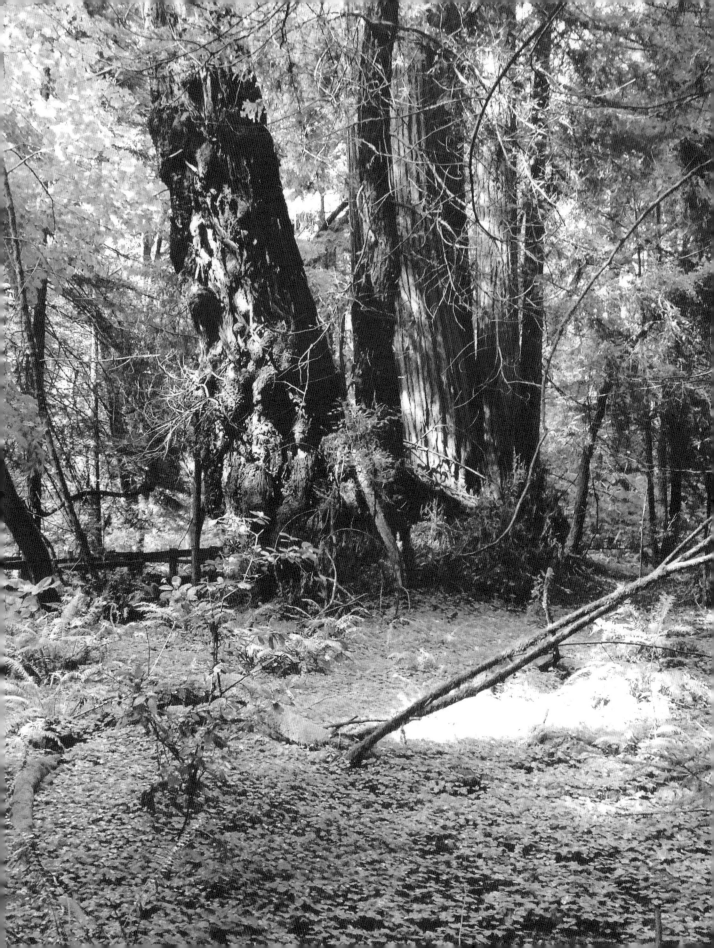

I

FOUNDATIONS FOR HEALTH

KNOWING YOURSELF IS THE BEGINNING OF
ALL WISDOM.

—ARISTOTLE

THE SYNERGY OF ALCHEMY

al·che·my /ˈalkəmēſ²

noun

1. *the medieval forerunner of chemistry, based on the supposed transformation of matter. It was concerned particularly with attempts to convert base metals into gold or to find a universal elixir.*
2. *a seemingly magical process of transformation, creation, or combination.*

Alchemy is a form of chemistry and speculative philosophy practised in the Middle Ages and the Renaissance and concerned principally with discovering methods for transmuting base metals into gold and with finding a universal solvent and an elixir of life.

The power of alchemy lays in its seemingly magical quality to transform matter. The mysterious philosopher's stone is, in fact, alchemy. The elusive missing piece to the philosopher's stone is *synergy*.

The *Oxford English Dictionary* defines synergy as: "the interaction or cooperation of two or more organizations, substances, or other agents to produce a combined effect greater than the sum of their separate effects."

For me, the logarithm for the *synergy of alchemy*, and one I have used over and over is quite simple:

$$2 + 2 = 10$$

Don't tell me you didn't learn that at school? Well, quite honestly, I didn't learn it at school either. I learned it through living. But I'm sure you did learn this one at school:

"The whole is greater than the sum of its parts"—Aristotle.

Well, that one my friend, is *synergy*.

In my world, synergy is required to make alchemy happen. So yes, 2 + 2=10, and this brave new world and this book are full of it.

---

2   "Alchemy," Oxford English Dictionary.

The synergy of alchemy allows us to combine tools and practices for deep transformation from dense levels of existence into radiant, golden, Mighty ones. I refer to tools such as liquid nutrition, detox, mindfulness, and inner questing as the keys to becoming whole again, radiantly healthy with a peaceful mind and a joyful heart, fully engaged in *sacred action*.

THE ALCHEMY OF WELLNESS

Remember that wherever your heart is, there you will find your treasure.

—*Paulo Coelho*

Wellness is more than just the physical expression of beauty and well-being that we seek. Wellness is activating the magnetism innate in living a soul-based life. Wellness is activating our ancestral memory to lead a life aligned with the Earth and the world around us. Wellness is activating the life-force energy that moves through us that is life, light, and love. Wellness is congruent action that comes from living from our highest potential. Wellness is our birthright as much as our duty, for the world needs your highest expression, and this life is but a precious gift providing an opportunity to seek it.

The journey towards wellness and radiant health is really a journey of alignment with wellness and radiant health, and with that space that already exists within us—for we are already whole. The journey of gathering the fragmented pieces of our selves through our heart connects us to our sacredness. The process of embodiment of our true nature and the emergence of our sacred heart consciousness are our compass, as we allow our inner light to shine down on our path towards unleashing our **mightiness**.

The power of radiant health lies not just in itself, but rather in its ability to spark our own evolution and be our inner map towards the self, and the road to our awakening to the wisdom of being Earth citizens.

Radiant health is the power you and I have to change what no longer serves us, and create new paths of peace in this brave new world. It is a path to making peace with your self, your body, your mind, your family, your culture, your community, your ecology, and ultimately with the God of your own understanding.

The alchemy of wellness has the power to activate your greatest potential and spark your own process of revolution, or rather involution, as you seek to express your own personal truths and your soul's purpose into the world. It demands that you take massive, imperfect sustainable action, for wellness is your birthright, and living in alignment with alchemy is your gateway to wholeness and happiness.

The future is calling, and the way forward is greatly supported by opening our hearts to the ancient. The ancient whispers and the future calls, and somewhere in between the spaces of your heartbeat, *you awaken to your own Mighty personal power for healing.*

FOUNDATIONS FOR HEALTH

But the real secret to lifelong good health is actually the opposite: Let your body take care of you.

—Deepak Chopra

Good health is something many people take for granted, something you think and hope will always be available. Until you find yourself suddenly without it.

Some of us awaken to the necessity of building a stronger foundation for health from a challenge or a crisis, of perhaps being brought to our knees. Others awakened to this necessity as a key tool into finding the expression of health and well-being we desire.

In whichever way you have awakened and arrived at this place, I honour your path, I honour you, and I invite you to bring a deeper sense of awareness to your process. I invite you to step into this brave new world with the curiosity of a child, open and willing to seeking new depths and levels of well-being.

Our foundation can only stand as strong as the roots that hold it. We are multidimensional beings and, as such, our foundation is also multidimensional. We must address each of the roots that make up our foundation to ensure they are strong and sustainable, and will allow us to rise and shine our light into the world through self-sustainable practices.

Our Foundation for Health has Five Roots

1. *Root down into the physical body and your greater body, Mother Earth,* through eating a light diet high in whole foods and fresh raw living foods that are life-generating, life-sustaining, and grown through authentic, sustainable, organic, soil-rejuvenative practices. Such a diet is composed of minimally processed living foods that are rich in minerals, friendly bacteria, and phytonutrients.

   You root down into your physical body by nourishing it with liquid nutrition, by claiming your magic and your mightiness through the ritual of detox and activating the cell memory of wellness within you.

2. *Root down into the emotional body* through mindfulness in stillness and in movement practices, deep breathing exercises, and self-inquiry practices that bring you back into the feeling body, into living with an open heart.

   You root down into the emotional body by engaging in life-supporting, regenerating practices of self-care, care of others, community, social relationships, and your relationship to spirit. You do this by instilling practices that facilitate the emergence of your true nature, that allow you to tap into your true self, and that allow you to live with an open heart.

3. *Root down into the mental body* through mindfulness practices that open you up to inner space of stillness, that anchor the mind in the body and allow you to connect to your higher mind beyond the ego. You do so by instilling practices that allow you to connect with grace, and with the God of your own understanding.

4. *Root down into the soul body* through alignment of body, heart, and mind, and the practices that keep you in alignment with your true self and raise your consciousness. You remember you are a soul having a human experience and reclaim your soul's mission, always benevolent by nature and always in service to others.

   You root down into the soul body through creating sacred space and stillness within, as well as through ritual and ceremony offered in sacred reciprocity. As you trust in the universal intelligence that created us, and in the awareness that we are part of a spiritual evolution of life on Earth, you will continue to anchor into your soul body.

5. ***Root down into the spirit body.*** As you root down into the soul body, you begin to rise towards spirit and, once you ignite your connection to the above, you begin to root down into the Earth so deeply as you *revolution* yourself alive.

   You root down into the spirit body through sacred reverent action, gratitude, and developing your spiritual practices. You anchor deeply into the spirit body through the ritual of detox, consistent and committed mindfulness practices, inner questing, and through committing to your own process of awakening.

Through developing and strengthening your five roots, you will be truly able to build a strong foundation for health, one that is not just simply living without symptoms of disease. The expression of optimal radiant health we seek begins and ends with the health of our physical cellular systems, and the health of our five bodies.

Good health of the physical body is necessary for us to host the health of the heart, mind, soul, and spirit we seek. But, it's often the challenges of the physical body that bring us to the awareness of the need to do the work around healing our heart, emotions, mind, and thoughts to create a more intimate and healthy relationship with our true self (soul) and spirit.

The stability of your foundation for health can only be as strong as the five roots that hold it. The flexibility of your foundation for health is directly connected to the depth and malleability of roots of the system.

Life expresses itself through laws, patterns, and systems. The alignment with the expression of health and wellness that you seek will require you to learn about your own system, and the remembering of the pattern of your true nature in alignment with the laws of nature.

ROOT CAUSES OF DISEASE

We cannot solve our problems with the same thinking we used when we created them.

—Albert Einstein

Root Cause #1: The misuse of your senses

Are your senses in charge of your body complex? Or is your high spiritual self or soul the master of your being? Have you developed enough awareness to bear witness to your body's sensorial feedback of how a particular experience makes you feel? Or do you keep putting your hands into the fire, hoping **this** time you won't get burned?

Your senses are constantly engaging with the world, and your body is constantly providing feedback about how this interaction makes you feel. Does the experience support your body? Does it nourish your nervous system? Does it leave you drained and fatigued? Does eating a particular food cause or exacerbate the eczema that is plaguing you? Are you still eating that food? You get my point.

Root Cause #2: Crime against your wisdom

Are you connected to your inner wisdom, your inner compass that can guide you through a healthier engagement with life? Or are you just running on autopilot and unable to hear the guidance of this inner wisdom above your thinking, ego mind, and the luring of the senses?

An understanding of Ayurveda—the healing science of life or conscious living that comes from the Vedic Hindu system (Part II, pg. 45)— can help guide you back into your wisdom, into being in alignment with the laws of nature. Once in alignment, you are now free to create and shape your body complex into the best sacred vessel you can possibly create, to allow the laws of nature to be expressed in a way that can lead to happiness, rather than disease. The pathway to reconnect with your inner wisdom develops the calibre of your character, your intuitive awareness of self, and your ability to hear and respond to that inner wisdom.

Root Cause #3: Time in motion

Excessive activity in the mind will cause you to age more quickly, and disturbances of the mind will actually cause you to age the fastest. Developing the ability to remain calm is vital to your healthy longevity; developing your ability to remain calm in the midst of trauma is key to your daily health, and will lead towards healthy longevity.

When you can get your Prana (life-force) centred in your being, you can begin to slow both time and the motion of time. This allows you to ground, heal deeply, pause and feel, and make conscious decisions in alignment with your Dharma (soul purpose) that lead to conscious sacred action, which will lead you further into happiness, and away from suffering.

The root cause of the three root causes: forgetting your primordial nature.

KISSING THE GROUND RUNNING

The strength of my Soul was born on the backs of moments that brought me to my knees.

—S.L. Heaton

Have you ever been brought down to your knees?
Have you ever kissed the ground running?
Have you ever been challenged so deeply that every fibre of your body has been shattered into a million pieces?
Has your heart ever been cracked wide open?

We lead busy lives today, lives disconnected from our selves and from *one another*. We have forgotten that we live in a world of systems, laws, and constant creation.

Massive numbers of people worldwide are kissing the ground running. Yet, we are also waking up to the ancient wisdom of deep nourishment, of right action to self and other, and of what it means to live in sacred reciprocity.

We are waking up to the sustainable systems we must put in place again, not only for our own individual survival, but for the survival of our species.

There are good reasons today why our bodies begin to fail. The system within has been inundated with as much toxicity and pollution as the environment around us, and our bodies can no longer sustain good health and well-being. The more we educate ourselves, the more we rebuild our inner systems, the more we show up fully for ourselves, the more we will begin to transform the challenge, we allow it to become our greatest teacher.

I know it can be tough. I know it can be frightening. But I also know that it's through the cracks in my heart that the light has come in. I know that as I begun to surrender to its call to deepen, change and evolve, my fall became a kiss, rather than a full impact crash-bang-Boom!

*If you are **kissing the ground running**, know that you have options. Know that you are powerful beyond measure and that you have the tools to not only transform your challenge but also begin to thrive again.*

DETOX, SHMETOX … OR MAYBE NOT?

If you don't take care of this the most magnificent machine that you will ever be given … where are you going to live?

—*Karyn Calabrese*

Detox.

It's a powerful word with such a vast meaning. Our great-grandparents never heard of it.
But you and I had better hear it, understand it, and do something with it.
Everything in the world exists in relationship. This is a universal law. Period.

Our external environment has become toxic and polluted with a vast array of chemicals, garbage, pesticides, herbicides, and plastics, due mainly to unaware human action, rooted more and more in greed. Because the universe we live in operates according to laws, your body and mine have now become a mere reflection of the state of affairs of this external environment, of our world.

The macrocosm is a reflection of the microcosm and vice versa. And though some efforts are being taken to reduce, recycle, and clean up our act in our immediate environment, we are **now** being asked (or rather demanded) to do the same in our inner temples.

We, as humans, have never before experienced the high levels of toxicity we are living with today. We've also never experienced the pandemic of disease we are experiencing today, either. As individuals, we can continue to turn a blind eye to it, or we can begin to take action towards healing our bodies, therefore healing our world, too.

Detox is not just a tool. It is a key step in our very survival. But in my world, I don't want to just survive, I want to **thrive**.

In today's world, it is key that you detoxify your system and allow your body to rebuild, regenerate, and rejuvenate. The good news is we live in this brave new world where you have access to amazing information, tools, and practices to do it safely, and in a way that will boost your whole system into thrive mode.

I invite you to find inspiration on these pages; to try the recipes, to seek new recipes, and to initiate some radical self-loving! I invite you to make it your intention to detoxify so you can *ignite your healing, transform your life,* and *spark your own revolution* into the best possible person you can be. Your *potential* and your *mightiness* await!

TOXICITY

It is no measure of health to be well adjusted to a profoundly sick society.

—*Jiddu Krishnamurti*

You and I have become toxic people, wandering without direction. We have lost our connection with our true north and to the land that sustains us, and along the way we've picked up all the garbage there was to pick up—the more the merrier.

You and I are full—oh so full—of this toxicity that has learned to hide in the dark corners of our bodies. This toxicity has found its way into our water, the air we breathe, the food we eat, and the soil upon which we rest our feet. It learned that our vision was limited and we did not see far enough into the future to understand the consequences of our actions. It learned to evolve, (for in life nothing is static) and now here we are: walking-talking-breathing-ticking-tacking time-bombs at your service, exploding every second with this or that disease.

Toxicity is the *missing well-known link to our current health crisis*, yet it is not really a missing link; it is, rather, a well-known fact, a causality of our current health crisis that's been proven by many. Many people prefer to just keep on avoiding the subject, hoping it will simply wash away and they can continue with "business as usual." But the reality is quite different. Toxicity in our environment has been proven to be responsible for driving animals into extinction. It has created more erratic weather patterns. In our bodies, the chemotoxic overload has been proven to break down the genetic communication system, rendering it unable to perform its code of conduct. So we mutate, we grow and expand in other ways, for life will find a way. It always wants to live and thrive, even at its own cost.

Toxicity was created first by ignorance, and then by mankind's lack of personal and ethical responsibility. Perhaps at the beginning of the Industrial Revolution, when changes began happening too fast to be able to cope with the increasing demand, men did not stop to think of the consequences. But now, now that science has proven the harmful cause-and-effect relationship between chemical pesticide and herbicide use, food colouring, additives, and preservatives used in manufactured food products, the toxic overload of greenhouse gas on our atmosphere, the toxic overload of the oil industry on our waters, the toxic overload of our consumerism society… Will we still try to deny its effect on our health and well-being? Are we still capable of looking away, as if it can never affect us?

Dear Mighty healer, we just don't have the time, nor do we have the global wellness to ignore it anymore.

The high toxicity levels being experienced today in the world at large are also being experienced within your physical body. Every food latent with chemical residues, food colouring, and genetically modified organism (GMO) manipulation will create a toxic build-up within your system. Every breath of air that is tainted with chemical or particulate pollution will add to that toxic build-up within your system. Every cell that is permeated with water latent with nitrogen, phosphorus, mercury, and so on, will create a toxic build-up within you and me. As you can see, these sources of toxicity are not hard to find—they are everywhere. You and I are bombarded with them from all directions, and our bodies are trying to cope as best they can.

When toxicity accumulates within our system, our body begins to break down. This is simply cause and effect, and logical. The problem is, most people have not yet made the connection between the expression of disease in their body and the levels of toxicity that have accumulated in that body through years of constant exposure. From the lead in our lipstick to the bleach used in our toilet paper and tampons, and everywhere in between. Yes, all that toxic garbage finds its way into our precious blood stream.

When our body's natural detoxification processes can no longer bear the burden, our cells and organs begin to accumulate and store this toxicity. In a desperate effort to clean house, our over-taxed system begins to burn our enzyme reserves. Our liver and kidneys begin working double shifts, without a break, or they simply shut down. Our energy begins to decrease, and we're often tired. We experience pain. We take drugs to relieve ourselves of this pain, creating more toxicity and masking the pain. But this pain is actually our body trying to tell us, indeed, yell at us … **you have a problem!** That we have fallen out of alignment, that we've lost our rhythm, that we've lost the integrity of our system and we're falling apart. But because we have lost our intimacy with our body, we don't usually get the message. We further detach ourselves from the problem. We take more drugs, which then begin to conflict with one another, creating a deeper state of imbalance and increasing the toxic load.

And that's just what is happening on the physical level. When your physical body becomes toxic, your whole-body system experiences it. Your mind, emotions, thoughts, and clarity of thinking, intentions, problem-solving ability, and hope for the future are all influenced by the toxic state of your physical body, as is your connection to your true spiritual self, and to your source.

Sometimes it is this very crisis of toxicity that will send us forward on our journey of realignment and deepening. It will ask you, as it asked me, to push beyond the existing boundaries of your diagnosis as you seek first to educate your self, and then, armed with new information, make your way to the very edge of both new and ancient wisdom—your brave new world. Here you will find tools, practices, and protocols that can support and ignite your healing in ways that are simply not available in your current belief system. This very crisis in toxicity will become your teacher, your guide into health and wellness, as you learn to create the right conditions to thrive.

MINERAL DEFICIENCIES

You can trace every sickness, every disease, and every ailment, ultimately, to a mineral deficiency.

—Dr. Linus Pauling, winner of two Nobel Prizes.

Mineral Deficiencies are the other missing, well-known link to our current health crisis. We all know about the importance of having enough mineral density in our body for proper function. Few of us realize the effects low density highly processed foods have in our body and the havoc mineral deficiencies cause in our well-being. We also know that if we eat a diet rich in mineral dense whole foods, we provide our body with the optimal fuel for health and deep healing. Mineral dense whole foods facilitate the appropriate mineralization within the body to create healthy and optimal gene expression, which protects us and our animal friends from disease.

So, as you can see, when you provide your body with highly mineralized, authentically grown organic foods, you can effectively turn on healthy and optimal gene expression in your own body. By consuming these kinds of foods, you can change the current terrain of your body to an optimal terrain, making it harder for disease to exist. It's easy to check the quality of your terrain by monitoring your pH values with a simple litmus strip (find more about this on pg. 95). When our pH is more alkaline, our systems are working most effectively and our terrain is in optimal, radiant health.

Minerals are needed for proper electromagnetic communication at a cellular level. They help reorganize and heal our DNA structures, and their frequencies. Minerals are needed for all levels of intra and extracellular communication and repair within our DNA.

Optimal mineralization at an intracellular level is key to optimal Radiant Health. Often, we expect to simply have radiant health, without finding the deep-rooted awareness that the health of our whole multidimensional body depends heavily on our cellular health.

Let's hold that thought for a moment as we go back to how we have become mineral-deficient in the first place, because this is not happening to just a few people here and there. This has become a global problem. Humans have become mineral-deficient.

One simple question might just answer our why … who is the new king of the world?

Any guesses?

Answer: The new king of the world is (drum roll, please…) ***convenience***—a.k.a. fast and processed foods, and their ultimate delivery system, ***the drive-thru.***

It's our habit of living fast and processed lives, away from nature (which has served us for so long) that has now caused us to forget our own true nature.

I have two more questions for you:

Where do we see more disease in the world?

Answer: In countries where the new king of the world, convenience, rules supreme.

And, last but not least … who is the new jester to the new king of the world?

Any wild guesses this time?

The answer is ***our own lack of awareness,*** our own ignorance and blind trust in the institutions, agencies, and government systems that were created to protect us and the quality and integrity of our health. This ignorance has been facilitated by the breaking down of our ancestral communities, along with the lineages that held and passed down the ancestral wisdom of our interconnectedness to all of life, and our interrelationship with all beings.

Sad, I know, and troubling, too. But it's extremely important to understand what has happened, because this allows you to seek the answers. To become aware. To reclaim your health, your vitality, your ancestral wisdom, and ultimately your freedom.

It makes sense that if our food is grown in mineral-deficient soil, it's only a matter of time before you and I are also mineral-deficient. But now it gets a bit more complicated. The food that most of us are eating is not just whole food grown in poor, mineral-deficient soils. The food most of us are eating has been so greatly modified it barely resembles food at all anymore. All sorts of chemical agents and food colourings have been added to our foods, along with ample amounts of harmful salts and sugars and unhealthy processed oils. Sadly, our bodies cannot recognize many of these ingredients, and have begun breaking down in their desperate attempts to digest them. With no way to either digest or eliminate these ingredients, our body then gives up and stores them away, deep into our cells, as toxicity. Then, when they come back out to play, well … it's not pretty.

The more a food is processed, the more we are changing its molecular structure away from the living systems code that our body understands so well. The further we remove ourselves from whole, natural, organically grown, minimally processed foods, the further you and I are taking our body away from radiant vibrant health.

The problem becomes this: how can we re-mineralize our body in order to return to radiant, vital, glowing health, if the soil in which our food is grown is mineral-deficient and toxic with chemicals? How can we gain access to these building blocks of health?

How did this happen in the first place? Was it just a minor oversight? It happened with the break in our ancestral lineages through war, occupation, and power domination. It happened when we no longer received and passed down our ancestral wisdom—that we are a part of the earth, and the earth is a part of us. As our lineages broke down, so did the wisdom of our ancestry. As these lineages, along with the bonds that connected us deeply to our roots of the five bodies, began breaking down, we began to forget; we began to fragment, and to lose our connection to our soul, to our source, and to our sacredness. We began to be at war with the earth, with the world, and ultimately with ourselves.

We no longer remember who we are. We no longer remember our natural rhythms and our essential nature. We no longer know how to thrive. We no longer know how to care and nourish ourselves deeply.

So these mineral deficiencies are not just in our physical bodies. We are deficient in all five bodies—physical, emotional, mental, soul and spirit bodies. We have become deficient in our hearts, for most of us live with a closed heart, unable to process our emotions, and unable to see ourselves in the eyes of the other. We have become deficient in our minds, for most of us live from a place of ego, and the subconscious mind is running the show. We have become deficient in our souls, for we have forgotten that our soul's purpose must be for the benefit of the all. We have become deficient in our spirit, for most of us have forgotten our connection to the pulse of life that causes our heart to beat, the part that is far greater than our body.

Key to our survival is the feeding or nourishing of all five roots (pg. 8) that sustain the five bodies so necessary for our well-being. Key to our survival is the reclaiming of the fragmented pieces of ourselves in order to reclaim our wholeness. We live in a world that is interrelated and interconnected; this is an immutable universal law.

So, where do we begin?

How do we begin to heal ourselves and our mineral deficiencies?

REMINERALIZATION IN THE 21ST CENTURY

Many things can prolong your life, but only wisdom can save it.

—Neel Burton

Today, more than ever before, we are experiencing the consequences of decades of ecological irresponsibility and ancestral wounding. You and I are feeling it, both in our minds and in our bodies, through our lack of personal connection to place, to each other, to the Earth, to spirit, and to our true nature.

There is a direct link between the state of our external environment, and the state of your internal one. The high rates of degenerative diseases—such as diabetes, cancer, auto immune diseases and so on—are not a coincidence or some random act of disease manifestation. They are a direct consequence of the toxic pollution in our environment, in the foods we eat, in the air we breathe, in the water we drink and bathe in, in the emotional imbalances we are experiencing, and in the high-stress environments we have created to work and live in. Today's rapid lifestyle leads to rapid (empty) solutions without much thought given to the need for deep cellular nourishment, nor to the nourishment of our soul. All of this is part of our lives in this twenty-first century, and is a direct causative factor in why so many people are so sick.

The forgetting of our ancestral wisdom through our ancestral wounding has given rise to living without the self-care and heart-nourishing practices that kept us connected to the land and to our hearts, that kept our minds in the present moment of creation, and that kept us in the awareness of our soul and our deep connection to spirit.

The proof exists; our soil is depleted, and our food no longer contains the depth and array of mineral and vitamin content that we need to thrive. The fruits and vegetables that travel to us from faraway lands are often sprayed with all sorts of chemicals to make bringing them across our border safe for our country.

But they look beautiful, so we eat them, along with all those chemicals. Sadly, our bodies don't know what to do with that heavy chemical overload. Yes. It IS overload. Your immune system suffers and you suffer. But as consumers, we remain in the dark as to what's really going on in our food supply, to what is really going on in our immediate and not so immediate environments. We are at a critical point where we can no longer ignore the elephant in the room; it's happening now globally, and people are getting sicker worldwide.

Our lack of emotional processing tools, our lack of mindfulness practices, and our spiritual void are equally powerful players contributing to the lack of health of our systems.

The number one tool for regaining our health, for regaining our sanity, our vitality, and our strength is *remineralization*. It is key to our longevity. Re-establishing our alkaline balance is the best way to reverse disease, to decrease inflammation, to regain our vitality, and to remember, at a DNA and cellular level, the wisdom that already exists within us. You and I have the ability to be a part of the solution. We have the ability to be a part of the shift and the change towards the regeneration of our soils, of our self, of our immediate environment and the world at large. We just have to start.

When you re-mineralize yourself, you are building your alkaline powers while both detoxifying and rejuvenating your whole-body system. You begin to feel better, you begin to shift both externally and internally, and you begin to understand, through experience, just how important this is for your longevity, and for the quality of your daily experience of life.

The fastest way to re-mineralize your body system is to include liquid nutrition in your daily life, clean up your diet so as to include a high intake of whole foods and living-plant-based nutrition and to reclaim your ancestral wisdom. Liquid nutrition is the essence of food—minerals and life-force energy—in a jar. A clean diet further assists in the healing and well-being of the body as it is alkaline forming and supports the body in its detox efforts and remineralization of the whole system. You are infusing and basking your whole body in exactly what it needs: minerals to cleanse and rebuild and life-force energy to re-establish coherence in your body, which will in turn awaken the seed of ancestral wisdom within you.

Reclaiming your ancestral wisdom is a journey best supported by mindfulness practices and by staying connected with our hearts through what I like to call the alchemy of inner questing. The process itself awakens in you the wisdom to live in balance, harmony, and sacred reciprocity. It also re-establishes coherent patterns of being by aligning your true essential nature with the natural laws of the universe.

By rooting down into the physical, emotional, mental, soul and spirit bodies, we create a stronger foundation for health. Our roadmap to wellness is through r**emineralization at the root level of our system.**

A CLEAN DIET

I choose to make the rest of my life the best of my life.

—*Louise L. Hay*

A clean diet is a diet that is pure, *rich in whole foods, and raw, living-plant-based nutrition;* it is a powerful solution in today's health crisis and it will lead to the awakening of your true primordial nature.

Its power is based on the understanding of the effects and deep awareness of how food affects your body complex, taking into consideration the alkaline/acid properties of food, the subtle energetic properties of food, the understanding that nourishment is provided to the body through your senses, and that food is more than the material form of that which you put in your mouth.

A key aspect of a clean diet is the biogenetic diet, which is composed of 30-50% life building, regenerating (bioactive) foods; and 50-70% life sustaining foods high in enzymes. It also includes up to 25% bio-acidic foods as a transition into a high plant-based diet, or as part of a high raw-living-food diet.

A clean diet:

- Is rich in whole, fresh, sun-ripened, enzyme-rich, organic plant foods.
- Consists of food that is alkaline building.
- Consists of food grown through authentic, organic farming practices, as local as possible.
- Emphasizes the biogenetic diet.
- Reflects a proper balance of the six tastes: salty, sweet, sour, pungent, bitter, and astringent. Sweet is the taste your body uses for rejuvenation; bitter and astringent are used for detoxification and purification.
- Includes alignment of proper portions of food according to your needs, proper food quality, proper eating attitude, proper time for eating, proper regime for eating, proper food combination for your constitution, time, and season, and proper preparation of food.
- Advocates that your main meal is usually at noon. Your last meal is best before sunset.

- Requires special attention be given to preparing a meal in order to enhance its quality with love and awareness.
- Builds on the power of resonance between the food you eat and its healing, building, rejuvenative, and regenerative powers.
- Is high in life-force. Takes into consideration the energetics of food, rather than just the conventional nutritional systems.
- Minimizes violence.
- Is light in essence: light eating and light natural food promote lightness of being and easy digestion, providing abundant energy.

A clean diet promotes:

- Health, vitality, endurance, calm, clarity, longevity, peace, love, joy, and spiritual inspiration.
- Purification of your bodily system. Deep detoxification and the rebuilding, regeneration and rejuvenation of your body's mental, emotional, and spiritual levels.
- Self-discovery and self-transformation.
- Your understanding and felt-experience of cosmic energy and your spiritual awareness.
- Strengthening the bio-electricity of your cells in a way that increases individual electrical potential, thus enhancing and strengthening your health, your electroluminescence, and your own life-force energy.
- Building your subtle organizing energy fields (SOEFs) (more on this on page 65).
- Organizing and rebuilding your body complex in harmony with the universal resonance of peace.
- The flow of the spiritualizing force in your body.
- Understanding diet as a way of consciously relating to the world.

A clean diet supports and sustains:

- Your meditation and spiritual practices.
- The alignment of your body, emotions, mind, and soul into a unified complex system.
- Your reconnection and alignment with your personal rhythms, rhythms of nature, natural forces, and universal laws.
- Your reconnection with Mother Earth, your soul's life purpose, and your inner ecology, and re-sensitizes you to be, act, think, and do in harmony with Mother Earth and all creation.
- The expansion of your awareness and consciousness from individual to global to universal being.

- Your becoming aware of the gift that is your life, and that an act of love really is to be of service to humanity.
- Your understanding of diet as lifestyle, and of lifestyle as a way of reclaiming your power and influence in the world.

A clean diet and lifestyle in today's world is key to:

- Balancing your body complex, attaining optimal health and longevity as you ignite your Mighty inner healer. The fast-paced, over-acidic-producing, chemical roller coaster ride of a life that has become the norm in today's world will drive you fast and furiously straight to the grave, without any grace.
- Reminding you to create purity within your body complex, through purification and cleansing practices, in addition to the power of growing, preparing, and eating your foods with spiritual awareness.
- Bringing coherence into your life as you shine your light into the world, creating peace, awareness, and consciousness within your life and the lives of those around you. It offers the tools you need to reach self-realization and enlightenment.
- Sparking your spiritual transformation. Creating peace by being peace. It brings you into alignment and harmony with your soul, with your mightiness, with Mother Earth, and with spirit. It facilitates the rebuilding of both your inner ecology and the Earth's ecology.
- Becoming that which you yearn, as you also become a more efficient and sustainable Mighty force of wellness in the world, and take on a more active role in the solution to our global crisis.

Heaven and Earth are calling. Your soul has heard the call; your Mighty inner healer is ready and eager to ignite your spiritual transformation as you power up your health!

13 TOOLS, TIPS, AND TRICKS FOR HEALTHY GENE EXPRESSION

I have all these great genes, but they're recessive. That's the problem here.

—*Bill Watterson*

Oh the gifts of growing young! Yes!

I know you have discovered some on your own. Isn't it wonderful to have tapped into the wisdom that exists for ***healthy gene expression?*** We don't have to age with sickness and degenerative disease. You and I can choose, instead, to age with grace and turn back the gene expression currently manifesting in our life. By changing the food you eat, your lifestyle, your thoughts, and the depth of your breath, attitude, and gratitude, you will begin to change the current gene expression manifesting in your life, and bear witness as your whole being begins to change. Your whole-body chemistry that affects each and every cell … can change! I don't know about you, but when I was not well, that seemed like a far-fetched dream. As I got better, I began to learn about healthy gene expression, and about changing the current terrain within my body to an alkaline, positive, structured, love-infused space!

Our genes contain the power to express health, or the power to express disease. And as science is proving, you and I have the power to control which genes we express through our diet and lifestyle. Yes, there might be a lineage of a specific disease in your family, but if you are aware of it, you can move away from the circumstances, nutritional and mineral deficiencies, lifestyle patterns, and habits that can activate that gene within you.

Life can be complicated. There are millions of diseases, causes, and conditions out there. If we became paranoid of each and every one of them, our life would be miserable, right? So, why not give it your best shot? Why not eat, drink, and be merry in the pursuit of great health! The truth is out. You can provide your body with the food and lifestyle needed for healthy gene expression. Yes, you can …

I chose to believe in my body's ability to heal and I still believe that. I chose to surrender my heart and open it wide. I chose to change. I chose to integrate and take the road less travelled.

13 Tools, Tricks, and Tips for Healthy Gene Expression

1. **Eat a majority of fresh, whole, local, and (as much as possible) organic, raw plant-based foods.** Put on your chlorophyll antioxidant-rich glasses! The world looks prettier this way because you begin to shine and glow from the inside out. When you feel good, your whole perspective changes! It will, because chlorophyll is liquid sunshine! It provides oxygen to your body in high quantities along with high-density phytonutrients, antioxidants, enzymes, and more. It literally has the power to revolution your cells alive!

   Most likely your vegetables and fruits will be annual foods, because their root system is relatively small. These foods contain within them the power of the present (what is currently present in your soil).

2. **Eat wild foods, wild foods for a wild heart.** Even if you don't know it yet, your heart longs to reclaim its wildness and connection to the rest of life. Wild food contains vital information for our survival, for our perception of connectedness and unity. Think of it—wild foods know how to survive exposed to the forces of the elements; no one is watering or weeding around them. Wild and bold, they are connected to all that is under the stars.

   Wild foods are perennials, so their root system is often deep, much deeper than our dearest annual vegetables and fruits. This enables them to provide us with a different variety of nutrients, minerals, and trace minerals from the depths of the earth, and they contain within them the power of the ancient forces.

3. **Eat foods with seeds and eat the seeds of wild foods. Eat the nectar of our world: bee pollen.** Seeds contain the information of growth, longevity, potentiality, wisdom of purpose, and wisdom for survival. Seeds contain the power of the future, the power of knowing one's place in the unveiling of the earth. Eating the seeds of wild food is simply eating Mighty superpowers!

   The sweet nectar of our world—bee pollen—is one of the most concentrated superfoods that we can eat. Why you say? Well, bee pollen comes from the flowers around where you live (hopefully), which again contains evolutionary information for longevity, the unfolding of our purpose, for living vibrant, radiant lives. It is the nectar of our world. An echinacea flower knows how to grow and be an echinacea flower. It absolutely can't be a daisy. When we eat bee pollen, we are not only eating a mineral- and vitamin-dense food, we are also eating the intelligence of "knowing" our identity the way plants know their identity. We are eating the nectar of the world, which inherently carries the intelligence of procreation and longevity.

4. *Drink your heaven on earth. Yes. Drink it. Liquid nutrition goes straight to your heart,* straight to your blood and to each one of your incredible cells, which make your incredible you. The optimal way to get high-nutrient-dense goodness into your body: juice it, smoothie it, liquefy it, and then drink it!

5. *Eat, drink, and be merry with your friend, turmeric.* Yes, I'm all about gathering the magic powers of the world onto me, and embodying those powers myself. Why turmeric, you ask? Well, think of the times we live in: we are all suffering from one type or another of inflammatory diseases, from arthritis, to any –itis, to any infection, to memory loss. Turmeric contains the Mighty curcumin, a powerful anti-inflammatory. Turmeric cleanses and purifies your blood, increases antioxidants in your body, improves brain function, and lowers risk of heart disease, just to name a few. From tea, to stir-not-fry, to tinctures, welcome your new BFF—turmeric!

6. *Grow your own food or get to know someone who does.* Even if it's just a pot of herbs on your windowsill, grow and get to know your food. Grow, get intimate with it. Grow, get your hands into the earth and feel how balancing, nurturing, and harmonizing it is, the great alkalizer!

When we think of alkalizing our body, we often think only of foods. But there's more to this equation than meets the eye. What you do, how you do it, and how you feel while doing it are all great practices of awareness and great alkalizers. When you grow your own food, there's a magical energetic exchange that happens, something that isn't often talked about. It's pure alchemy! It doesn't get any more local than that!

As you take care of your garden and spend time making it your sanctuary, it begins to respond to you, to shift and structure itself to your needs. It begins to show you the way of the wild, the way into your natural self. So, it's not just about growing food. It is about the shift in awareness that happens as you grow your food. Last but not least, there is absolutely nothing better tasting than your own home-grown food!

If you can't grow some of your own food, or your green thumb is just not happening, no worries. Just get a pot of soil and put your hands in it. Feel how good it feels to come back to the earth. I'm kidding. Get to know someone who grows food. Visit a local farmers market. Get to know your farmers. Connect with the hearts of those who grow your food. Connect with the food at its source. If you can, visit a farm, get a community-supported agriculture (CSA) membership and begin to taste the real taste of fresh food.

7. ***Take time off. Yes. Lights out. Electronics off. Noises off.*** Even if it's only ten minutes here and there, or a day, or if you can, more! Go for it. How can you truly grow yourself young while in the midst of constant stimulation, constant noise, and constant busyness?

    You can't. It's that simple. Nature has shown us time and again that to maintain a healthy expression of your genetic code you must follow its patterns of information, which, by the way, are stunningly beautiful. You must live in resonance with those patterns. When you do, you take your health to another level, for true health is not simply the absence of disease. It's the full expression of your soul manifesting itself through your body in this life.

8. ***Get outside: walk barefoot on the earth.*** Ground yourself through earthing (more on this on page 266). Yes, touch the ground. How does it feel? Cool? Soothing? Caring? Supportive? Getting outside into nature calms our whole nervous system. Not only are you breathing cleaner air, but you also begin to commune with nature. You begin to release stress, take in clear, vibrant energy, clear your head, feel your heart, and reconnect with the one and only—Mighty you.

9. ***Breathe deeply into health and mindfully move your body.*** Breathe. Witness. Pause. Feel. Consciously Move. Flow. Evolve. Live. Surrender. Heal.

10. ***Set time aside to be in silence daily. Connect with your heart. Connect with your inner smile.*** When was the last time you felt your heart beat? Yes, I know you know your heart beats. But when was the last time you felt your heart beat with excitement for life, for the dawning of a new day, the smell of a garden or a forest, for that which you're passionate about? When was the last time you allowed yourself to show your heart? Can you still feel the sunshine from in there? When was the last time you knew what your heart wanted? When was the last time you made it happen?

    What are you grateful for? What are you thankful for? What tickles your soul with sheer joy? What nurtures you deeply?

    Meditation is my way of connecting with my heart on a daily basis. It is my time to disconnect from the outside world and for tapping into my inner sanctuary and connecting deeply within. It is a gift I give to myself. What will your gift to yourself be?

11. ***Use rituals for detox, self-care, and deep nourishment.*** To be our healthiest expression, our bodies must have sources of deep nourishment, beyond just the food we eat. A mineral-deficient body can never express itself in health. A broken heart must be nourished into

loving again. An unfulfilled soul must pursue its fullness. In order to achieve longevity, we must detoxify our bodies yearly (the spring season is best) and must continuously care for ourselves through ritual. Wellness is a series of actions and everyday rituals that build our well-being.

12. *Get your beauty sleep.* How many all-nighters can you pull in a row before you (as my son would say) feel like total crappolla? Our body was designed to balance its rhythms while we sleep. We harmonize, integrate, release, assimilate, and dream our dreams so that we can get up and make them happen. When you shift your sleeping habits, your natural rhythms get disturbed. Your chemistry, hormonal balances, and body processes begin to fail, one at a time, until perhaps you begin to notice that your lifestyle plays a bigger role in the state of your health than you might care to acknowledge.

13. *Engage with the world in sacred reciprocity.* See yourself as a part of the whole. Be in relationship with, rather than ownership of, your body, the space you inhabit, other people, and the earth.

As you can see, what you choose to do and what you choose not to do will have great impact on the health of your gene expression through your body, mind, heart, and soul.

> *What do you choose?*
> *What do you consciously not choose?*
> In which ways do you choose to revolution yourself alive?

ESTABLISHING A HEALTHIER RELATIONSHIP WITH FOOD

Ask not what you can do for your country. Ask what's for lunch.

—*Orson Welles*

By the way, how is your relationship with food?

Do you eat when you are truly hungry? Or, do you eat out of habit, or when you are sad or stressed? Do you create a ritual around eating? Or are you always eating on the run? Do you pray over your food? Do you offer gratitude for the food that will nourish your body, and turn into vitality, health, and beauty within? Do you prepare you own food? Are your senses in touch with the food of your sustenance? Just observe without judgement. Simply become aware of what is true for you right now.

Our relationship with food is also a process. I like to think of it as a process of courtship. Can you begin to fall in love with the food you eat? Rather than just seeing it as a foreign substance that fuels your body, can you begin to see it as one of the vehicles through which the intelligent life-force energy enters your system? Can you fall in love again with the art of deeply nourishing your body?

Our ***relationship with food*** greatly varies according to our culture of origin. It is embedded with tradition, with cultural practices and expectations. Though you may not be giving it too much thought or attention at this time in your life, food is at the core of your being. Have you ever tried changing someone's diet before they are ready? Or not eating at the right time before your loved ones got HANGRY?

Yet, can you come into a healthy relationship with food, not just ownership? Food was meant to be whole, home-grown, home-prepared, and home-cooked. Food was meant to be a complete source of deep nourishment, and to keep us in relationship with the cycles of the Earth.

Yet this global, 24/7, all-you-can-eat drive-thru approach to food has distorted our once-healthy relationship with food. Today, most people are not even aware of where their food comes from. They don't know how food is grown, nor are they really interested in the current food industry practices of GMOs, preservatives, and herbicide-laden foods that are killing us as a species, and causing so many expressions of dis-ease. Did you know the acronym for the standard American diet is SAD? Food for thought, isn't it?

Let's come back to turning within, and noticing how a particular food makes you feel. Let's come back to sitting as families around the dinner table, to talking and sharing with each other about our day—away from all devices, away from the TV. Let's come back to home-cooked foods, eaten at regular times, and shared with people we love.

Let's come back to being in a healthy relationship with our food.

LIVING SOIL = LIVING SOUL

To forget how to dig the earth and to tend to the soil is to forget ourselves.

–Mahatma Gandhi

Once you begin to nurture and nourish your roots, you naturally arrive at what feeds them, the soil in which they grow. Is our soil living? Is it deeply nourishing us?

The quality of the soil where your food is grown will directly affect your expression of health. Food is not just fuel for your body; the food you eat has the potential to be both the source of your greatest health or of your greatest disease.

Strange as it may sound, soil is part of our foundation for health. Not only is the earth the ground you stand on and root into, but it is also the very source that feeds all, that feeds you.

Soil is alive. It is full of microorganisms ready to engage with each other and all of life to bring more life to fruition. The ecology of the soil is a living ecology, feeding and building living systems, which of course continue to emerge and feed other living systems.

The Earth herself, who provides all you and I need to thrive, and to *evolution* ourselves alive, contains within Her the power of alchemy. All the nutrients we need exist within Her vastness, from every mineral, micro and macro nutrient, enzyme, and antioxidant, to the life-force energy we need to re-establish the field of coherence and health, to the SOEF[3] systems (more on this on page 65), they all come from Her. Plants provide the synergistic process of transforming these life-sustaining nutrients into angstrom-sized molecules[4] we can absorb; they distil, if you will, Mother Earth's code/life-force/SOEFs into our own energetic language so we can assimilate, harmonize, and rejuvenate ourselves to be of service to Her own evolution.

Can you see perhaps just how interconnected and interrelated we are with the soil and the earth? Can you perhaps recognize that our own personal crisis and the crisis now facing our earth are part of each other?

---

3   SOEF, Subtle Organizing Energy Field.
4   "Angstrom (Å), unit of length used chiefly in measuring wavelengths of light, equal to 10–10 metre, or 0.1 nanometer. It is named for the 19th-century Swedish physicist Anders Jonas Ångström. The angstrom and multiples of it, the micron (10^4 Å) and the millimicron (10 Å), are also used to measure such quantities as molecular diameters and the thickness of films on liquids." — https://www.britannica.com/science/angstrom

We each have our own unique story of emergence, of unfolding, our own evolution of consciousness. We each have our own unique healing that begins and ends with the soil/soul of Mother Earth, with loving our living body, our foundation (our soil), the eternal within us (our soul as an expression of the soul of Mother Earth) and the process connecting them both: our life.

And so we begin to shift … to a deeper connection to the limitless self: our own soul. We begin to shift our choices, our habits, our needs, our desires, our thoughts, our actions, and our awareness of our responsibility. We begin to reclaim our food sovereignty. We begin to understand what constitutes a living system, why they are healing, and why they are our foundation and the key to our evolution.

> *By definition, living systems are* open, *self-organizing systems that have the special characteristics of life and* interact *with their environment. This takes place by means of information and material-energy exchanges.*
>
> —*Elaine Parent*

Living systems theory brings back into our awareness the fact that **all life is interconnected, interrelated, and expresses itself through systems of patterns that repeat themselves and engage with each other,** from the expression of a single cell to the magnificence of our universe. The health of the system can only be as healthy as its subsystems. We therefore owe it to our self to nourish our subsystems properly, for the expression of radiant health we seek begins in the very structure of our cells, and beyond that, with the health and life present in the soil—that place responsible for growing the very food that nourishes our cells.

The soil of the earth is also the soul of the earth. To heal ourselves, we must repair and heal the soil and the soul of the earth. We must reclaim our food systems, and integrate the three ethical responsibilities of permaculture: care for the earth, care for people, and fair share. Ethical responsibility goes beyond just permaculture; it is the backbone of living in sacred reciprocity and the key to our healing. Only then will we stop the cycles of violence to self, to each other, and to Mother Earth, which have been programmed and deeply rooted into our belief systems and our current political-economical systems.

On a personal level, there is much you and I can do to be a part of the solution. You can start growing your own small but Mighty garden. You can buy your produce from local farmers. You can join a CSA farm share. You can even grow sprouts from the comfort of your windowsill and enjoy the benefits of what an active soil and soul regenerator will do for your healthy gene expression.

EARTH'S CONSCIOUSNESS | UNIVERSAL CONSCIOUSNESS

For so long we've considered the Earth as just a big dead ball of dirt. It shocks us nearly out of our minds when we discover we're involved within something that moves. Copernicus said the Earth moved: he meant that it moved around the sun. When we say the Earth moves, we mean the whole process is alive. The Earth moves. In a sentence that is the heart of our cosmic revolution.

—Brian Swimme, PhD, The Universe is a Green Dragon.

You may already know there are different levels of consciousness and that consciousness evolves into different levels of awareness. You may also know of the universal consciousness that connects us all, and that while we are all individuals, we are also part of the greater whole.

You may also know that our individual consciousness has a map (if you will) of goals and lessons to learn while here on Earth. Yet this individual consciousness is still part of the universal consciousness that governs the universe. We are all expressions of this universal consciousness, and it seeks to constantly know and experience itself—through us. It seeks to expand through our bodies, through our minds, into our hearts, reminding us along the way of our true nature.

As the universe expanded, it created the right conditions for Earth and other planets to exist. Unbeknownst to many, our Earth and all the planets are alive and conscious beings. The first goal of Earth was to create itself as a crystal, a magnifier of universal conscious energy, in order to continue to expand its awareness. As the Earth's awareness expanded, it created the right conditions for humanity to come into being. You and I (humanity) are the product of Earth's seeking to express itself.

We are made of this Earth and to it we shall return. Our bodies, too, contain crystalline forms (pineal gland, bones, and so on), allowing them to remain in relationship with the Earth, and be able to connect and "download" its ancient wisdom.

Yet we are also made of spirit dust (universal consciousness), which also continues to seek expression. And because we are crystalline forms, we too can tap into the wisdom of the universe through our soul, and so remember who we truly are.

And so we will forever be made of Earth and spirit dust. The Earth's consciousness and the universal consciousness will always run their rivers through us, continuously shifting our perception and our awareness into higher levels of consciousness.

As we begin to awaken, we discover the truth: that ***we are always in relationship.***

You and I are always in relationship to everything and everyone around us, to the universe, the planets, the Earth, the elements, ourselves, each other, to the realm of energy and the world of the unseen.

The Earth's consciousness awakens in us as we begin to include more fresh, living, raw foods in our diet, in particular liquid nutrition, and as we begin to use ancient tools and practices for self-development. It is this awakening that deepens your relationship with self, other, and the Earth and transforms it into sacred relationship.

The pathways to your inner source are many. Yet we live in this brave new world with incredible access to information. Time is quickening, and you and I are being asked to show up like never before.

Because liquid nutrition is the essence of food, because we are transferring life-force energy that is inherently intelligent, your body begins to remember your inner wisdom, your true nature, and you begin to awaken from the dream of separation and disconnect, of us versus them, of *business as usual.*

Because ancient tools and practices for self-development give us protocols for integrating the mind-body complex, the ancient becomes the future and we have a guide at hand for the journey ahead.

Being in sacred relationship awakens in us sacred action, through which you and I engage our Dharma or soul's potential in service to the world.

There are many paths to awaken into sacred action. Ancient traditions knew the path to self-liberation is one of union. Union with the God of your own understanding—spirit, source, God, the great originating mystery—union between your body, emotions, mind, soul, and spirit.

There is great power in what you do, and also in what you don't do, in your life. The way in which you engage in relationship shapes your own healing journey, shapes your life, the world, and the future of the seven generations to come.

THE NEED FOR EVERYDAY RITUALS IN THE MODERN ERA

Any ritual is an opportunity for transformation.

—Starhawk

A **ritual** is a ceremony or action that is performed in a customary way, specific to given cultures. Rituals are actions with intentional symbolic meaning, undertaken for a specific cultural purpose, such as the passage from childhood into adulthood. Rituals may be religious or secular in nature. They may be repeated seasonally, monthly, or daily as a way to bring you back to your centre, to your inner source. Rituals reconnect you with your sense of belonging, with the present, as you honour the ancient, for humanity as a species has been involved in ritual since the beginning of our time here on Earth.

We lost our connection to *ritual* when we began to lose our sense of home. War, invasion, occupation, and displacement have been the main causes for the uprooted-ness of our collective sense of belonging to a place. Massive migrations due to political and economic instability have also uprooted our sense of relationship to our ancestral homelands, which in time disconnected us from the rituals of our ancestors and our connection to the land.

We live in a global world where our sense of belonging to a particular place is no longer rooted in our relationship with the land, with the elements, or with the world of the unseen, in the way it had been for our ancestral lineages. Most of us are not even connected to the food systems that sustain us, never mind the spirit of the land that nourishes our souls.

We live in an era of distraction. We live in the era of advanced technologies that are supposed to make our lives better. Yet many of us live in deep isolation from each other, from community, from the earth, and even from the self. We live in an era of fragmentation and busyness, living a fast life in the fast lane. So many of us are constantly stressed out, and lack the tools, practices, or time to effectively wind down. We are in ten places at once, yet in none of them at all, for we were never fully present in any of those ten places. We are always concerned about the future, or painfully reliving the past.

Knowing there is a problem, but lacking the awareness of exactly what that problem is, we are constantly seeking our solutions externally, effectively giving away our power to achieving that which can heal our fragmentation. The truth is, the only way home is to look inward and walk the inner path to the self.

We have options. You can choose *to live in the brave new world I've been speaking of. But living in this dimension demands courage; it demands that we take a good look at ourselves and become present in our bodies and with our lives. It demands that we make a conscious choice. It demands your awakening and a change in your actions.*

Living in the brave new world also demands that we begin to self-care, and care for others in sacred relationship in the ways our ancestors did, through *everyday ritual.* Everyday ritual is as simple as daily brushing your teeth, or as elaborate and sensorially rich as a summer solstice ceremony on the land. You get to choose.

I encourage you to craft your own rituals for radical self-care that will spark and ignite the alchemy and synergy of wellness within you. The rituals of liquid nutrition and detox, and the rituals of mindfulness practices and inner questing are all rituals for well-being. Practised regularly, they will enhance your connection with that inner space of sacredness, and open you up to living in gratitude through feeling grace.

It is through ritual that you begin to consciously reclaim the fragmented pieces of your self, and along with it your personal power. Through ritual you begin to reclaim your life and come into full embodiment of who, and what, you truly are.

Through ritual, we come to deeply honour each other, the elements, Mother Earth, and our soul, having a human experience. Through ritual, you begin to give back, to "feed" and nourish the world around you. Through ritual, you begin to create beauty in the world, a positive mind, and life-affirming actions that lead you to create peace.

You and I are made of earth and spirit dust. The ancestral wisdom within us is screaming to be liberated, to be honoured, to be heard, to be acknowledged, to be remembered, to be made whole.

Living in the modern world has a lot of advantages, too. So perhaps, just perhaps, we can bring the best of both worlds together and reunite, through ritual, our separation, our fragmentation, and our isolation, to weave the most complex web of all: the web of embodiment of our full potential in this lifetime. Here and now, in sacred relationship to all beings, in all dimensions, through sacred action.

YOUR ROADMAP TO WELLNESS

All you need is the plan, the road map, and the courage to press on to your destination.

—Earl Nightingale

There are two things you need to know when creating a road map: where you currently are, and where you want to go. The more you become aware of your current condition, the health of your inner terrain, and your current tendencies, the easier it is to carve your inner map at the same time you are creating your road map to radiant health. Yes, going about it in the dark might be fun for a day or two, but creating awareness of your path will lead to quicker results, and a more conscious quest altogether.

Knowing where we are can sometimes be a challenge in itself. You may know the symptoms you are experiencing, but not necessarily the root cause. You may know the outer expression, but be unable to fully understand the reason behind it. You may know the condition, but be unaware of the language your body is using to tell you what it needs. You may be experiencing a lot of emotions as you try to decipher your body's code. You may find yourself stuck along the way to radiant health, leaving you unsure of which way to turn, unsure of which tools and practices or supplements will be most beneficial for you, or unsure if there is even any hope for you at all.

Dear beating heart, there is always hope.

As you journey on your quest of alignment with the alchemy of wellness, know that you are unique; know that your quest and mine and that of your cousin will all be different, know that your path to ignite your mighty inner healer will be your own. And that you, only you, know yourself best, deep within the boundaries of your skin.

Every roadmap has a few stops or key portals along the way that will deeply transform us. These stops or portals, or tools, practices, people, and belief systems have their purpose. They become pillars; they become your foundation along your journey of *becoming* and *awakening* to your true nature, your personal truth, and the essence of who you really are.

Your **roadmap to wellness** has, along the way, three key pillars that will become the foundation for your deep transformation.

These pillars are ancient rituals. They have been used for thousands of years to heal the body, transform the mind, and open the heart into a more inclusive and intimate experience of ourselves and the world around us.

The Three Pillars of Wellness

The three pillars along your roadmap into wellness are:

- Pillar #1: *The ritual or Sadhana of liquid nutrition and the ritual of detox*
- Pillar #2: *The art of mindfulness*
- Pillar #3: *The alchemy of inner questing*

When used together, great **synergy** will awaken and powerfully transform you, if you gift yourself the opportunity to show up for the journey. Together, they are the pathway to your inner source. Together, they are your journey home.

The journey towards deep healing, radiant health, and your personal revolution will awaken the *hope activist within*. The hope activist within is the higher self in each of us that believes in the possibilities, that is willing to take matters into its own hands and try, try, try it all. It is a call of the soul.

Although your journey or quest may at times feel like a very long roller coaster ride, please know that you have the ability to face yourself, your emotions, your mental landscape, and your spirit, and dive within. Our greatest challenges always turn out to be our greatest teachers.

Anchor into gratitude along your roadmap to wellness—the conscious choice to be grateful opens the door of our perception to other possibilities; it is the lifejacket we put on as the plane heads down for a crash landing. Connect with your heart now, and choose to be grateful for what is *already* in your life that brings you closer to wellness. Then dive within to face the challenge. It's when you stand and face your challenges, or your shadow, that you gain access to your greatest light. Know that the hope activist in you is a health warrior of peace, your main coach and guide along your roadmap.

You don't have to reinvent the wheel. You just have to be willing to get the wheel moving again.

INTO ME YOU SEE (INTIMACY)

It is an absolute human certainty that no one can know his own beauty or perceive a sense of his own worth until it has been reflected back to him in the mirror of another loving, caring human being.

—John Joseph Powell

Intimacy can be defined as a close, familiar, and usually affectionate or loving personal relationship with another person or group. In the social sciences, we think of it as closeness, openness, vulnerability, and transparency. Within the practice of shamanism—the ancient healing tradition that connects us with nature, our true nature, and all of creation—we like to pronounce it giving greater dimension to its meaning: ***into me you see.***

Into me you see is the art of living present to who you truly are, present to self and to other in sacred relationship. In order to really live in such a deep state of openness and vulnerability, you must first be able to accept yourself completely, love yourself completely, and show up for yourself completely. It is a process, and part of our quest and journey home. And on some days, some emotions and some traumas are more easily seen than others.

We cannot offer our deepest truths to the world if we have not yet grasped them ourselves. You cannot offer yourself to another if you haven't offered yourself to your self. You cannot live in the alchemy of wellness if you are not willing to be the alchemist.

Being human is embracing our nature as a story, and at the core of every great story there is a plot and usually a challenge, which the main character of the story (you and me) must overcome, move through, surrender, release, transform, and accept in order for our hero to drive the story forward. You and I are in the midst of our own hero's journey.

The process of creating intimacy with your self begins by looking at your own story with great honesty, self-compassion, transparency, and humility.

The process of creating intimacy with life begins by showing up for your self, and being in "right relationship" with your self. By doing your physical, emotional, mental, and soul "work," you will eventually open up to the gate of spirit. You must look honestly and willingly at what and whom you carry in your heart and in your mind. This work requires us to look at our shadow, at our densities, and at our baggage in order to truly see each aspect of ourselves. To be surrendered to, released, transformed, and integrated by each one of us.

Acceptance is a funny thing. I see my shadow; I see the baggage I created for myself in this life, and I also see the baggage I inherited from the seven generations past, and I honour my path of evolution through it. Acceptance is about bringing compassion to your own humanity and your own process.

Acceptance is not about fixing or changing that dark aspect we don't like, or hiding it by stuffing it deeper into the closet. The journey of healing and reclaiming the fragmented pieces of your self demands that you see yourself, that you honour yourself, that you allow the emotions to be expressed, for the very word emotion is really "energy in motion."

Intimacy demands that you give yourself the sacred space to do "the work." That you honour your path and your process and show up, because if we can't show up for ourselves, how can we ever really show up for others?

Intimacy demands that we be present. Present to your breath, to your heart, to your mind. ***Into me you see*** will force us to look at our loneliness, at our need to feel loved and accepted by others, at our vulnerability, and at the honesty through which we present ourselves to the world. These are all such important steps in your process of claiming your mightiness.

In time, the more you practice intimacy with the self, the more it will begin to simply be the way we are in relationship with others. It is all a choice we make, one that takes commitment, and constant nourishing.

Into me you see will bring you face to face with your process of involution. I spoke about it in my opening words, "Forward or, Rather, Inward."

The process of involution is the journey through which we "revolution" ourselves alive. It is the quest through which you move through the old patterns, belief systems, disembodied actions, and thoughts, as you surrender, release, transform, and accept your very process, in order to allow for the expression of your true potential (mightiness) in this world.

The journey of involution is the awakening to your own humanity and to the compassion with which you must tend to your heart and whole-body systems in order to *heal*. "Birthing" ourselves with great transparency in this world is not easy. As we wear our heart on our sleeve, we must also build up our inner resources of self-compassion, boundaries, centredness, and grounding. We must constantly stay "connected" within, and know ourselves. We must constantly show up.

The journey of *involution* is a *spiral*, forever an opportunity to awaken from our *sleepwalking*. For some of us, life is living us rather than us living life. Sleepwalking can be great, but once you awaken to the truth that you are *powerful beyond measure*, that you can create your reality, and that you can engage with the world in deeper more meaningful ways, you can never go back to "sleep." We can never go back to not being in touch with who and what we truly are. We can no longer continue to numb ourselves with our addictions—like food and drink, or whatever our addictions might be, for they, too, will demand to be seen.

Intimacy is perhaps one of the most precious gifts you can give to yourself along your roadmap to wellness. The gift of a life lived to your best potential.

OPENING UP TO GRACE

Grace has been defined as the outward expression of the inward harmony of the soul.

—William Hazlitt

Grace can be defined in so many ways, but here is how I personally feel about it. Grace is moving, acting, and living from the place of your highest self and potential. Grace is deeply connecting to your inner space of awareness, sacredness, and reverence. It is simple to see and yet harder to achieve, until we begin to instil rituals for everyday living.

Since grace connects to potential, it is often associated with God or divine spirit. In many religions, a person finds their potential through connecting to that which is greater than themselves; to that higher level of potential that is often labelled as God, source, the universe, or similar terms.

Grace need not necessarily be a religious experience. Opening up to grace will, however, open you up to your own higher self or spirituality, and the ways in which you are in relationship with yourself and with the world of divine spirit.

The journey up to higher levels of potential is really a *journey in and through*. If you only go up, you will leave your body, and well, I don't particularly want to leave this beautiful life just yet. Rather, it's by going *in and through* that you get to experience and embody your sacredness, your gratitude, your sense of belonging, your connection to the great web of life, your interrelationship with source and all that is—and your grace.

As we deepen our relationship to self, to the world around us, and to the world of spirit, we begin to anchor into the core of our core, our centre. We begin to expand back from the innermost sacred layers of our heart and mind, towards our bones, muscles, skin, and whole body, into our actions. This process of expansion, once rooted into the inner space of sacredness, becomes our graceful living, for it awakens in us the call to act with kindness and compassion both towards the world and more profoundly towards our selves.

The seed of self-compassion towards our own humanity is a big step in our healing and along our roadmap to wellness. The seed of compassion towards others' humanities is also a big step in the making of peace with our stories, with our traumas, and with our health crises so that we may begin to make peace with the journey and truly rebuild a stronger foundation for health.

Grace cannot be bought or sold or bottled up, for that matter. It can only be given and received. It is an offering from the deepest realms of our hearts to life itself for the opportunity to be alive, here, now.

Today, what do you want to feel? What do you want to gift? What do you want to receive?

POWER UP YOUR HEALTH

The most important kind of freedom is to be what you really are. You trade in your reality for a role. You trade in your sense for an act. You give up your ability to feel, and in exchange, put on a mask. There can't be any large-scale revolution until there's a personal revolution, on an individual level. It's got to happen inside first.

—Jim Morrison

Your body will behave in a way that will cause either happiness or suffering. So how do you get your body complex to create more happiness and less suffering? Answer: you become aware of the root causes of your suffering, and then choose to take a different action, one that will have a different consequence, and directly influence your path towards creating more happiness in your life.

The three pillars of your roadmap to wellness have the power to deeply transform you—from every cell in your body to the ultimate transformation of your consciousness through the journey of awakening.

It's well-known that as we age we start losing some of our water content. As the years pass, we begin to contract in both body and mind. You can also experience this when living a very hectic busy lifestyle, when you are stressed and when your nervous system is unable to cope with the demands in your life.

The obvious protocol for moving against contraction is expansion. In your body, the most powerful tool for creating expansion is liquid nutrition; in your mind it is Mindfulness practices, and in your heart it is inner questing. When engaged, these practices enable you to begin reversing contraction and the effects of aging in your body, mind and heart, and tap into key protocols for longevity. You are not only transforming your physical body, you are also bringing in more flow to the emotional and mental bodies, and the expansion of your spiritual transformation.

While liquids in general have no definite shape, they do have a definite volume, and the ability to take the shape of their container and still maintain that volume. In our specific case, liquid nutrition is filled with nutritional density, which then begins to cause a chain reaction shift in your container — your human body. Mindfulness practices opens up sacred space within us, and inner questing fills us up with new possibilities for ourselves.

Your initial reason for pursuing Radiant Health might have been sparked by a physical desire or challenge, but as you journey on you will discover there is more to this body than its physical form. We are more than our emotions and inner landscape, more even than our spiritual relationship to self and the God of our own understanding.

We are, here and now: an expression of an evolution in consciousness.

As we continue to journey up into the world of heaven, into the world of spirit, we realize that in as much as we are reaching UP we are also reaching IN. We come to realize that the world of spirit resides both in the world of heaven, across the vastness of our Earth, and deep in the back corners of our very own hearts.

The journey up to connect with the divine layers of your existence and become whole again, demands that you create that inner space to connect deeply with the divine or grace within you. It demands also that you deeply nourish the roots of your five bodies. The more you carve sacred space within, the more your path of awakening to spirit will build greater resonance in your body, healing all your relationships to Self and Other.

For when we realize we are soul — a Divine Spiritual being — having a human (earthly) experience, we will open to the pathways in which spirit is constantly moving through us. The Great Originating Mystery/ God/ Spirit/ source, is the totality of the highest level of life-force consciousness that is always seeking expression through our bodies.

Expression, creative movement in our world, expansion into right action for the benefit of all, are all by-products of being In-Spirited (inspired); infused by the touch of grace.

To heal means to become whole again. Our journeys of deep healing are our journeys to reclaim our wholeness through reclaiming the fragmented pieces of ourselves. This is the journey of involution, the spiral movement through our five bodies that awakens us into living in sacred interrelationship and reciprocity with all of life.

As you commit to your journey of deep healing, you will begin to ***power up your health***. You will begin to create a new, more solid foundation from which you can now integrate tools and practices to nourish, feed, and strengthen the roots that are creating the stability of your foundation for health.

As you commit to your journey of involution, you will ***ignite your transformation***—and your life—with a new-found power and trust in your personal process of awakening.

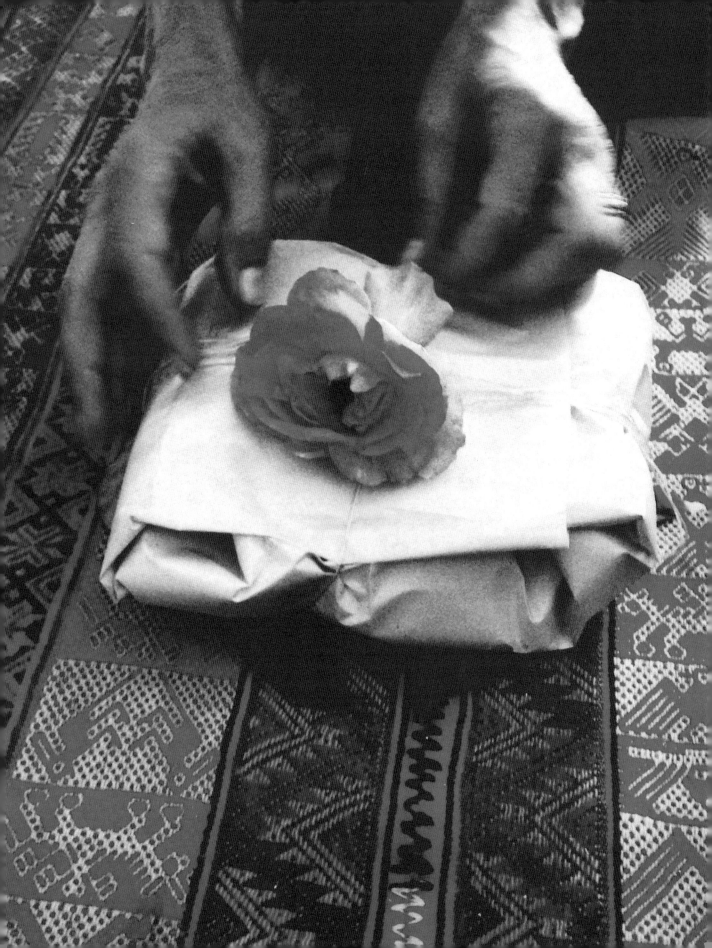

II

THE ANCIENT AS THE FUTURE

You didn't come into this world.
You came out of it, like a wave from the ocean.
You are not a stranger here.

—Alan Watts

LIFE-FORCE ENERGY

There is a vitality, a life force, an energy, a quickening, that is translated through you into action, and because there is only one of you in all time, this expression is unique.

—Martha Graham

Life-force energy is the vehicle through which ***pure un-manifested cosmic consciousness*** vibrates, pulses, and moves into form. Life-force energy is consciousness in movement. It is inherently intelligent, benevolent and healing in nature. It always seeks to flow. Invisible to most of us, we can sense it through our sensory organs. It animates our physical form and flows through, within and around all beings, all of life.

All apparently empty space is rather full of invisible life-force energy. Life-force energy has different names according to different lineages, but they all address the same invisible, life giving, animating, healing energy that supports and increases the body's natural self-healing abilities. It is also sometimes called universal energy.

Life-Force is known as ***Prana*** to the Hindu, ***Chi*** to the Chinese, ***Ki*** to the Japanese, or ***Aka*** to the Egyptians. These ancient traditions recognized that the free flow of intelligent, pranic energy is essential to a life of health and happiness, and they each developed systems and sciences to help the energy flow freely through the human body. Acupuncture, Reiki, Tai Chi, Qi Gong, and Yoga are all systems that enhance the flow of Prana/Qi in the body.

Within your body lies an intricate web of channels through which Prana or life-force energy flows. Known as ***meridian channels*** in Chinese medicine, or ***Nadis*** in the Vedic system (Hindu lineage), these channels can become blocked—affecting the flow of life-affirming healing energy through your systems, and impacting the health of your whole body. These channels can become blocked due to poor diet, lifestyle choices, stress, emotional and mental blocks, physical and/or emotional trauma, and so on.

When you consciously choose to tap into the innate intelligence of this vital healing energy, you can:

- Deepen your sense of well-being
- Shift from disease to health

- Transform blockages in your organs or any part of your bodies
- Gain vitality
- Cause the feeling of well-ness to shine so brightly others will begin to notice
- Begin to move in the direction of your Dharma (soul purpose) and away from the direction of your karma (cause and effect)

When this life-force or Prana is disturbed within your body; when you and I have interrupted the flow of this intelligent force within us that really wants us to thrive—the opposite happens, and disease settles into the body complex. That's when your journey (and mine) back to remembering and reconnecting with Prana begins, through the laws of cause and effect (karma).

Each lineage and ancient tradition developed its own ways to commune, enhance, and consciously guide life-force energy in and out of the body, in order to enhance and deepen the healing of the body. The following are tools and practices you can use to enhance your personal connection to your own life-force energy, and deepen your own healing:

- Eat a clean diet of foods that are high in frequency (fresh, organic, local)
- Drink your juices, smoothies, and elixirs!
- Do periodic liquid feasting
- Focus on conscious breathing
- Engage in meditation or contemplation
- Get a good night's sleep
- Spend time in nature—walk a forest trail, hike, canoe, or otherwise visit the natural environment
- Get sufficient physical exercise
- Do mindful movement practices such as yoga, tai chi, Qi gong
- Practice positive thinking and affirmations
- Do something you love, and ignite your passions
- Practice self-care rituals
- Connect with the emotions of gratitude and joy
- Practice loving kindness and compassion
- Take time to laugh!
- Release toxic thoughts and toxic relationships

A LIFE OF SYSTEMS

As long as we are not living in harmony with nature and our constitution, we cannot expect ourselves to be really healed. Ayurveda gives us the means.

—David Frawley

The universe is a very well-organized system that thrives on structure, patterns, and, yes, more systems! The following laws are universal, and bring subtle matter into form and manifestation, from the pure cosmic conscious state into the density of our human physical reality. These laws allow you to live in harmony with the laws of nature.

1. ***All matter is an energetic manifestation of pure cosmic consciousness through different ratios of the five Elements.*** The five subtle Elements form the basis for all things found in material creation, from atoms, molecules, and minerals to food and life forms. Each contains its own unique ratio of the five Elements. The five Elements are the foundation of the universe (macrocosm), and the psychosomatic existence of man (microcosm). The five Elements are Ether (Space), Air, Fire, Water, and Earth.

2. ***Law of the macrocosm (the universe) and microcosm (man).*** This law states that every element, natural force, and principle that exists in the macrocosm also exists within you, within your body-mind-emotion-soul system (microcosm). Any changes or disturbances that affect the macrocosm will have a similar effect on the microcosm, and vice versa.

   To heal one, you must address the other, for you and I are all interconnected and interrelated.

3. ***Because each individual is made of the five Elements in different ratios, we all have a unique constitution.*** The quality and quantity of "nourishment" for radiant health that each person needs, according to their own constitution, is different. You must come to understand your own unique constitution, in order to create the right conditions for maximum cellular energy and expression of health through your body.

When you are able to align the current expression of the elements that are moving through you with the unique ratio of the Elements at the moment of your birth, when you are able to see into the depths of your emotions with honesty and create space in your mind for awareness, and when you are able to connect with your soul and with spirit, then true alignment with radiant health and with pure cosmic consciousness will happen.

In deepening your awareness and understanding of the five Elements, you are able to deepen your connection with spirit, the divine, pure cosmic consciousness, through your true self, soul.

EVERYTHING IS MADE OF THE FIVE ELEMENTS

Ayurveda is the science of life and it has a very basic, simple kind of approach, which is that we are part of the universe and the universe is intelligent and the human body is part of the cosmic body.

—*Deepak Chopra*

All ancient cultures had, and have still, an elemental relationship with life, for they understood the pathway of the manifestation of consciousness into the world.

Everything in the universe is composed of the five Elements, from the stars above to the particles of dust below. The five Elements are the foundation and basis for all that exists. They are the foundation of your health, and understanding them intimately is the path to remembering your primordial nature, and the deepening of your healing.

The five Elements are the *dynamic forces* through which life-force energy or Prana moves via a process of densification, from the subtle into solid matter. It is a process of distillation and vibration, pulsation and movement, and not just movement. From the most subtle (incomprehensible by the human mind) to the most gross physical expression, pure cosmic consciousness is always seeking *expression and manifestation*. All matter is an energetic manifestation of cosmic consciousness, through different ratios of the five Elements. Each one of the Elements is a representation of a different state or quality of energy or matter.

A change in one Element affects the others. It is the bonding of these Elements that causes the universe to emerge and exist in manifested form.

Ether is the original element in its most subtle form. It contains within it the manifestation of the idea of space, the *universal vibration*—which creates the sacred vessel or container to hold that which will come into being or existence. Yogananda defined Ether as "the medium through which light travels." It is the channel that contains the river of your life.

Air is Ether in movement, and consists of both Ether and Air. It contains within itself the manifestation of the idea of movement, within the sacred space created by Ether. Air is the force that gives rise to motion and movement.

Fire is Air through repeated friction. It consists of Ether, Air, and Fire. It contains within itself the manifestation of the idea of illumination and passion, through the movement created by Air and within the sacred space created by Ether. Fire is the force that gives rise to heat and transformation.

Water is Fire condensed by heat. It consists of Fire, Ether, Air, and Water. It contains within itself the manifestation of the idea of life, the idea of flow, and the idea of nurture within the passionate illumination created by Fire, within the movement created by Air, within the sacred space created by Ether. Water is the force that gives rise to flow and fluidity.

Earth is the solid mass created by the cooling of Water. It consists of Water, Fire, Air, and Ether. It contains within itself the manifestation of the idea of form and structure, within the flow and nurture of life created by Water, within the passionate illumination created by Fire, within the movement created by Air, and within the sacred space created by Ether. Earth is the force that gives rise to solidity and stability.

Your body is composed of the five Elements in different ratios that create three main different constitutions (page 59), yet are unique to each and every person. The senses are the channels of the individual soul; they are the way through which you interact with all of life. Through the senses, you experience the world and come to know yourself.

Through our senses, pure un-manifested cosmic consciousness found its way onto living life on Earth. It reminds you, through your soul or higher self, of your own pulsation, or your interconnection with all of life, and of your sacred journey back to source itself: pure cosmic consciousness.

Your identification with yourself, or what makes up your self—the practices, patterns, and actions you identify with—will either create greater harmony, or will bring about greater dis-harmony or disease.

Understanding how the Elements are currently moving and expressing themselves through you will be key to igniting your Mighty inner healer. Are the five Elements expressing themselves in their fullest potential of vitality or stress? Are they expressing themselves through Love or isolation? Are they expressing themselves in harmony or disharmony?

THE POWER OF THE ELEMENTS IN YOUR DAILY LIFE

Ayurveda teaches us to cherish our innate-nature –"to love and honour who we are," not as what people think or tell us, "who we should be."

—Prana Gogia

The Elements are the root source and foundation of the power of radiant health. The more you begin to be in an intimate relationship with them, the more you can draw on their power to access deeper layers of healing, and deeper layers of radiant health. Following are insights for seeking a deeper space of alignment with the elements in your everyday life.

Ether

Ether is the medium through which sound is transmitted. The ear is the sensory organ of hearing. The organ of action for Ether is the mouth.

Ether is the seed, the space, the container, the core that holds your true north. It can also be seen as the womb of all creation.

Deep listening, your ability to speak your truth, your ability to hear your essential self, your ability to create space within and for yourself, your ability to connect with the space of sacredness within and in each other, and your ability to tap into the field of your potential, are all related to the element of Ether.

Have you taken the time to hear yourself lately? Have you taken the time to know your truth? Are there currently practices or tools in your life that allow you to listen deeply to your soul as you anchor into the sacred space within your heart?

You heal Ether within you with your voice, or by tuning in to the sacred sounds found in nature. When you anchor into the inner space of sacredness, wisdom, grace, and love. Your sense of home.

Air

Air is related to the sense of touch. The sensory organ for touch is the skin, the outermost layer of our body, and how we present ourselves to the world. The organ of action for Air is the hand.

The Element of Air is present as thoughts and ideas rise. It is the beginning of the action and movement in a particular direction.

Are you in tune with your path of movement and action into the world? Do you love the skin you are in, or do you resist your body's wisdom? Do you feel safe or do you feel threatened by the world around you? Are you able to accept that within your skin lies an irresistible, magical world, known to some, ignored by most, that has the ability to enrich your life, connect you to the god within, and the wisdom to explore your inner world beyond your mind, beyond your heart, into your soul?

In today's world, we are seeing an excess of the Element of Air. The busyness, the fast and constant movement (without clear direction) towards outside sources of gratification, self-worth, validation, identification, and so on. As a species, we are moving so rapidly our nervous systems have little chance to find our true passions, and the flow that would allow us to create from an ecologically responsible foundation for movement.

You heal Air within you, the force of movement, when you begin to bring awareness and mindfulness into your movement, into the ways you touch others and are touched by the world. When you ground and anchor your mind into your body, and connect with stillness.

Fire

Fire is related to vision, and the eye is the sensory organ of vision.

In your life and in your body, Fire is the main element of your digestive system, the spark of your passions and the inspiration in your mind. It is the force of heat and transformation.

How are you digesting your experiences? Are you assimilating them? Are you allowing your heart to feel your passion? Are you allowing your body to feel your heart? Are you allowing yourself to spark yourself alive? Is your Fire burning in sustainable ways, or are you burned out? How are you feeding your Fire? How are you igniting your transformation? Are you willing to spark your own revolution?

Do you have a clear vision of your potential and your roadmap to wellness? Can you trust in your vision, dreams, and inner guidance to walk towards your inner truth? Can you see into your own habits/thought patterns/shadow and beyond their limitations, accepting them as lessons, as teachers along your path to inner freedom? What steps are you taking to move towards your highest potential and mightiness?

You heal Fire within you, the force of heat and transformation, when you add just enough Water (flow) and just enough Air (movement) to the flame of your inner fire. Most of us are dealing with fires that are burning us out with inflammation and adrenal fatigue, because we've run ourselves into exhaustion. So, can you pause, and consciously add the right amount of love to ignite your passion and right action (mindful sacred movement) for living a fulfilled life? Can you do this while stoking your inner fire in just the right way so as to transform your stress and anger into radiance and illumination?

Water

Water is related to the organ of taste, the tongue being the sensory organ of taste. The organ of action for Water is the sex organ.

The main principle of the Element of Water is transportation and flow. How are you flowing through the rivers of your life? Can you allow yourself to flow with your challenges? To flow with your resistances? To flow with your present moment? Or do you check out?

Can you stop and taste your life? Can you stop and taste your journey? Can you slow down enough to savour the moment? Can we begin to slow our lives down to taste the gifts of life?

Can you commit to showing up and releasing that which keeps you stuck, that which binds and twists your heart, so the healing energy can move through you freely and you can hear your own voice and your purpose?

Water is also related to the sex organ of action. So, yes, the ways in which we interact and express ourselves sexually are related to the expression of Water, but it doesn't stop there. Water is related to the womb of creation. What are you creating? What is emerging from the depths of your being? What are you giving life to? These are all questions and aspects of ourselves that are in relationship with the Element of Water.

You heal Water within the flow and fluidity of your body complex when you begin to examine the ways in which you are not flowing and what is keeping you stuck. When you begin to pause, feel, and taste your experiences as to better integrate them. When you get out of your own way and instil practices that enhance the anchoring of your mind into your body so you are grounded in your flow, rather than running madly and uncontrollably through the rivers of your life. When you align with your purpose and consciously define what you are giving life to.

Earth

Earth is related to the sense of smell, to the sensory organ of your nose, and your ability to again, stop and smell the roses. The organ of action for Earth is the anus.

Earth is what gives your body system and your actions form and stability. It is also your foundation, the ground you stand on, root into, and stand tall on.

Earth, to me, is also the element of rooting one's self to our ethical self. Your sense of smell is one of your most powerful senses, with the ability to take us back beyond the boundaries of space and time. It is the element of rooting down to ancient times, to the recognition that we must honour the ancient relationship with Mother Earth to your own body, in order to find peace within. To begin to act from a place of peace, and from a place of the universal, rather than individual consciousness.

As you align with the Earth element, how stable is your foundation? Does it reflect your current belief system? Is it truly supporting you or can you see the cracks that are not holding you up? Can you stop, pause, and feel? Can you stop and smell the roses? Can you re-evaluate your foundation as to power up your health, ignite your transformation, and spark your revolution? Of course you can.

Are you aware of your conscious power of choice, action, creation, and their consequences? What are you choosing and creating in your life? What would happen if you held your intentions in your heart and made them the foundation for your actions, creations, and manifestation in the world?

Who are you dedicating your manifestation to? Who are you building your life for? What kind of footprint are you creating? What kind of impact are you leaving behind?

Earth is the solid manifestation of all the elements. It also brings you full circle back to Ether: your sacred space. Can you be a part of the creating of a world where the sacredness of humanity comes first? Can you be a part of the creating of a world where human rights are respected and are the foundation that hold the sacred space within you where you will develop, grow, and experience your journey? How solid is your integrity? How solid is your foundation? Can you build one based on ecological and social responsibilities?

You heal Earth within you, within the solidity and stability of your body complex, when you begin to stop and smell the roses. When you pause and bring joy into your life, you metaphorically emit the fragrance of roses from your body. You heal Earth when you work on your ability to poop daily, to eliminate the toxicity of the day, to release the weight of the past and engage in a more conscious relationship to that which gives your life weight and form.

As you see, there is great potential for igniting your Mighty inner healer by anchoring into the awareness and the symbolism of the power of the elements. When you have moved into disharmony and disease, it's the opposite quality to the symptoms of your disharmony that will bring about the greatest healing.

Understanding the elements and how they are currently expressing themselves in either balance or disharmony is key to reclaiming your health, further igniting your healing and creating a stronger foundation for health.

Understanding the relationship of the elements with your sense organs and organs of action, and your ability to power up your health by shifting, cleansing, and using your senses and organs of action in a new way will revolutionize your life and gift you with the power and the healing that comes from deep alignment with soul and universal consciousness.

Take a moment to write down the symptomology of your disease or disharmony, even if it's subtle. Then, begin to place your symptomology into the different qualities and expressions of the elements, and you will discover quick ways to address them that will empower your healing. Guaranteed.

You begin to heal when you choose to begin.

THE SEED OF YOUR UNFOLDING AND THE HEALTH OF YOUR INNER TERRAIN

To thine own self be true.

—William Shakespeare

We are all born with the *seed of our unfolding* already within us. This seed is your constitution at birth, and contains an imprint of your talents, tendencies, and weaknesses, along with your lessons while here on Earth. It is the design of your individual nature. This seed is composed of the five

Elements in different ratios, and is unique to each one of us. It is this seed you must constantly strive to come back into alignment with, in order to experience radiant health and well-being.

Although you and I and the rest of the world are all different, according to Ayurveda or Ayurvedic medicine—the healing science of life or conscious living that comes from the Vedic Hindu system—there are seven main seeds or constitutions. There are really three main **constitutions or doshas (vata, pitta, kapha),** which are combinations of the five Elements, but most of us have a dual constitution as the seed we were born with, meaning two of those constitutions are higher in expression than the third. You could also potentially be tri-doshic (expressing all three main constitutions in close balance of each other.)

In Ayurveda, the word dosha means literally that which disturbs things. Dosha is really the tendency to go out of balance within your body in a certain way.

- Ether and Air give rise to the vata dosha.
- Fire and Water give rise to the pitta dosha.
- Water and Earth give rise to the kapha dosha.

Constitutional medicine is at the heart of Ayurveda or Ayurvedic medicine.

The seed of your unfolding is the seed of your creative potential, and you must nourish it. For your seeds to grow healthy, strong, and vibrant, they require your inner terrain to be fertile, nutrient-rich, healthy, and balanced. This inner terrain is your present condition, the current expression of the ratio of the five Elements through your body system today.

The more you are able to bring your inner terrain into alignment with your own unique seed at birth, the more you will be able to heal deeply and shift away the symptomology you may currently be experiencing. It is by understanding your current terrain, those ratios of the elements present or absent within you, that you can provide yourself with the proper quality of nourishment required to bring your system back into balance and alignment with your unique seed and live a radiant, vibrant, healthy life.

To achieve radiant health, you must journey within to seek and understand that your inner rhythms are both inspired and controlled by the outer rhythms of the elements. To achieve Elemental balance, you have to bring out and engage the "honesty mirror" with an open heart. You must explore what each Element means to you, how it exists within you, and how to then "play" with the outer rhythms of the Elements, and engage in radical self-care until you find balance with the existing ratios of Elements within you.

At birth, the seed of your unfolding contains your creative potential, yet the Garden of Eden you seek to express into the world requires the right soil, the right amount of light, rain, Elements, and spirit dust for life to blossom and flourish.

If you are interested in discovering your own Ayurvedic constitution and how to bring it back to balance through food and lifestyle, I highly recommend the book and work of one of my teachers: Ayurvedic Tongue Diagnosis[5] by Walter "Shantree" Kacera, as well as The Idiot's Guide to Ayurveda[6] by Sahara Rose Ketabi. Both of these books are well worth your time. In the reference section at the back of this book, you will find a list of other Ayurvedic books, resources, and wisdom I have found very helpful along my own healing journey.

Disharmony or disease can be broken down into its qualities, and these can then be related back to the qualities of the Elements. By working with the Elements, you can bring your systems back into balance. Through your symptoms, you can determine if it's a vata, pitta, or kapha state of imbalance. If you use the tools—including food, lifestyle routine, exercise, and meditation that bring that particular constitution back into balance—you'll be amazed at the results. Dis-ease is never just an isolated symptom. The expression of disharmony is always a result of the disturbance of food intake, or lifestyle, or your emotional and mental landscapes and/or your relationship to divine spirit.

By focusing on the Elemental expression of your current state, you can develop a healthier relationship with your disharmony. So, rather than being disempowered by the depth of the current disturbance in your body complex, you can be empowered by the journey. Begin to look at the symbolism and the qualities of your symptomology. It is quite the enlightening process.

Take a deep breath. Pause and feel. Breath deep again. Know you've got this.

---

5   Walter "Shantree" Kacera, Ayurvedic Tongue Diagnosis (Twin Lakes, WI: Lotus Tree Press, 2006).
6   Sahara Rose Ketabi, Ayurveda (Idiot's Guides) (New York, NY: Penugin Random House, 2017).

STOKING YOUR INNER FIRE

Vitality! That's the pursuit of life, isn't it?

—*Katharine Hepburn*

The quickest way to heal is to *pause, feel, and reset* by anchoring the mind in the body. You must anchor the Prana of your mind to reconnect with your inner wisdom. This enables you to bring your actions into alignment with your wisdom and true nature through the proper use of your senses. *The quickest way to remembering your primordial nature is through stoking your inner fire.*

Your **inner fire** is the metabolic power that keeps your digestive forces working; the spark that allows the flow and continuity of processes in your body to happen. It controls your body temperature, your immunity, your awareness, your thoughts, your mind, your health, your energy, and, therefore, your life! It's important to understand that your inner fire is not just present in the digestive system, but is the activator in every metabolic process of your body at a cellular level. When you truly understand this, you understand the importance of your inner fire being strong. Your inner fire is also the metabolic fire that powers your sacred fire, your soul, and your sacredness. It is the spark that fuels your life's purpose; your journey of self-discovery towards your fullest potential.

In opposition to it, we have the **toxicity** that builds within the body. According to Ayurveda, digestion is the cornerstone of health. As dis-ease or dis-harmony move into your body, your inner fire begins to diminish or unbalance your ability to digest, metabolize, and assimilate the life-force in your food is greatly affected, and internal toxicity begins to build, creating imbalance, more dis-ease, and more dis-harmony. On the other hand, the natural by-product of a balanced inner fire is vitality.

The quickest and most effective way to burn off inner toxicity is to balance or increase the power of the digestive fire, your heat and metabolic forces, your connection with the divine, and your own sacredness, and to increase the all-encompassing multidimensional sacred forces of your inner fire. Your inner fire literally burns off toxicity because a strong, balanced inner fire allows you to fully and completely digest, absorb, and assimilate what you ingest (not just the food you eat); therefore, there is no creation of toxicity. Your inner fire also boosts your immune system by destroying any harmful organisms and toxins.

At an emotional level, having a balanced inner fire and digestive power allows you to move through your experiences without a strong attachment to them or to the emotional responses they cause. You can remain *in the flow* and allow the movement of the energetic digestive powers to digest and absorb, then release what is not needed. You are able to stay connected to what ignites your passions and the voice within your heart that is soul.

At a mental level, having a balanced inner fire allows you to develop self-awareness, builds perspective, and further allows you to have a calm and balanced mind, which also allows for the flow of life to move through you freely.

At a spiritual level, having a balanced inner fire allows you to tap into your soul's purpose, building your digestive spiritual power and bringing alignment and congruency back into your life, and removing the veils of spiritual toxicity.

In Ayurveda, rebalancing the digestive fire is a fine-tuning act of connecting with the rhythms of nature and of your body. Understanding your constitution is key to rebalancing your digestive fire. The more you understand your constitution and how it is out of balance, the more you get out of your own way, the more alignment you will have in your life, the stronger and more balanced your digestive power and your inner fire will be, and less toxicity will be present in your system. When your digestive fire is balanced, you feel nourished, full of life, and vibrant. You are able to receive and integrate life's nourishment into all aspects of your body system. When your digestive fire is weak or too strong, toxicity can get hold of your body, emotions, mind, soul, and even your connection to spirit.

The detoxification processes your body uses to activate your inner fire and get rid of toxicity are the feces, urine, and sweat mechanisms for eliminating waste. When these detoxification mechanisms are working efficiently, they move the whole bodily system towards optimum health.

Your body's main channels for interaction with the external environment are through the food you eat, Prana or breath, and water. They, too, bear a huge impact on the activation of your inner fire, and the toxicity production of your body.

An inner-fire balancing program *builds vitality* in the body and consists of the following aspects:

- The physical food you eat, digest, and assimilate
- Everything you consume, digest, and assimilate through your mind, emotions, soul, and spiritual body
- Remembering your sacredness and your divine connection to the *ancestral sacred fire* by aligning your rhythms with the rhythms of nature

The alignment or remembering of all aspects is key to the enhancement of your inner fire for the whole-body system, regardless of the constitution.

Some tools and protocols you can use in your daily life to balance your inner fire are:

- Eating a diet rich in living-plant-based nutrition (a clean diet)
- Using the six tastes to further bring balance into the body (pungent, sour, salty, sweet, astringent, bitter); in particular, using the pungent taste to burn off toxicity
- Applying caution, and the awareness of your constitution, season, age, and so on to prevent creation of further imbalance by the overuse of a taste
- Using herbal bitters such as aloe vera, neem, gentian root, barberry, and goldenseal
- Juice fasting/feasting
- Deep breathing
- Exercising and movement
- Meditating
- Inner questing

As you can see, you will be learning all about the power to balance and rekindle your inner fire throughout this book! How awesome is that!

You may think of stoking your inner fire as mainly stoking your digestive fire or the fire in your belly, but it's much more than that. It's also about reconnecting and awakening the fire in your heart and mind, and stoking your ancestral sacred fire, your soul, your connection with the divine, and your connection with your mightiness.

Stoking the fire of your soul through deep nourishment is as important as eating and drinking the right foods for your constitution, for you are not just a physical being, you are soul, a multi-dimensional divine spiritual being in a process of self-discovery and spiritual unfoldment. When your digestive and sacred fires burn brightly, you are able to align yourself more deeply with the divine, and allow your mightiness (divine life's purpose) to come forth and express itself through you. Stoking the fire is a constant journey of bringing sacredness back into your life and aligning yourself with peace to be peace embodied.

ACTIVATING YOUR COGNITIVE MEMORY

The sixth sense is at the core of our experiences. It is what makes experiences out of events.

—Henry Reed

Cognitive memory is your ancestral memory, your sixth sense, and it lives in your gut. You experience it in those moments of déjà-vu, in those feelings of deep inner knowing that are beyond time and space. It allows you to connect and ignite your remembering of who you are. It is your inner guide.

By deeply nourishing the five roots of your foundation for health, which nourish your five bodies, you are rebuilding your connection with your cognitive memory. By engaging with the world through sacred action, you reconnect with your ancestral knowing, your ancestral lineages, and that aspect of your self that is eternal.

To connect to your cognitive memory, you must awaken and rebalance the element of Ether (space). The practices that heal or awaken our awareness of Ether are sound—in particular sacred sound—breath and silence.

Sacred sounds are the sounds found in nature, mantras (word specific sounds), or sounds created to awaken, harmonize and open specific portals within your body system. Sacred sounds are pathways for healing body, heart, mind, soul, spirit and have been used by many cultures to connect us to the Elements of the universe through our body. Sound has the power to rebuild and harmonize your energy body and the space within you. Your energy body and inner space are directly connected to your essential ancestral cognitive memory. Our lack of exposure and connection with nature, in particular, to the sacred sounds of nature, has caused us to lose our connection to our ancestral cognitive memory. We are living in the midst of a collective amnesia.

Breath: Deep breaths connect you to the Prana of pure cosmic consciousness. Breath not only brings oxygen into your body, but it also brings life-force energy along with it. It is the process through which you are being breathed in and out by the power of life itself. Your breath animates, inspires, and ignites in you your vibrancy, your aliveness, and your connection to the feeling body, to your own wisdom (both ancestral and personal), and to spirit. The life-force energy in the breath is filled with the universal intelligence that informs your cognitive memory.

Silence: In understanding *silence* you begin to know the power of quieting the mind and sitting in the self. You can access the depth of silence in your meditation practice or by spending time in nature. The more you train your mind to bask in *silence*, the more you begin to experience great mental and emotional clarity, and along with it clarity of vision. Through the fullness of silence, you re-awaken to the tapestry of the ancestral field that has always held you, weaving cognitive memory into your heart and using it as your compass forward.

Your understanding and relationship to the five Elements deepens your roots into Mother Earth and anchors your journey into your heart, your Mighty heart. These five Elements also keep you connected and anchored into the cognitive field of memory, as you remember your mightiness.

SUBTLE ORGANIZING ENERGY FIELD (SOEF)

When SOEFs are energized, they develop a more structured and defined organization that better maintains the form and function of the human system. This energizing reverses entropy. It is this property of the SOEFs that reverses the aging process.

—David Wagner and Dr. Gabriel Cousens,
Tachyon Energy: A New Paradigm in Holistic Healing.

As you already know, your body is composed of five body systems, and you've gotten to know your physical form. Surrounding this physical expression is your subtle luminous energy body or field. This luminous energy body has been called many things through the ages and the varying traditions, but one thing remains constant: you *have the ability to affect your luminous **SOEF** and vice versa.*

It is believed that dis-ease first starts in the disorganization of your energy field and, through a process of distillation or materialization, it comes into the physical body. In his book, *Spiritual Nutrition,* Dr. Gabriel Cousens writes at length about the process of materialization of your subtle luminous energy field. He also explains your ability and opportunity to organize and affect this subtle luminous energy field through the consumption of fresh raw living food.

When you consume ***liquid nutrition,*** you are consuming the *essence* of fresh raw living foods, already patterned and coded perfectly for your whole-body system to understand it without the need of an interpreter. It has the power to deeply nourish your system from the cellular level up, reorganizing the expression of coherence or health in your system through repairing, rebuilding, rejuvenating, and regenerating your energy field, not just your physical body.

The power of liquid nutrition extends beyond the physicality of losing weight, and the health and radiance of only your physical body, into the unseen world of subtle energy. It extends into the quality and clarity of your thoughts, into the awareness of your emotions, and that of your subtle luminous body. Perhaps not now, but soon enough, it will reveal itself to you.

The ancestral wisdom of your lineage holds, at its core, practices for the health of the field of coherence around your body. Both mindfulness practices and inner questing are tools to continue to build, integrate and awaken you to your SOEFs.

Mindfulness practices anchor your mind in your body and into the present moment. They re-establish the natural rhythms of breath and brainwave patterns for you to access greater clarity and coherence in everyday living. They allow you to reconnect with your intuitive self and the wisdom of your lineage. They allow you to develop self-compassion, and compassion towards your own humanity.

Inner questing practices allow you to normalize your inner conversation. They allow you to consciously see what is currently present, what is creating the state of dis-ease, consciously release what no longer serves your process, consciously upgrade your operating system, consciously transform, consciously surrender, and consciously integrate as you rebuild the field of coherence in and around your body, and begin to live in greater coherence.

QUANTUM HEALING

Quantum healing is healing the body-mind from a quantum level. That means from a level which is not manifest at a sensory level. Our bodies ultimately are fields of information, intelligence and energy. Quantum healing involves a shift in the fields of energy information, so as to bring about a correction in an idea that has gone wrong. So quantum healing involves healing one mode of consciousness, mind, to bring about changes in another mode of consciousness, body.

—Deepak Chopra

The *quantum field* is the field of energy and physics; the field of consciousness and its journey into form.

Quantum healing is a two-direction process of igniting your Mighty inner healer.

1. *The first direction is the healing that occurs as you journey from form (Earth–body) into consciousness (Ether–soul).*

It is a pathway of involution towards your core that leads to extension in the body system. As you anchor into the five roots, integrate your journey, and rise up, you begin to activate and ignite your whole-body system. You begin to lengthen as you reach up to the sky and rise. As you shift the fields of energy information into greater alignment and coherence, you begin to create space within your body, sacred space to hold yourself, with self-compassion and self-love as you reclaim your power, your truth, your self, and of course, your mightiness.

2. *The second direction is expansion and expression of radiant perfect health as you now move from your integrated core into the outer layers of your system again.*

This second direction of quantum healing holds on to your growth, your shifts in the pathway of your involution and the extension you have created in your body, as it now travels from a more awakened level of consciousness (Ether–soul) into great levels of coherence and health in form (Earth–Body). This second direction moves from the core of your core towards the outer layers of your skin and beyond.

In quantum healing, you integrate all the systems that constitute your body, for the depth of the healing you seek resides in all aspects of your self, not just in one particular area. The expression of disease in your body is affected by your emotional state, mental state, awareness of soul, and spiritual connection. How often have you heard that *the manifestation of disease in the physical body is a cry of the soul to align itself with its spiritual nature?* Your crises and challenges always come from a spiritual condition, and are always an opportunity for a spiritual awakening.

The entire field of quantum energy is malleable to your thoughts, emotions, presence, and intentions. It is a field of resonance and vibration, one you can access as you align your conscious mind with your *super conscious soul,* and as you enrol your subconscious mind in your process of evolution for your highest good.

THE JOURNEY HOME

A man travels the world over in search of what he needs and returns home to find it.

—*George A. Moore*

The journey home is the path to your inner source. It's the path of remembering of your true nature that is primordial.

Your journey home is your path to the space deep within that brings forth your sense of belonging, your sense of well-being, and your sense of love and of engaging with life through sacredness. It is the pathway that leads you to connect deeply to the eternal aspect of yourself that animates you into longevity, and which allows you to be in relationship with the part of yourself that is immortal.

The journey home is different for each of us, for home is a different place to us all. We are all unique and, in your uniqueness, your sense of home will vary from mine. Yet the quality of our sense of home is the same.

The journey home is your journey of involution, your path of healing, of becoming whole, of aligning your body-mind-emotion-soul-spirit bodies with universal cosmic consciousness and with the mightiness you came here to express and be, always benevolent in nature.

The journey home is your path of deep healing and personal revolution that leads to radiant health and well-being.

So I ask, when you close your eyes:

- What does home feel like?
- What does home smell like?
- What does home taste like?
- What does home look like?
- What does home sound like?

Take the time to explore with your senses your feeling of home. The more intimate you become with it, the more it will nourish your well-being. The more it will both guide and ground your journey. The more it will become a part of your heart compass, guiding you along your roadmap to wellness.

THE ANCIENT AS THE FUTURE

The future has an ancient heart.

—Carlo Levy

The laws of the universe are eternal. ***The ancient is the future. The future is the ancient.*** The universal laws of your unfolding and your becoming exist in constant motion and will continue to carve your sacred path. But are you creating the best sacred vessel you can to allow the laws of nature to express themselves through you? Can you use the ancient wisdom that lives within you as the foundation for your future self to stand on? Can use your future self as a vehicle for the ancient wisdom to come alive again?

Knowledge is learned. Wisdom is remembered.

The ancient wisdom was born out of the consciousness of the Masters. It is here, alive within you, in your ancestral lineage, in your DNA, ready to be remembered and awakened, ready to help you elevate. The ancient can teach you much about your path of alignment with radiant health, your path of personal evolution and self-realization, but are you able to slow yourself enough to listen, and deeply feel its wisdom?

The ancient has the power to spark culture into creating new realities. In today's modern world, an era of disconnection from the multi-dimensionality of your body, of disconnection from your sacredness and your wholeness, the ancient is your foundation to reclaim your ecological self and through it build a sustainable future. The power of radiant health lies in the reclaiming of all the fragmented pieces of your self: ancestral self, essential self, ecological self, emotional or conscious mental self, sacred self, intuitive self, and the cosmic self. Your radiant health is the quest for your becoming whole again.

What kind of future are you creating now?
Are you still gathering the fragmented pieces of your heart?
What kind of foundation are you building for your self and for the generations
to come?
Do your actions stop with your life, or are they eternal in their consequence?
Do you already have what you need to be the change you seek in the world?
I trust you know the answer.

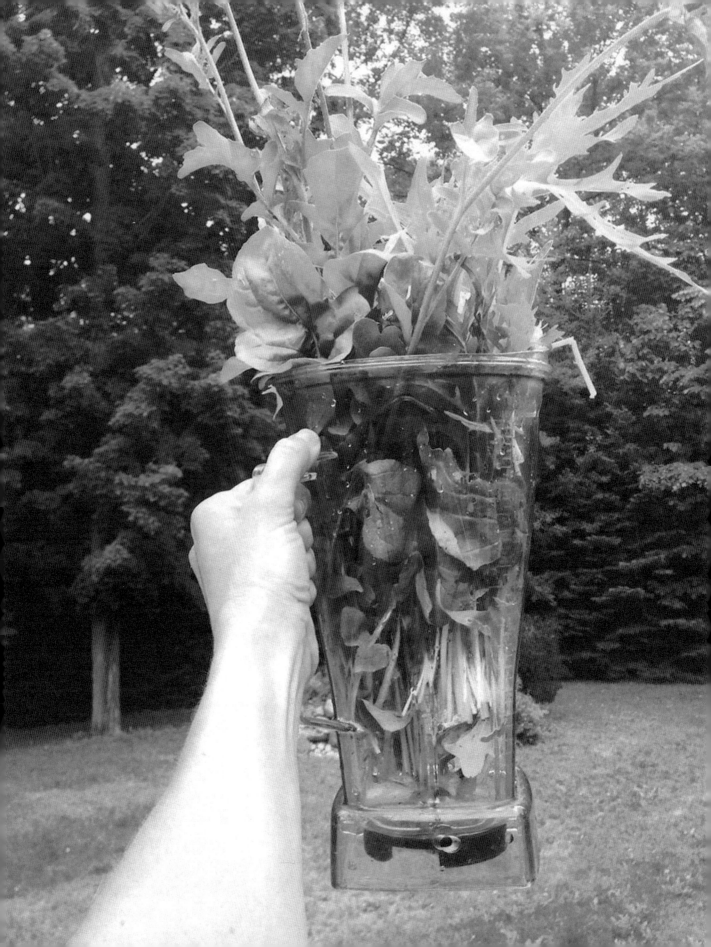

III

LET YOUR INNER SHINE GLOW WITH THE POWER OF LIQUID NUTRITION

WHEN THE HEART IS ON FIRE, LIGHT COMES
FROM WITHIN.

—TANIA SILVA

DO YOU LIKE GREEN JUICE AND HAM?

I do NOT like them!
I do not like green juice and ham…

But what if you knew green juice had double super Mighty powers?
Would you like it then?

I would not like it now,
I would not like it then,
I would not like it in my house,
I would not like it at your house,

I would not like it here,
I would not like it there,
I would not like it at a Starbucks,
I would not like it annyyyywwhhere!!!

… Wait, what? Double super Mighty powers? What did you just say?
You and I are living at the best of times. We are also living at one of the most challenging times for our health and the health of society. Somehow, something is failing us. We live at the best of times because we have available to us incredible tools, technologies, and sources of information to facilitate our own healing and our capacity to express our best potential. On the other side of the coin, we are being challenged by an epidemic of disease that surrounds us in all its forms.

As you become aware of the connection between your health and your habits, your emotional landscape, the foods you eat, your lifestyle, and the levels of toxicity in your immediate and not-so-immediate environment, you will come to understand that the pursuit of radiant health can be a long and complicated one. Yet because we live at the best of times, we have available to us incredible tools and technologies, both simple and complex, to facilitate the remembering, awakening and igniting of your Mighty inner healer, as well as facilitate your journey towards radiant health, and support you in maintaining it.

You may or may not have heard of the green juice revolution, but perhaps smoothies have made their way into your house and into your heart. Or, perhaps you are new to all this, so welcome! It's a brave new world, and one where it's clear your actions have great power to build your own road towards greater health or disease. The choice is yours—and we can no longer afford to remain unaware.

Though disease in its many forms may apparently manifest suddenly, it actually takes years to build internally. To quote Dr. Max Gerson, *"Disease can only exist in the body if two conditions are present: toxicity and mineral deficiencies."*

Please read that again.

Let's take a look at the first condition: **toxicity**. Are we living in challenging times, where toxicity has skyrocketed? Do we find that our water, our air, and the soil where we grow our food is not as clean as it used to be? Are the overall levels of heavy metal toxicity in our bodies a lot higher than the generations that came before us?

Let's take a look at the second condition: **mineral deficiencies**. Is it possible that our bodies are not getting what they need? Is it possible that because of the poor soil quality we have today, food, in general, is lacking in the full mineral diversity needed for our bodies to thrive? Is it possible that because, as a society, our diet has shifted to one of mainly processed foods, we are also facing mineral deficiencies?

It is, in my opinion, all very possible. Having healed myself from elevated heavy metal toxicity that was causing numbness on the right side of my body, *I know this:* we have the ability to address both toxicity and mineral deficiencies, and heal ourselves from the cellular level to the tip of our nose! The journey ahead is non-linear. It's a process that might require us to change, but as change is the only constant in life, that is a good thing. *Change—though sometimes challenging—forces us to grow, to see ourselves, and perhaps to reach our best potential.*

I also know that **liquid nutrition**—fresh-pressed juices, smoothies, and elixirs—is the fastest and safest way to address both toxicity and mineral deficiencies. The art of including fresh juices, green or not, smoothies, and elixirs into our diet provides the body with the tools and technologies needed to address our present condition *at its root cause.*

The super Mighty powers of liquid nutrition are anchored on what I like to call its *dual action properties.* Liquid nutrition allows you to cleanse and detoxify your system at the cellular level. At the same time, you are providing your cells with a vast array of mineral density to restore your body from the ground up by repairing, rebuilding, rejuvenating, and regenerating your system. Though there is no magic pill, there *is* a magical process, for when you begin including liquid nutrition, be it a fresh juice, smoothie, or elixir, you will feel change start to happen from the inside out.

We all lead busy lives and I know that changing your habits and your relationship to food is not an easy task. Yet I also understand the *law of addition:* as you begin to add new habits into your life that better support and sustain you, what no longer serves you simply gets left behind. As you add liquid nutrition to your current diet, you might just find yourself craving a healthier diet than the one you currently follow. You might find yourself inspired by a new exercise routine, or our new-found commitment to get outside and walk in the nearby woods.

What I'm saying is this: whether you eat ham or not, fresh-pressed juices, smoothies, and elixirs are here to stay. They have the power to revolutionize your body, your heart, and your mind. I invite you to welcome them into your life—for if you try them, you might like them and if you like them, you may just be a part of the greater liquid nutrition revolution. And that just might change your life.

THE POWER OF LIQUID NUTRITION

Breathe more than what you drink, drink more than what you eat.

—*Shantree Kacera*

You've heard about it, you've seen your friends try it, you've been getting closer and closer—as if standing at the edge of the hill on tiptoes, ready to jump, waiting for the winds of change to take you over the edge.

So what is the craze ,you ask? What is this thing called liquid nutrition? Why is it "da cool" thing to do? What is its power, and what kind of power does it infuse into us? What is juicing and smoothing? Why now? Why me? Why should I bother anyway? All fair questions. But if you are here, there's a good chance your heart already knows the answers.

Liquid nutrition has the power of restoring your vitality, repairing your nutrient deficiencies, and re-mineralizing your body and rebuilding a stronger foundation for radiant health in your life. Liquid nutrition contains three main pillars, and all three need to be utilized to maximize the potential of what this new foundation offers.

The three pillars of liquid nutrition are:

1. Juicing
2. Making smoothies
3. Making elixirs

Each pillar contains a variety of tools and benefits, and each works in its own way to help you and I blossom into a new state of well-being and radiant health.

Juicing is the art of adding fresh-pressed, living, unpasteurized juices to your diet. For more healing and greater alkalizing, fresh-pressed green vegetable juices are recommended. Juices are the essence of living food in liquid form; all the fibre is removed from the vegetables/fruits, leaving only high-nutrient structured water full of minerals, enzymes, oxygen, and life-force. Because it is a fibre-less liquid, your body does not need to digest it; it's as if the foods we juice are pre-digested, thus freeing a lot of energy for the needed detoxification, cleansing, repairing, and rebuilding processes. Juicing helps liberate key nutrients and enzymes from the tough plant cell walls, allowing your body to receive and easily absorb most of the nutrition. Fresh-pressed juices are the number one alkalizer!

Smoothies, in particular green smoothies, have won the hearts of many as they contain fibre that acts like a broom on your insides, sweeping away all toxicity, particularly in the large intestine. Smoothies are also great alkalizers, but in comparison to juices, they are digested by the body due to their high fibre content. Smoothies or blended foods are great for us, as a big part of the digestive process has been pre-done for you by your blender, so your body has an easier time digesting them—without expending lots of energy!

Elixirs, on the other hand, are medicinal infusions of love; they are your immunity rebuilders. They are often based on tea infusions from medicinal herbs, wild edibles, and herbs steeped for our well-being. They can be synergistically combined with a variety of superfoods to enhance the healthy gene expression of your core, but they have the Mighty power to do that on their own. They are fascinating in that by consuming them and getting to know them, we begin to get in touch with our own ancient plant wisdom, with the process of emergence of the heart and the emergence of universal consciousness through us.

Liquid nutrition is the process of integrating nutrient-dense fresh-pressed living juices, smoothies, and elixirs into your daily life for healthy gene expression, for longevity, for radiant and vibrant health, and for the emergence of your Mighty sacred heart. Liquid nutrition is a process, a tool to let your inner shine glow, and for remembering your body as a living sanctuary. It is a tool to reclaim your health, your ownership of your body, your sacredness, your ecological self, your radiance, your clarity of thought and action, and your responsibility over your life and the earth. It is a tool for understanding the nature of your mind and the possibilities that exist for making the life of your dreams the life that you live. Liquid nutrition is an ally in the awakening of your mightiness.

You see, food and drinks are not just what we put into our mouths a few times a day, with no consequence or effect on your system. What you eat and drink has the power to revolutionize your consciousness and the consciousness of the planet. The depth and variety of mineralization available to your body system through what you eat and drink can lead you down two very distinct paths: the path to radiant health (mightiness) or the path to disease. Yes, I realize there are other factors affecting us, too, but this one is key to your well-being.

You are born to thrive. Your body wants to live and grow and evolve, and your heart wants to emerge. They know their purpose even if you have forgotten. Can you remind yourself of your journey? Can you reconnect with what it means to have a clear bond with your heart, your mind, and your mission? Can you take responsibility over your ecological self, and reclaim your sacredness along the way? Everything is interconnected.

What is happening in the world at large is also happening inside our body. The environmental mess we are in globally is reflected in the large numbers of autoimmune disease, cancer, diabetes, and so on that humanity is experiencing as a collective at this time. Our inner terrains are collapsing; we cannot sustain ourselves on this road. It is simply impossible. But we do have options. Yes, you might be required to change your ways. But if you have the courage to make that change, you'll start to see the fruits of your labour: you will begin to feel better, to be more vibrant, to flow with life-force energy, and to inspire yourself and those around you to live more coherent lives.

This is not just about me or you. It's about **all of us**. Each individual experience of change and healing results in a collective change of consciousness and transformation into a new era of peace, respect, sustainability, responsibility, love, and evolution. One juice, one smoothie, one elixir at a time. *So, let your inner shine glow!*

HISTORY OF LIQUID NUTRITION

No matter what it is you're looking for, you can probably find it at the bottom of a green smoothie glass.

—Britt Brandon

Although fresh-pressed living juices and smoothies seem to have been caught on a wildfire of popularity, and it seems like juice bars are opening up on every other block, they are, in fact, not a new invention. But there certainly have been plenty of recent innovations in the field of liquid nutrition.

Early documented evidence of people juicing for health can be found on the Dead Sea Scrolls dating from 408 BC to 70 AD. It is described in the scrolls as: "*A pounded mash of pomegranate and fig resulting in profound strength and subtle form.*"

Through the centuries, juicing for healing was actually made through pestle and mortar, grinding and pressing the mash through linen or cloth to extract the essence of herbs and plants thought of as medicinal, to be used both internally and externally. One of the best-known users of liquid nutrition for healing was the Greek founder of modern medicine, Hippocrates.

From the 1920s to the late 1950s, German scientist Dr. Max Gerson used fresh raw living juices in combination with a vegetarian diet to treat his patients suffering from tuberculosis, heart disease, kidney failure, and cancer. He first began to experiment with diet and fresh raw living juices because he personally suffered from severe migraines. Through treating one of his patients with migraines in this way, he discovered he was also able to treat tuberculosis. He went on to further study the effects of diet on our health, and founded The Gerson Institute, which still operates today in San Diego and Mexico.

In 1936, Dr. Norman Walker published the book *Raw Vegetable Juices*.[7] He studied and immersed himself in the lifestyle of what he called living foods. His work was key to the development and understanding of raw foods and fresh living juices as a tool for vibrant health. The Norwalk Juicer became the world's best juicer, and is still considered the best in the world. Developed by Dr. Walker, it's a two-step juicer. First, all the raw vegetables and fruits are ground to a fine, moist pulp. Second they are passed through a hydraulic press, which extracts the juice from the pulp

---

7   Norman W. Walker, Raw Vegetable Juices: What's Missing in Your Body? (Betonville, AK: Norwalk Press, 1970).

by pressing them under high pressure. This two-step process allows the juices to contain as much as 50% high-nutrient density and will produce 25% more juice from the same amount of raw produce than other juicers.

The Norwalk Juicer is the one used at The Gerson Institute. Then, in 1954 the Champion Juicer was invented—the world's first masticating juicer.

Between 1960 and 1980, the power of juicing was introduced to the American public through the work of people like Bernard Jensen, Jack Lalanne, and Jay Kordich. In 1961, Ann Wigmore and Viktoras Kluvinskas founded the Hippocrates Health Institute, which became the face of the alternative health care movement in the USA. It has evolved into an educational centre for health and healing, successfully treating disease through a raw food diet and high quantities of fresh raw living juices. Today, the Hippocrates Health Institute still operates in West Palm Beach, FL.

In 1987, Dr. Gabriel Cousens, founder of the Tree of Life Centre in Arizona, published *Spiritual Nutrition and The Rainbow Diet*.[8] He revolutionized dietary consciousness by shifting the materialistic–mechanistic paradigm of nutrition into a spiritual one, recognizing that living food and liquid nutrition have the power to detoxify, repair, regenerate, rejuvenate, and heal our whole-body systems at the DNA level, as well as at the subtle energy level. This approach to nutrition has the power to raise our vibrations and our awareness, and therefore shift our consciousness.

In 2004, Victoria Boutenko created the green smoothie. Her book *Green for Life*,[9] revolutionized the health movement. Victoria and her family used raw foods and green smoothies as the foundational tools to heal themselves of life-threatening diseases they developed after immigrating to America from Russia in 1990, and adopting the standard American diet (SAD). In her search for deeper health, she created the green smoothie, and returned to our social awareness the power of including fibre and chlorophyll as part of our liquid nutrition.

Over the last twenty-five years, David Wolfe—health, nutrition, and natural beauty expert—popularized the use of superfoods and elixirs as tools for deep nourishment, healing, radiant health and longevity. His book *The Sunfood Diet Success System*[10] introduced greater awareness to the public about the power of raw foods.

Many others have walked the path and been a big influence on the discovery of the power of liquid nutrition. These are only a few whose work, tools, and principles have guided my journey

---

8 C: Cassandra Press, 1987)
9 Victoria Boutenko, Green for Life (Berkeley, CA: North Atlantic Books, 2010)
10 David Wolfe, The Sunfood Diet Success System (Berkeley, CA: North Atlantic Books, 1999).

into liquid nutrition, and whose words and actions have awakened in me the desire to understand its powers.

I would say this about the history of liquid nutrition: there has been a shift in consciousness about the power of liquid nutrition to regain our health, to be the fountain of youth, to be the elixir of life … the elixir of immortality … the philosopher's stone.

Although its synergy still lives in the world of the mystical and magical, you and I, here on this earth, have the opportunity to create a little heaven within our own body to act as a conductor of the cosmos through the emergence of our Mighty heart. All this is facilitated by the power of liquid nutrition to nourish your whole being with the evolutionary vibration and information to be your own fountain of life, by being the conscious alchemist of your own life, and thus continuing to assist the world's shift in consciousness.

THE PURPOSE OF LIQUID NUTRITION

---

*Remember that every single green drink you create is an investment
in your quality of life — now and always.*

—*Kris Carr*

There are many purposes for integrating liquid nutrition into your diet. As you begin to include more liquid power into your life, you will begin to change and revolutionize yourself from the inside out. As you alter the terrain of your cells into an alkaline state, you begin to re-mineralize yourself, detoxify old wounds—and old piles of undesired friendly organisms (UFOs) that have made your precious body their home.

As you detoxify you re-mineralize, your symptomatology perhaps won't be as strong or maybe won't last as long, as you are now rebuilding yourself from the ground up. You simultaneously detoxify, repair, rebuild, rejuvenate, and regenerate! One drink at a time. By bringing the essence of life in liquid form into your body, you are rapidly and massively changing, enlivening, and infusing your cells with vitality, and activating not only your healthy gene expression, but also the expression of longevity in your life.

As you begin to include more liquid nutrition in your diet, you'll begin to feel better—more alive, more radiant, more vibrant, more energetic, more enthusiastic—and you'll able to more easily cope and deal with challenges. Your relationship to self and others will change because you've shown up for yourself; your body begins to trust you in a different way as you begin to trust yourself. And so the world begins to shift—and simultaneously your view of the world begins to shift.

You begin to sharpen and fine-tune your senses. You begin to connect with deeper levels of your intuition, with the voice within, and with the essence of your potentiality, and a clearer emergence of purpose begins to appear. Your senses sharpen, if you will, because you are not spending as much energy digesting your food, leaving more nutrition readily available to absorb and use for detoxification, repairing, rebuilding, rejuvenating, and regenerating. Very impressive!

Our five senses are the way we gather information from the external world, as well as the way we deliver our internal information to the external world. The clearer and sharper your five senses are, the clearer and more effective your communication will be—with both the outer world and the realm that exists within you. Your five senses provide you with the information you need to interpret, make sense of, and interact with the world around you, in synergy with the world within.

Remember (again) when I spoke about the root causes of disease? Do you recall what the first root cause of disease is? (See page 8, if you want to take a peek.)

The first root cause of disease is the misuse of your senses. So, mighty reader, through liquid nutrition, you have an opportunity to address the first root cause of disease—at its source. Whoa! Powerful! The more you sharpen your senses, the less you will misuse them, the more you will power up your health, ignite your transformation, and (yes!) spark your revolution. Period.

Also, remember reading about the Elements, their relationship with your sense organs, and your ability to fine tune their expression of harmony or disease by shifting the action of the particular sense organ? (See page 54 if you want to take another peek.) Again, liquid nutrition is one of your strongest allies in your ability to shift, and bring balance and harmony into your life.

Liquid nutrition is an activator and a facilitator of that sense and heartfelt clarity. It's a portal, a gateway to the journey from your mind back into your heart, and through to your spiritual connection to self, to community, to others, to your wholeness, to universal intelligence or the god of your own understanding, back through to the heart as the emergence of the Mighty sacred heart, now living in conscious relationship with both the seen and unseen worlds, to all *life,* including living in conscious relationship with Mother Earth, our original source and the foundation of our existence.

The Mighty sacred heart is that space within that is universal truth and love. The cleaner and more aware you are of the power of your senses as the bridge between your current self identification and the ancient wisdom that lives within, the more you will be able to be of service to yourself, your immediate community, humanity as a whole, and Mother Earth.

With great purpose comes great responsibility. It's important to identify and be specific about the intention behind cleansing the sense organs. I believe your intention will greatly support the outcome of your cleanse and the clarity of the unfolding that naturally happens.

It's important to be honest with yourself. And whatever the answer is for you, it is perfect for you. It's all good. We are all unique, and it's by recognizing and tending to your own uniqueness that you will begin to integrate your self back to wholeness. Your journey is yours, so cherish it.

Intentions are the seed for manifestation, so what is it you want to manifest through the cleansing of your sense organs? What is it you want to manifest by incorporating liquid nutrition into your life? What are you searching for? Can you be your most true expression of your potentiality, right here, right now?

My intention for incorporating all three pillars of liquid nutrition into my life began in the midst of a healing crisis. It began because I truly believe our body has the innate ability to heal itself; we just have to understand what it is trying to tell us.

My intention for including liquid nutrition on a daily basis, and as part of monthly and seasonal detox, is the awakening of the Mighty healer in me, the purification of my entire body complex (physical, emotional, mental, and spiritual bodies), clarity of mind, awareness of soul, depth of purpose, a deeper experience of who I really am, and a deeper connection to spirit, inner peace, spiritual freedom, and ultimately enlightenment.

Take the time to inquire within. What are your intentions? What is your purpose in aligning yourself with the powers, purposes and mightiness of liquid nutrition? Remember all is good, anything goes … just be true.

LIVING SYSTEMS CODE OF LIQUID NUTRITION | PRINCIPLES AND PROPERTIES

There are living systems; there is no living "matter."

—Jacques Monod

In life, there are always many great systems at play that rule our existence. These systems contain within them principles and properties for life, as we know it, to exist. These systems create the sacred container through which all life exists, yet as we shift in consciousness and in awareness, new life systems come into place with the potential to advance your own evolution, as well as the evolution of the planet.

What I call the living systems code of liquid nutrition can be broken down into the following principles and properties:

1. Made with fresh raw living organic foods and superfoods
2. Cleansing and rebuilding dual action
3. High enzymatic power
4. Building your alkaline powers
5. Structured living water
6. Conscious drinking
7. Vibrational resonance

1. MADE WITH FRESH RAW LIVING ORGANIC FOODS AND SUPERFOODS

The food you eat can be either the safest and most powerful form of medicine or the slowest form of poison.

—Ann Wigmore

Fresh raw living foods contain the most minerals and vitamins of any food. Not only that, when consumed with as little processing as possible, or when processed below the temperature of 115°F, there is little loss of vitamins and minerals. Your body cells get a chance to bathe and indulge in a rich environment of minerals and vitamins necessary for your well-being. Minerals and trace minerals are the basic building, health-maintaining, detoxifying, and rejuvenating substances that your body needs to continue to build up to better health, to be disease resistant, and to journey on towards longevity.

The mightiness of liquid nutrition lies entirely on the principle that it is made with fresh raw living foods and superfoods. The power of liquid nutrition is the essence of the power of these fresh raw living foods to be a foundation for radiant and optimal health, and a founding principle in the healing journey should we have lost our way. Liquid nutrition results from the history of the evolution of the awareness of diet, in particular how a diet of fresh raw living foods can be a foundational stone in our health, and in our experience of life as a vibrant, interconnected consciousness seeking to express itself.

As you begin to introduce more fresh raw living foods and superfoods into your diet, you will begin to increase your awareness of not only *what you are eating/putting into your body, but also what you are* not *eating/putting into your body.*

This shift and progression in awareness will lead you to the impact, power, and recognition of the importance for organic food to become one of your sources for deep nourishment.

Authentic organic Agriculture is a step forward in the reclaiming of your inner and world ecology, and it plays a key role in the sustainability and healing of the planet. It is a step towards reconnecting with the Element of Earth to bring much needed balance to our modern societies. It is a step towards producing high-quality health-building food without the use of GMOs, irradiation, or toxic chemicals (pesticides and herbicides).

Authentic organic agriculture should involve the practice of the growth of multi-crops, which re-mineralize the earth, providing much-needed nutrients to our topsoil. It's a more ethical, aware, and humane practice for food production, and for animal growth. Through eating organically grown foods, you become aware of the connection between the foods you eat, and your health and vitality. You begin to recognize the power of your choices, and the power you have as an individual to change a culture addicted to the convenience of processed foods. You begin to recognize food as something far more powerful than just what you put into your mouth a few times a day. You begin to recognize the part you play in the current ecological mess our planet is in, and you begin to take responsibility for what you can do locally (because we can do a lot) and the footprint you choose to leave behind.

Living plants grown through authentic organic methods are the foundation of the living systems code of living and liquid nutrition, and of fresh raw living foods. They are at the core and root of your well-being and, yes, your mightiness.

Living plants grown through authentic organic methods are highly mineralized sources of sun energy, information, frequencies of consciousness, and electromagnetic frequencies for your body to assimilate, integrate, and thrive. Without them, the biochemistry of your body begins to fail and you cannot survive, never mind heal. Without them, you cannot engage fully with life and develop to the best of your potential. Without them, our bodies begins to atrophy and die.

Minerals are the foundation of life. This is a known fact. All life on earth, including human life, is composed of minerals, and requires minerals on a continual basis to survive, thrive, and heal. It is a known fact that the state of our health can be traced back to having sufficient minerals, or a lack of them. It is a known fact that the minerals, enzymes, and life-force found in our living foods are destroyed by cooking in high heat or with rancid oils. It is a known fact that most animals eat living plants as the foundation—if not all—of their diet. We just seem to have forgotten.

The role of living plants is to convert the minerals found in living soil, through the energy of the sun, into ionic or "Angstrom-size" minerals for us to absorb. They are the "middle man," or perhaps a better analogy would be, they are our "distillation process" between pure raw cosmic energy and cosmic energy that has been distilled or transformed into a language or code that our body can understand.

The role of living plants is to also provide your body with:

- Friendly bacteria that will protect you from infections from pathogenic bacteria, viruses, fungi, and parasites
- Phytonutrients you and I need for optimal health. Plant-based proteins, fats, carbohydrates, fibres, enzymes, and complex nutrients found only in raw or minimally processed live foods
- Adaptogens that assist you and me in adapting to life's demands and everyday living
- Antioxidants that assist your body in getting rid of free radicals, but also in reversing the process of oxidization that literally "rusts" your body from the inside out

It is safe to say that humanity is now experiencing the advanced, destructive effects of the Industrial Revolution. For those of us who can see and have awoken to the brutal reality of deep pollution, greed, and the manipulation of nature, we can see that our health and the health of the planet have both been compromised by the practices that developed from the unconscious industrialization of our systems.

The unconscious mass production of food by huge commercial factory farms and factory processing has caused the quality of our food to deteriorate so badly the human race is now declining in health globally. But not many are wanting to see it, nor are they wanting to follow other more conscious and sustainable systems that have begun to manifest as a result of reclaiming our health (of body/emotions/mind/spirit), our ancestry and heritage, and our planet in ways that will provide sustainability for generations to come.

Note: Even though choosing organically grown food is important, I understand that organic produce is expensive, not always available or accessible, and sometimes just not possible. But there are ways to eat cleaner foods without breaking the bank. The following are some suggestions I personally follow:

- Invest in buying organic foods such as leafy greens, as well as the *dirty dozen* foods listed here, which are most heavily sprayed:

Apples	Pears
Celery	Potatoes
Cherries	Strawberries
Grapes	Spinach
Nectarines	Sweet bell peppers
Peaches	Tomatoes

- Know your fifteen clean conventional (non-organic) foods that suffer the lowest pesticide use:

Asparagus	Kiwi
Avocados	Mangos
Broccoli	Onions

Cabbage	Papayas*
Cantaloupe	Pineapples
Cauliflower	Sweet corn*
Eggplant	Sweet peas (frozen)
Honeydew melon	

Per the EWG—Environmental Working Group, a small amount of sweet corn, papaya and summer squash sold in the United States is produced from Genetically Engineered (GE) seed stock. If you want to avoid GE produce, buy organic varieties of these crops.

- Visit a farmers market and get to know your farmers! Many farmers are not certified organic farmers, yet they are growing food in natural ways, with minimal use of pesticides and herbicides. Supporting them continues to support the reclaiming of our ethical responsibilities towards our individual bodies and our greater body: Mother Earth.
- Invest in a CSA membership or weekly food basket. CSAs are seasonal or year-round farm memberships that support the local farming economy. On a weekly basis, you will receive a basket of local seasonal produce in exchange for your financial support of the farm. It's a great way to support your farmers, and get to know the heart, soul, and soil of the people who grow your food.
- Grow your own sprouts at home!
- Grow a small garden in the summer. You will be amazed at the amount of produce you can enjoy from your own small garden.
- Purchase fruits and vegetables that can be peeled if non-organic.
- Above all, eat and drink with the awareness of love. Any fresh produce is better than processed food and will begin to build your body up.

2. CLEANSING AND REBUILDING DUAL ACTION

We must always change, renew, rejuvenate ourselves; otherwise, we harden.

—*Johann Wolfgang von Goethe*

Fresh raw living food nutrition, and specifically liquid nutrition (juices, smoothies, and elixirs), has the ability to both cleanse and rebuild your body at a cellular level. It literally flushes your whole system with high-density nutrients, cleaning out all that inner toxicity at a cellular level, and nourishing those cells with oxygen, high-octane nutrients, and life-force.

Liquid nutrition has the potential to rebuild your DNA and turn off disease gene expression. Because raw food does both simultaneously—it cleanses *and* rebuilds—I call it the ***cleansing/ rebuilding dual action.*** Raw foods, in particular liquid nutrition, have the power to also repair, regenerate, and rejuvenate your body at a cellular level. It is truly pure synergy at work.

Are you beginning to see why it has the potential to be the philosopher's stone?

Knowing this, you can then emphasize one action or the other, depending on where you are on your journey. For example:

- You can introduce ***juice fasts*** into your lifestyle, as a way to deepen the cleansing action, and create a deeper sense of spiritual purpose and clarity
- You can introduce ***juice feasts*** and ***smoothie cleanses*** into your lifestyle as a way to deepen your rebuilding action, feasting and bathing your body with nutrient density, allowing mineral and nutritional deficiencies to be addressed. These will, of course, also detoxify your body
- You can use high dosages of superfoods, probiotics, and food enzymes to go even deeper and force a major rebuilding, repairing, rejuvenating, regenerating change within your cells
- You can juice fast just one day a week, to give your internal organs a break, and let them focus on spending their energy repairing and rebuilding
- You can add specific raw foods to rebuild, and place more emphasis on superfoods, sprouted nuts, seeds, and greens

Life-force means the energy that is able to create life. Raw living foods have their life-force almost intact, and thus transfer it to us when we consume them. This life-force is not just the physical accumulation of the right minerals, vitamins, enzymes, and so on, but a field of energy that builds upon your health and sustains, detoxifies, and regenerates your whole-body system into the future. This life-force is what gives you that inner vibrancy and vitality that makes you shine, and honours within you the force that gives you life.

When you prepare a juice, a smoothie, or an elixir, you are distilling this life-force into its essence; a liquid power shot of the vibrancy of life with the ability to express your highest and purest living potential!

3. HIGH ENZYMATIC POWERS

Enzymes are a true yardstick of vitality. Enzymes offer an important means of calculating the vital energy of an organism.

—Dr. Edward Howell, father of food enzyme research in the Twentieth century.

Ann Wigmore, founder of the Hippocrates Health Institute and mother of the raw-foods movement in America, says that "enzyme preservation is the secret to health."

Dr. Edward Howell, food enzyme researcher, taught two key concepts about enzymes:

1. Enzymes are living, biochemical factors that activate and carry out all the biological processes in the body, such as digestion, nerve impulses, the detoxification process, the functioning of the RNA/DNA, repairing and healing the body, and even thinking.

2. The capacity of an organism to make enzymes is exhaustible.

Enzymes are energized protein molecules, and necessary for your body's every function. There are three types of enzymes:

1. Metabolic, which activate all your metabolic processes
2. Digestive, in charge of your digestion processes
3. Food enzymes

Enzymes are the cornerstone of health, and a major reason why fresh raw living foods are deeply healing, detoxifying, repairing, rebuilding, rejuvenating, and regenerating. All vitamins, minerals, and hormones in your body *must have enzymes to function properly.* As we age, our body's ability to produce enzymes declines naturally, more so if it's been under the stress of having to process cooked and denatured foods for most of our lives.

Imagine, if you will, enzymes as the team captains. They know the treasure map of your body in ways no one else does, and lead the way to vibrant health and longevity where "X" marks the spot. Imagine, if you will, enzymes having the ability to act like Pac-Man, eating away all the debris and cellular toxicity that's been allowed to build within your body.

Powerful. Now imagine that, as we age, and because we've been eating a diet low in enzymes, your team captain (enzymes) begins to get lost and is unable to deliver the treasure of radiant health, because it no longer has the strength, ability, or the numbers to play its favourite Pac-Man game, allowing toxicity to build within your system and simply take over.

Fresh raw living foods are the highest in food ***enzymes***. Nature is wise, and has provided the enzymes necessary to digest particular foods—within the foods themselves! This is of key importance in the maintenance of your own enzymatic levels, as well as the proper functioning of your digestive system.

Most diseases begin with a weakness in your digestive system, due to many possible causes. But if your system is weakened, and you become aware of the power of enzymes to heal, rejuvenate, and rebuild your digestive system, you can easily understand how to use this vital tool to your advantage. Enzymes are health activators; I like to think of them as my *health activator warriors.* They are pure potential, and work both on a physical and energetic level.

When plant enzymes are taken as a supplement or, even better, when you drink your liquid gold (because it is full of enzymes), particularly on an empty stomach, they boost your immunity by cleaning house, by clearing the toxicity that becomes a burden to your liver and internal organs, and by purifying your blood and bringing oxygen rich nutrients into your cells.

When you drink fresh juices, smoothies, or elixirs, this high-enzymatic power found in fresh raw living foods is absorbed rapidly because you are consuming liquid nutrition, which your body then uses to create the best possible conditions for vibrant radiant health.

Food enzymes are destroyed when food is cooked above 115F. There are two ways of maintaining optimum levels of enzymes in your body: the first is by taking enzyme supplements, the second, and the one I prefer, is through drinking liquid nutrition and, even better, doing it on an empty stomach.

Some of the benefits of taking enzymes, both supplements or through fresh liquid nutrition on an empty stomach, are:

- Stimulates the immune system
- Shatters crystalline deposits
- Breaks up cholesterol deposits
- Increases white blood cell size and activity
- Increases the surface area of the red blood cell, enabling it to carry more oxygen to all parts of the body
- Aids in the digestion of proteins
- Aids in the assimilation of fats
- Aids in the reduction of bacteria
- Aids the assimilation and elimination of toxins
- Aids in the elimination of yeast (*Candida albicans*)

4. BUILDING YOUR ALKALINE POWERS

No disease, including cancer, can exist in an alkaline environment.

—*Dr. Otto Warburg*

The acid-alkaline balance of the body is key to good health. Our ***pH*** is a measure of hydrogen ion concentration; a measure of the acidity or alkalinity of a solution. Understanding what makes your pH more acidic or more alkaline is key in staying balanced and healthy, or in regaining our health, should we become ill.

Within your body, a pH balancing act is continuously at work to maintain homeostasis. Homeostasis is the tendency of the body to seek and maintain equilibrium within its internal environment, even when faced with external changes. The pH of our blood is very sensitive to this dynamic homeostasis, and the body's innate intelligence will do anything to protect the fine balance of the pH range in our blood. The normal blood pH is 7.35—on the alkaline side of the scale. Balancing your pH and rebuilding a more alkaline environment within you is the process of re-mineralizing yourself alive! Simple, and profound.

pH balance is measured using a scale from 1–14, with 7 being the neutral (middle) point. Your goal when we check your own pH balance is to be as close as possible to a measurement of 7. The pH scale is not a linear one; it's a logarithmic scale in which two adjacent values increase or decrease by a factor of 10.

Anything under 7 is considered an acidic terrain. The lower the number goes towards 1, the more acidic the terrain by a factor of 10, the higher the toxicity levels are in your body, and the more we are creating the breeding grounds for disease.

Anything above 7 is alkaline, and this is what we strive for. Now, if we become over-alkaline, that too has its consequences, but these days, with our lifestyles and stress levels, it's pretty hard to be over-alkaline. So if your urine pH this morning was 6, that's ten times more acidic than your goal of being 7. If it was 5, that's 100 times more acidic than your goal. You get my drift.

The pH measurement of your urine (in particular our first morning's) reveals the state of health of your whole bodily system. A first morning urine pH reading of 6.8–7.5 is considered ideal. The pH measurement of your saliva (away from food) mirrors the health of your blood and your enzymes, as is a first morning saliva pH testing of 7.0–7.5. Both will vary dramatically, depending on the foods you eat, the drinks you consume, your breath, and your lifestyle. We can remain in health by consuming a diet that is 70–80% alkaline and 20–30% acidic for our physiological types.

It has been scientifically proven that a diet high in plant-based foods creates alkalinity in our body, and a diet rich in animal protein of any kind—including dairy, along with sugar, caffeine, and processed foods—will create acidity in the body. Acidity is the first step in the buildup of inner toxicity, and inner toxicity results in a breeding ground for a whole wide gamut of diseases. Oxygen cannot be delivered to our cells within an acidic environment. Due to that lack of oxygen, our body is unable to distribute and absorb nutrients as efficiently, creating further acidity. Eventually all the systems of the body begin to malfunction and break down, and chronic diseases, autoimmune disorders, and cancer manifest themselves in this acidic environment.

On the other hand, an alkaline body environment supports the overall system by providing ample amounts of oxygen and nutrients to your cells, and thus to your whole system. Your enzymatic, immunologic, and repair mechanisms all function best in an alkaline environment. Alkaline foods are able to neutralize the body's natural acidity and build up our alkaline reserve, which is needed to neutralize the extra acidity and stresses our bodies are experiencing today.

The cell *pH* of a body in health is alkaline. In disease, the cell pH is below 7.0 (acidic). Our body produces acid as a by-product of normal metabolism. If your body is not able to release this acid through your detoxification systems, an acid build-up begins to form. Our body tries to balance this acid build up by "borrowing" minerals from our alkaline reserves, and eventually becomes exhausted because our body does not create alkaline reserves. Soon it becomes too acidic and begins the process of disease and dying. Your alkaline reserves are only built by the intake of alkaline-forming foods, alkaline-forming lifestyles, thoughts, emotions, actions, and your ability to connect with the harmonious rhythms of nature.

As Gabriel Cousens explains in Chapter 3 of *Conscious Eating*, the food we eat will either make us more acidic or more alkaline, depending upon our dominant system.

This is a huge revolution in our thinking, because now we have the knowledge to understand that it's not only the foods we eat that are causing extra acidity in our body, but it is also how your body metabolizes those foods that creates either acidity or alkalinity in your body.

Eating a vegan, or raw, living vegan diet will still create less acidity than if one was to eat a diet rich in animal proteins, sugar, and processed foods, but it is crucial for the rebuilding of optimal health to understand your dominant system, and to understand which foods will build alkalinity within you.

Generally speaking, fruits and vegetables—being rich in alkalizing minerals such as calcium, magnesium, potassium, sodium, selenium, and iron—are considered alkalizing foods. They are great detoxifiers and regenerators. They cool and soothe inflamed tissue, and heal and enhance cellular function. Generally speaking, animal proteins, dairy, processed foods, sugar, and even vegan protein (grains, seeds, nuts and beans), are considered acidic foods. Foods rich in acid-forming elements such as phosphorus, sulphur, chlorine, and iodine are considered acidic foods.

Acidic foods slow, inhibit, or stop the detoxification process. They tend to be inflammatory and mucus-forming and become free radicals, causing tissue damage.

Foods grown through commercial factory-farming practices, full of pesticides, herbicides, chemicals, in poor soils, and with poor ethics, lead to extra acidity in our body. Your body does not know what to do with them, so they get stored into your tissues and cells, creating further acidity and building the inner toxicity of your body. It's a dangerous road that unfortunately sooner or later leads to disease and disharmony.

Foods grown through organic farming practices deliver greater nutrition, and don't leave a residue of un-identified toxic substances within us. They are more like the food past generations ate and, depending on the person's choice—either a standard American diet (SAD) or a diet that includes higher plant-based foods—will either create acidity or alkalinity in the body. But generally speaking, they contain more "organic minerals"—a synonym for alkalinity. Having said this, organic foods that are picked green and then must travel the world to get to us don't deliver as much nourishment as locally grown food, nor are they as alkaline-forming.

Furthermore, the term "organic" can have a very loose definition in other parts of the world, so we can't really know how truly organic that apple or pear or tomato might be. Something else to consider is the processing of the organic foods in our country and if (or not) they are being sprayed against different bugs that may be on them. We simply don't know.

Foods grown through authentic organic agriculture are the best and most alkalizing foods for several reasons: they are grown locally in repaired soils, they are filled with most nutrients because the farmers care and love what they do, they are filled with most energy, nourishing our Subtle Organizing Energy Fields (SOEFs), they are part of the solution in creating peace in ourselves and in the world, and they build our connection to spirit. Know where your food comes from; better yet, grow your own!

Exercise: Purchase pH strips at your local health food store. Test your first morning urine and saliva to monitor your pH, and record them on the chart provided below. As well, get curious about how food affects your body, and how you are feeling. Measure your pH after eating certain foods, and begin to create the solution to your own puzzle by finding the answer to your own riddle. Also, note how stress, mood, food choices, exercise, deep breathing, and meditation all affect your pH.

TIME	SALIVA PH VALUE	URINE PH VALUE	FOODS EATEN	FEELING	NOTES reflections on physical heath, emotions, stress levels, etc.
Upon rising					
After breakfast					
After snack					
Before/ after lunch					
After snack					
Before/ after dinner					
At bedtime					

Get curious about how your body functions. Witness your changes throughout the day, through just perhaps doing a mindfulness practice, or yoga. Witness your body as you eat different foods and hold space for your findings. You can find a downloadable printout of this chart on my website: www.natyhoward/resources

My pH can change one whole number with only doing my meditation and deep breathing practices first thing in the morning, without having drunk or eaten anything. That's *powerful!*

5. STRUCTURED LIVING WATER

Life is water dancing to the tune of solids. Without that dance, there could be no life.

—*Albert Szent-Gyorgyi*

Fresh raw living foods are highest in structured living water!

This structured living water in fresh raw living foods is healing because it has been patterned by the elemental forces of nature to be readily absorbed by your body, and its information is readily understood by your energetic system. It is magic at work: it is hydrating, grounding, and the most important element of the human body.

The term *structured living water* comes from the nature-coded patterns that whole living foods and water have. Therefore, structured living water is the healthiest water your body can have, and found naturally in everything Mother Nature creates—as long as we integrate it into our lives in its natural state.

Structured living water is water that contains within its molecules the vibration of life. It is life-force energy organized in a way that your body, your genetic code, can understand. It is water that has been structured by and with sun energy, life-force, and elemental energies to serve as a decoder of the process of life, as a delivery system of nutrition, oxygen, and nourishment to all your cells, and as primary medium of resonance to the frequency of healing cosmic energy.

Structured living water is primordial, as it contains information for the healthy expression of your genetic code. Structured living water contains the history of our evolution, and the living systems code for this next chapter in our evolution. Structured living water is the medium of our consciousness. Our body is made of this structured living water, and this structured living water is what we need for our well-being. Structured living water is water that springs from the depths of Mother Earth herself, charging itself energetically for your ultimate well-being.

Structured living water carries higher energetic frequencies that match the energetic frequency of our genetic code, and it has the power to heal and reorganize the corrupted cells in our systems. Its nutritional energies address the subtle aspects of your body, inclusive of the physical (body), mental (mind), emotional (heart), and spiritual body.

Structured living water has at its foundation the evolution and expansion of your consciousness, the alignment of your life with your true nature, your own emergence through your heart, the information needed for your own personal revolution and shift to greater awareness of universal law, and of your own clarity of purpose and certainty of heart.

Liquid nutrition is, essentially, the incorporation of high amounts of this structured living water into your diet. Because we are using fresh raw living foods, naturally high in structured living water, there is a natural transference into our body of this essence of life.

Think of it as the anti-virus software on your computer, repairing the code of this most magical tool of action: your mighty body!

Spring water is the ultimate structured living water. It has not been processed, bottled, or altered in any way. It is nature's gift, the way it was intended. The way our ancestors drank it hundreds of years ago.

When we consume spring water that is coming from the source, the core of Mother Earth, bringing forth not only pristine nutrient density, but also information coded into its very own molecular pattern, we begin to transform our own core at lightning speed.

Think of it; cold spring water emerges from the earth, usually at the top of a mountain or hill. It has defied gravity to make it so, it has let go of the heavier densities (toxicity) to be able to do so, and it contains the *code* on how to do it. You and I are drinking this code, therefore transferring this information on *levity* or lightness,[11] and defying gravity, which is key information for our longevity. You are now transferring the information of how to let go of heavy densities and toxicity out of your body, so that you too can emerge, but this time, into an ethical, ecological, responsible relationship with the Earth.

Spring water begins to shift that which vibrates at lower resonance out of your body, creating room for a new resonance and coherence to now exist. It begins to feed your body, not only physically but also energetically, creating an energetic roadmap for your personal and global healing as much as for your own expansion of consciousness.

Along my healing journey, I have experimented with many tools. Some have been greater and more beneficial to my journey than others. Living spring water is right at the top, and it's one of those things you may just have to discover for yourself.

---

11   Spring water works on the principle of levity and levitation, lightness, as it is constantly defying gravity in its quest to emerge at the earth's surface. The Merriam-Webster Dictionary defines levitation (from Latin levitas "lightness") as a verb: "to rise or float in or as if in the air, especially in seeming defiance of gravitation."

It is fairly easy to find a natural spring near you. Here you go!
www.findaspring.com
Find it. Gather it. Drink it.
Feel the revolution from the inside out.

6. CONSCIOUS DRINKING

Your health is what you make of it. Everything you do and think either adds to the vitality, energy and spirit you possess or takes away from it.

—Ann Wigmore

When you choose to include liquid nutrition as part of your everyday life, you are making a conscious choice. You matter. It matters.

You matter. That is a big part of your conscious choice, for as you have read, there is Mighty power in adding liquid nutrition into your life. You are taking the time to nourish yourself deeply, and to provide yourself with the best prevention and healing action there is. You are taking responsibility for your own state of health, and reclaiming not only the health of your multidimensional body, but also your ecological self, along with your responsibility in being part of the solution to our planetary crisis.

To eat and drink consciously is to bring into your awareness the quality, the quantity, purpose, energetics, thoughts, emotions, intentions, and consequences of your choices and the food you eat and drink. Eating consciously is a choice you and I make, and that choice takes into consideration the efforts, energies, economics, thoughts, and environmental responsibilities that we and others have taken to grow, produce, create, and prepare our food.

To drink and eat consciously is about tapping into your own inner wisdom of a deeply nourishing soulful existence. To drink and eat consciously means to tap into your body compass and listen deeply for what you need, and for how you can nourish yourself deeply.

It matters because if not us, then who? Who will be a part of the inner revolution of self? Who will recalibrate your heart compass and bring sacredness back into your life? The joyful state of being in a deeply respectful relationship with all sentient beings, with both the seen and unseen worlds, and with your own self?

If not I, then who will guide my own transformation and evolution in consciousness?

If not I, then who will take responsibility over this body, over this life, *my body, my life?*

If not I, then who will live a life with grace and clarity of purpose, as allies along the journey to the Mighty sacred heart?

If not I, then who will?

7. VIBRATIONAL RESONANCE

Resonance happens when your mind and heart come into sync.

—*Ravindra Shukla*

Everything that exists, both seen and unseen, exists because it has a ***vibrational frequency.*** From the subatomic particles in the mountain to the subatomic particles within each and every one of your cells, you and I are all made of vibration. Vibration is a condensation of energy from the most ethereal to the densest form, and it varies in intensity and frequency according to the state of manifestation. All beings, all things that exist—seen or unseen—vibrate at different frequencies and intensities. This is the structure and language of the universe.

The sun shines its vibrational frequencies upon the earth, the living plants receive this information and transform it into the different minerals and nutrients needed for their (and our) survival. When you eat a diet composed of high amounts of fresh raw living foods, you are receiving all that vibrational energy and information into your body, therefore transferring not only the material nutrient density of the living plant, but also the subtle vibrational frequencies. By eating a diet rich in fresh raw living foods, whose vibrational frequencies have not been corrupted, and incorporating liquid nutrition into your lifestyle, you are able to raise your own vibrational frequency and begin to tap into the awareness of vibrational resonance.

Our life, and everything that constitutes our life, is so because of our current state of vibration. When your vibration begins to rise, you begin to change from the inside out, you ripple out, expanding from your core towards the outer expression of a new wave of being. It's very similar to when you throw a pebble into the water and its vibration sets off ripples in the body of water that move out and away until we can no longer see them, yet they have affected the whole body of water at a subtle level. As the frequency of your vibration rises, you begin to root down into your most inner essence, remembering your truth and your interrelationship with the source of all life: universal consciousness.

For his book *The Hidden Messages in Water,*[12] Japanese scientist Dr. Masaru Emoto was able to microscopically photograph the transformation of the molecular structure in water from different sources when exposed to human words, thoughts, emotions, sounds, and intentions and activated by the frequency of vibrations of those thoughts, emotions, sounds, and intentions.

Dr. Emoto's work revolutionized the idea that our thoughts, vibrations, and intentions can change the physical structure of water. He is one of the most important water researchers the world has known.

We can see in the photographs, the water that was infused with the vibrational frequency of prayer and love and gratitude is of shinning beauty, while the water exposed to ill thought (lower vibrational frequency) is deformed. The subatomic particles, the elementary particles, and aspects of water are able to change their outer visible expression because of the rate of vibration at which the specific water samples were oscillating.

---

12   Masaru Emoto, The Hidden Messages in Water (New York, NY: Atria Books, 2005)

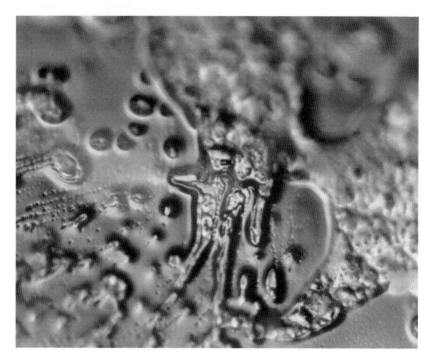

Water exposed to the written words "You make me sick, I will kill you"

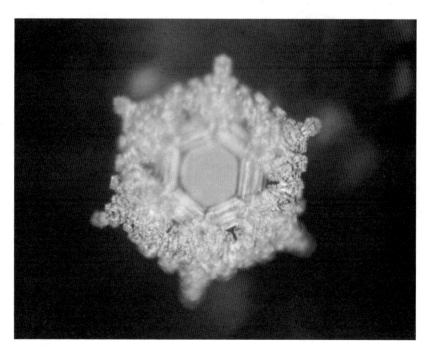

Water exposed to the written word 'Love & Gratitude'

Microscopic photographs of ice crystals by Dr. Masaru Emoto.
© Office Masaru Emoto, LLC

These images come from Dr. Masaru Emoto's water experiments and are proof that our thoughts, and the vibration carried in and delivered by our thoughts, affect the patterns of the water molecules and of our state of health.

The most important message we get from his work is this: the vibrational resonance of our thoughts and emotions is capable of shifting the shape (expression) of matter (our physical bodies). Dr. Emoto's experiments were performed on water and we are able to bear witness to the effects of loving thoughts and emotions, meditation, and prayer as compared to ill thoughts, emotions, and pollution upon water.

Your body is composed mostly of water! Therefore, the quality of your own thoughts and emotions about yourself will greatly affect the shape (expression) and energetic well-being of your body. As well, the quality of your environment, both nature and the people with whom you surround yourself, and the quality of their thoughts and emotions, will also greatly affect the shape (expression) of your body towards health and coherence, or towards disease and disharmony.

The other important message we get from Dr. Emoto's work is the importance of the vibrational frequencies stored in the structured water of the food we eat and drink, and its power to affect, heal, or debilitate our whole-body systems.

So as you begin to feed your body higher vibrational frequencies like those found in fresh raw living foods and liquid nutrition, your subatomic particles, your elementary particles must then also be able to change their outer seen expression and their outermost subtle expression.

At a cellular level, atoms and molecules assemble to form the elementary particles that make up each and every one of your cells, and allow them to do their job. But what would happen if you changed the quality and rate of vibration of the food you are feeding your cells with? Is it possible that if you feed your cells a higher vibrational frequency, their elementary particles will be able to change their seen and unseen expression, thus being able to manifest greater health at a cellular level, which amounts to an expression of greater health throughout you whole-body system?

It is here at the elementary particle of the cellular structure that change begins. It is here where cells begin to resonate together to form an ocean of rippling pebbles of new-found awareness, consciousness, and health. It is here where the expansion of your awareness begins, one vibration at a time, one juice, one smoothie, one elixir at a time. It is here where fresh raw living foods and liquid nutrition have the power to change, infuse, grow, and regenerate your body. It is here where the biggest shift can happen, and where we begin to remember who we really are, as soul.

*When one or more cells begin to vibrate at higher rates of frequency, the whole organism begins to reso-
nate with that new wave of frequency; thus, your thoughts, emotions, ecological and spiritual awareness
begin to change.* When you, as a living entity, begin to resonate at higher levels of vibration, you
too act as a vibrational resonance activator for your family, community, and the world at large.
This process is called entrainment.

Vibrational resonance is one of the universal or spiritual laws that govern every aspect of the
universe, and one of the laws by which our world and the entire cosmos continues to exist, thrive,
expand, evolve, and emerge.

HEALTH BENEFITS

A healthy outside starts from the inside.

—Robert Urich

There are many health benefits to including liquid nutrition in your lifestyle:

Physical Benefits:

- Blood purification
- Stabilizing weight
- High enzymatic bioavailability to the body
- Sensorial clarity
- Prevention of acute and chronic disorders
- Fastest way to change the inner terrain of your body, and to aid in detoxification and lowering of inner toxicity
- Fastest alkalizer (especially if you do green juices)
- Aids in revitalizing and stabilizing of inner glands and hormones
- Improves digestion and absorption of nutrients
- Anti-stress tool
- Promotes better sleep
- Aids in breaking addiction patterns
- Creates overall feeling of whole-body wellness

- Aids in deep cellular nourishment, the building block for whole-body radiant health
- Aids in the repair, rebuilding, and regeneration of your DNA
- Enhances life-force within your own body
- Gets you drinking structured living water, which is in essence liquid sunshine coded to ultimate perfection for your body to understand and use. Structured living water also contains vital information in the form of specific molecular patterns that your body needs to survive and thrive
- Dual action; aids in remineralization of your body, and in detoxification (lowers body toxicity)
- Full of life-force energy from the earth

Emotional Benefits:

- Provides emotional clarity and flow of emotions, both current and past
- Aids in the release of habits and/or patterns that no longer serve you and in the release of old belief systems, old wounds, and old emotional traumas that hold you back
- Allows deeper emotional intimacy to self
- Permits deeper emotional availability to others
- Provides deeper source of commitment to your Mighty sacred heart—the space within you that is truth and love
- Because you begin the process of anchoring your self in your heart, you begin to make choices and act from a place of love rather than a place of fear
- Improves clarity of purpose, rooted on self and worldly ecological responsibility
- Facilitates the emergence of the sacred consciousness with the awareness of the universal law of interconnectedness.
- Improves clarity of purpose rooted on self and worldly ecological responsibility

Mental Benefits:

- Improves mental discipline
- Improves clarity of thought
- Creates awareness of your thought patterns, habits, and addictions
- Creates overall feeling of mental clarity
- Facilitates the process of quieting the mind
- Improves clarity of vision of your life

Energetic Benefits:

- Enhances, rebuilds, and repairs your energetic circuitry, your energy body
- Enhances your awareness of your energetic body
- Enhances your awareness of the sacred within, and the sacred within all
- Enhances your awareness of the energy field of the earth
- Enhances your awareness of the understanding that you are a part of the universe, the earth, and life beyond your body

Spiritual Benefits:

- Enhancer of the understanding of life-force as your ultimate source of spiritual nutrition
- Spiritual enhancer of your connection with grace and the god of your own understanding
- Activator of your spiritual and karmic evolution
- Tool for evolutionary consciousness transformation
- Serves as a portal to the world of quantum healing
- Gatekeeper into the inner spaces of deep nourishment and deep healing, where you can spark your own revolution and ignite your inner healer
- Ignites your heart into sacred action, and sparks your awareness of earth's consciousness

As you can see, the physical benefits of liquid nutrition are but the side effects of a deeper process of transformation being facilitated within ourselves. And yes, I do understand that for some of us it can be a big shift in thinking and in lifestyle. But I also believe and understand that big changes generally happen one step at a time, one drink at a time, one glass or jar of liquid nutrition at a time. Once a week, perhaps, once a day, perhaps, until you are ready to commit at a deeper level to your greatest expression of health, one fresh raw living juice, one smoothie, one elixir at a time! Come on! Are you ready? I know you are.

Ultimately, liquid nutrition allows you to bring greater coherence into your whole-body system, *shifting* you from chaos (disease) into greater order (harmonious radiant health).

Liquid nutrition allows us to connect with the greater consciousness that moves through us. It connects us to the greater network of intelligence that exists in the quantum field from where you can access the inner space of deep healing, and shift your body into radiance.

CHLOROPHYLL

I don't think I'll ever grow old and say, "What was I thinking eating all those fruits and vegetables?"

—Nancy S. Mure

If there is one magic word to remember along this journey to optimal health, that one magic trick that once understood, you know it's pure scientific healing with a few extra ounces of charm because it works so well, it is **chlorophyll!** It is, in essence liquefied, sunshine. Consuming chlorophyll helps us detoxify, cleanse, and build our blood by delivering a nourishing bath of nutrients currently *missing* from our everyday Western diet.

Here it is: the molecular structures of chlorophyll and hemoglobin are very similar, differing only in their nucleus; chlorophyll has magnesium as its nucleus, where hemoglobin has iron. Hemoglobin is the structure that carries oxygen in the human blood. Chlorophyll has been shown to help boost hemoglobin production, and is also high in oxygen content, which helps deliver more oxygen to the blood, facilitating recovery from ailments and disease. Having high oxygen levels in your body helps support a healthy body. The magic? Because of their similarity in structure, your body knows exactly what to do with chlorophyll, and where to do it.

Some of the benefits known to chlorophyll are:

- Alkalizes your blood and your body
- Cleanses and rebuilds your blood
- Effective against *Candida albicans*
- Encourages healing
- Promotes healthy digestion by maintaining intestinal flora and stimulating bowel movements
- Promotes healthy iron levels
- Powerful antioxidant and anti-aging element
- Reduces inflammation

Why is it the missing link? *Simply because it is missing from our Western diet.* Our current Western diet is heavily based on grain, animal products, and dairy, along with the fast food and highly processed foods that have become the norm. Most people no longer have the time, nor the interest in preparing meals using whole ingredients, and we are bearing witness to the rapid increase of disease in our society.

As you have read, chlorophyll is the cornerstone of our vitality and health, and a key protocol for our longevity. It is not a totally forgotten link yet. We are certainly beginning to recognize that it has been missing, and it's time to reclaim it, and along with it our health.

FRESH RAW LIVING GRASS JUICE

Wheatgrass juice is the nectar of rejuvenation, the plasma of youth, the blood of all life. The elements that are missing in your body's cells-especially enzymes, vitamins, hormones, and nucleic acids can be obtained through this daily green sunlight transfusion.

—Viktoras Kulvinskas

Fresh raw living grass juices are the extraction of the liquid essence from a young blade of grass. They are about 70% chlorophyll, making them "Queens of Health." Grass juice is the mother of all superfoods, queen of all living juices, if you will, and often overlooked as it literally grows in our backyards, not from some faraway exotic lands. This is the best vitamin and mineral supplement you can ever get. As it becomes a part of your life, it will become a continual source of your well-being, rather than another supplement to keep you going.

I make an emphasis on it being **fresh raw living grass juices,** because here is where all its power lies. When you drink it fresh, you get the enzymes, bio-electricity, and vibrant nutrition that is still within the juice and that we so want! When you drink grass juice, you gain access to the tiny nutritional elements, which are essentially pre-digested, making it easy for your body to assimilate and utilize the plant's life-force energy. *The nutritional constitution of any fresh-pressed juice will begin to change within twenty minutes of its making.*

You are transferring the life-force (bioelectrical current) energy of this powerhouse of a plant to your system. Your body will use it all to cleanse, rebuild and rejuvenate itself. Research shows these powerful nutrients can also prevent DNA destruction, and help protect us from the ongoing effects of premature aging and cellular breakdown. Research also shows that only living foods and juices can restore the electrical charge between the capillaries and the cell walls that boost the immune system. Remember, life always wants to thrive and heal. But we have forgotten how to get out of our own way so the body can use its natural intelligence to do so.

Yet I also understand that we live very full and dynamic lives. As a result, there are some Mighty companies who grow different grasses, cold press juice them, vacuum seal pack them, and flash freeze them so you can enjoy the benefits of fresh living grass juice in the midst of your busy life. There are also some pretty Mighty dehydrated living grass juice powders out there that are worth your time. Get to know these products, and find one that suits your needs.

Some of the better known grasses are wheatgrass and barley grass:

Fresh raw living wheatgrass juice is the juice from the young wheatgrass blade, harvested when at the peak of its chlorophyll, protein, and vitamin concentration, before the grass produces any grain. It is slightly more bitter than barley grass.

Fresh raw living barley grass juice is the juice from the young shoots of the barley plant, harvested when at the peak of its chlorophyll, protein, and vitamin concentration, before the grass produces any grain. It has a milder taste than wheatgrass.

Both grasses provide a high source of chlorophyll, and both contain a wide range of nutrients, including vitamins (A, C, E, K, and folate), minerals (calcium, iron, magnesium, and potassium), antioxidants, and amino acids.

A mix of grasses will provide you with the broadest nutritional intake.

Some of the benefits of consuming grass juice are that:

- Its high chlorophyll content helps oxygenate your blood
- It helps to inhibit the growth of disease bacteria
- It increases energy
- It aids digestion
- It relieves constipation
- It improves health of skin, hair and nails
- It balances the pH of the body to promote excellent health and immunity
- It increases red blood-cell count; cleanses the blood, organs, and gastrointestinal tract; and, stimulates metabolism
- It stimulates your thyroid gland
- Assists in circulation of the lymph system

- It may help reduce the damaging effects of radiation, courtesy of the enzyme superoxide dismutase (SOD), an anti-inflammatory compound
- It detoxifies the liver, thyroid, and blood from heavy metals and chemically neutralizes environmental pollutants

COLD PRESSED FRESH RAW LIVING JUICES

Food is a dynamic force that interacts with humans at the physical body level, the mind-emotional level, and the energetic spiritual levels.

—Rabbi Gabriel Cousens M.D., founder of The Tree of Life. Spiritual Nutrition Six Foundations for Spiritual Life and the Awakening of Kundalini.

By choosing the type of dynamic force—and its state—that you activate your body with, in this case, fresh raw living juices high in mineral and nutrient density, you activate the dynamic forces of assimilation, detoxification, purification, rebuilding, repairing, restoring, rejuvenation, and regeneration within you that facilitate deeper nourishment to each and every one of your cells. Keep in mind that because juices contain a concentrated essence of the foods juiced, when we use high-sugar vegetables and fruits, the sugar content of the juice will be high.

Fresh raw living juices help us rebalance any mineral or nutrient deficiencies that can be causing body, mind, emotional, and spiritual imbalances. Fresh raw living juices further enhance, balance, and support your physical and sensory health, calming and facilitating a pure state within your body, a pure state of mind and emotions, as well as having the power to enhance your spiritual connection.

When you juice, you are literally extracting the essence from the vegetables and fruits, which is in essence liquefied sunshine, pure life-force. Life-force is everything. It is the foundation and quality of our existence. Without it we cannot thrive, and we spend our lives trying to recover it, even though most of us are unaware that it is life-force we are in search of.

The quality of life-force energy that moves through you determines your individual consciousness, and empowers your every action towards both self and the world. You have a choice when it comes down to what kind of life-force energy you surround yourself with and put into your precious temple: your body.

Liquid nutrition has the power to affect and shape the quality of your body, mind and soul, the quality of your life, the quality of your thoughts (your awareness), the quality of your experiences (your perspective), the quality of your health (your well being), and the quality of your relationships to self, community, environment, and ecological responsibility (awareness of the consequences of your actions).

The life-force in your juices directly affects your consciousness, your awareness, your ability to activate your Mighty inner healer, and your ability to transform your life.

SMOOTHIES, GREEN OR NOT, HERE I COME!

Blended green smoothies are a simple and delicious way of accessing the healing properties of greens.

—*Victoria Boutenko*

Smoothies are a sweet or savoury way to add nutritional density into your life. They consist of blended vegetables and/or fruits along with water or milks (dairy or non-dairy) to create a beautiful array of awesome-tasting greatness. The power in smoothies is two-fold: first it is liquid nutrition, second it contains the alMighty one, **fibre!**

Oh so dear to us, fibre has also been slowly and not so slowly falling to the sides of our standard American diet (SAD). Yet fibre is the broom that cleans your body from the inside out. It is the bulk that pushes toxicity out and creates room for better nutrient absorption and assimilation. And I'm not just talking about your intestines. It goes all the way down to your cellular structures. So I say, *Broom the excess away and give power to the fibre*!

Smoothies are also a great alkalizer, especially green smoothies, a wonderful pre- and post-workout replenisher.

We live in the era of the fast food revolution, and smoothies are an answer to reclaim the path of the whole food revolution. Fresh homemade smoothies, in general, use whole food ingredients.

Yes, fresh homemade, with fresh ingredients and drunk soon after you have prepared them. They are powerful allies in our journey to greater radiant and vibrant health.

Smoothies are a great way to integrate vegetables to the diet of the fussy eaters in your life, for instance your beloved spouse who is not ready for the green revolution, yet might start to see your inner shine glowing and want some of this for himself. It is a process. From my own experience, everybody loves a sweet, refreshing, brain-tickling smoothie. They may not know at the beginning that along with your blueberry power smoothie you have sneaked in some added kale, seaweed powder, plant-based protein powder, bee pollen, and even goji berries! Or they might. Eventually, they might ask that all of those added bonuses be an integral part of their smoothies!

Smoothies are also great because you can add in all sorts of superfoods, and blend in all sorts of extra Mighty powers. You can combine sweet fruit with greens to make green smoothies, you can combine all sorts of delicious savoury ingredients to make delightful raw soups, you can make them into ice creams, you can serve them to those you love who might not be quite ready for a fresh green juice, with great confidence that they too will love them—especially when you add a hint of magic superfoods, (seaweed, chlorophyll and the like) as secret ingredients. I love it!

ELIXIRS

Tea is the elixir of life.

—Lao Tzu

How long has it been since you gave yourself a letter of love? Really, how long?

Would you like to? Because you can—give yourself a letter of love. Okay, Great!

Elixirs, for me, are just that: liquid letters of love. The synergy that happens when we combine herbs, wild edibles, medicinal mushrooms, and superfoods with structured living water is equal to a blissful experience of heaven on earth: a liquid letter of love to each and every one of your cells, so good it may just make your brain tickle and do a happy dance. It is that good.

Elixirs are powerful tools for bringing into your body the mineral grace of herbs, wild herbs and edibles, medicinal mushrooms, and other superfoods that may not be as tasty when eaten in their whole form, yet are just so powerful when their whole form is infused in water or made into a tea, or combined with other ingredients that make them shine with your taste buds, and cause their medicinal personalities will aid your body with vitality, radiance, and longevity.

Elixirs are builders of your immunity. They are one of the main vehicles through which the wisdom of our plant allies travels to the most inner aspect of your being to spark your heart revolution. They awaken within us our noble essences.

There are many ways to brew your home brew. Here are a few that have become my favourites.

Tea Infusions & Overnight Infusion. The art of combining one or more herbs, medicinal herbs, wild herbs, or edibles in a cup or a jar, in particular the more aerial aspects of the plant: seeds, leaves, and flowers. Add hot water and let them sit for five minutes, a few hours, or overnight while the herbs are infusing the water with their goodness. Some of us like our infusions light, others like them stronger, so play with it. Once you know where you stand, drain and strain the herb mixture, and drink the water throughout the day. Or, you may use this water as the basis of your more complex elixirs, smoothies or tea decoctions. Some of the herbs, medicinal and wild herbs and edibles are:

Alfalfa	Mugwort
Basil	Oat Straw
Cleavers	Plantain leaf
Clover	Rosemary
Dandelion	Stinging nettle
Fennel seeds	Marshmallow
Horsetail	Mint
Motherwort	Yarrow leaf and flower

Tea Decoction. The art of making stronger infusions, generally using herbs, medicinal and wild herbs and edibles, in particular their roots, as well as medicinal tree barks, and medicinal mushrooms that need a longer simmer to access their nutrient dense beauty. They can be drunk on their own or serve as the base for the ultimate elixir. Some of the more common ingredients for powerful tea decoctions are:

Astragalus root	**Ginseng root**
Burdock root	**Goji berries**
Cat's claw (bark)	**Pau d'arco (bark)**
Chaga mushroom	**Reishi mushroom**
Dandelion root	**Schizandra berries**
Don Quai root	**Turmeric**

The Ultimate Elixir. Use infusions or tea decoctions to serve as a base and build a liquid super power. Usually superfoods are added to the mix, either warm or hot, for maximizing our nutrition and our absorption of their bounty. Just imagine your home brew of pau d'arco, cat's claw, chaga and reishi mushrooms, cacao leaf, and goji berries that you have strained. Place your brew in the blender while still nice and hot and add more magic to the mix with superfoods such as cacao, bee pollen, more goji berries, a hint of seaweed powder, maca, lucuma, turmeric or mesquite powders, and raw honey. Blend with a touch of love and you have prepared the ultimate elixir. When I add a touch of coconut butter or homemade almond or nut mylk, I have gone to heaven on earth. You can join me there!

Brews. These are fermented teas such as homemade kombucha, jun, water kefir, and rejuvelac. I know, most people don't consider brews as part of the elixir category, but by now you should know that I'm not most people. I consider them to be an elixir because these brews are very powerful, often made from the herbs, wild herbs and edibles, medicinal mushrooms, and superfoods that place them in a class of their own, and because of the fermentation process itself. Brews are higher in enzymes, and a powerful source of pre- and probiotics for your gut health. So, you see, not such a stretch after all. And, yes, I did say homemade. There are some wonderful companies in the market now offering really phenomenal products, so if you don't want to make it yourself, seek one that is as ethical as they claim to be. Then go ahead and drink up!

Broths. Though not your traditional elixir, I have included them here because they are so mineral-rich and nutrient-dense, and because they have the power to nourish your system so deeply. Broths have been used in ancient cultures to sooth the body, in particular the gut, to build immunity, and to replenish our systems.

THE SADHANA OF PLANT MEDICINE WISDOM

The flower doesn't dream of the bee. It blossoms and the bee comes.

—*Mark Nepo*

Plant medicine wisdom *inherently contains within itself the ancient wisdom of healing.* Plants know their purpose on earth. Plants know what minerals they need to grow into the best expression of themselves, and when in trouble, they are known to communicate through the mycelium (tiny mushroom) web that exists underneath the soil, and either gift what they have in abundance to another plant ally, or send out a request for what they need. It's simply brilliant. Kind of like borrowing or giving that one cup of sugar to your neighbour.

Plant wisdom inherently contains the enzymes necessary for your body to digest that particular plant. They contain not only their particular mineral wisdom, but they also contain the wisdom of the five elements, of the sun and the moon and the stars and of the wind, of being in inter-relationship with the world around them, in great harmony. They also are key to the awakening of your immunity.

Plant wisdom connects you and me with the very essence of Mother Earth and our source energy. So when you include plant allies into your liquid nutrition, you are absorbing all that wisdom, from the most known of their minerals to the most subtle of their effects upon your body. Including plant wisdom becomes the art of truly nourishing your body with the intelligence of Mother Earth herself.

One of the fastest ways to include plant allies into your everyday life is through making them key ingredients in your fresh-pressed juices, smoothies, elixirs, and teas. Variety is key, and of course as local and organic as possible. As you become more confident in your own process and your body begins to detoxify and rebuild more efficiently, this brave new world will continue to expand and present to you new possibilities and new depths of healing. You might even find yourself drawn to learning and including more wild foods into your liquid nutrition! These are wild times.

Now I want to introduce to you the concept of *sadhana*. Traditionally, sadhana is the art of gifting our hearts with complete reverence as a spiritual practice. For me, sadhana is not limited to the time of when you or I, are in our meditation, yoga practice, or prayer, but rather it is the art of living in reverence.

I invite you to approach your relationship with plant wisdom in this way: *with complete reverence.* Keep a journal beside you, and note the small and not-so-small changes that begin to happen within you and around you, as you change your way of action in the world. I thank my plant allies for the wisdom they will impart upon my body, and the radiant health they will assist me in shining.

I invite you to approach your relationship with liquid nutrition as one of sadhana, one of devotion to self, to your own journey of healing as you power up your health, ignite your transformation, and spark your personal revolution.

THE RITUAL OF LIQUID NUTRITION

Your health is an investment, not an expense.

—Unknown

Now that you are familiar with the practice of sadhana, I invite you to see liquid nutrition as a practice that has the potential to become an everyday ***ritual for wellness,*** if possible, for you.

It is by taking the opportunity to bask in high-density nutrition that you will truly gift your body the medium and means to upgrade your inner terrain into the fertile grounds where true health and healing can blossom, and grow strong into wellness and longevity.

The ritual of liquid nutrition begins with a commitment to self to use liquid nutrition a certain number of times per week perhaps, or even better, daily. It begins with a conscious choice; it is one of those I do towards the self. I do, and *I will show up for myself like never before.*

Here we go. Close your eyes. Breathe deeply. Place your left hand on your heart, your right hand on your lower abdomen. Breathe some more. Pause and feel. How do you feel? How are you feeling right now? What is it that you truly desire in your heart? Whether it is wellness, radiant health, healing, or the shifting of an emotion, allow this desire to expand from your heart towards your entire body, from your core towards the boundaries of your skin. Expand … breathe … feel …

I invite you to feel into the wellness the breath brings into your body. I invite you to feel into the possibility of the life that awaits you. I invite you to feel that you are powerful beyond measure, and though the journey up to this point may have been very challenging, it has also developed your resilience and your character. It has prepared you for you to become aware of your soul purpose. It has awakened you to your true nature.

I invite you to pause and feel next time you are having some awesome liquid nutrition, and truly feel how it nourishes you, how it supports you, how it soothes you. I invite you to be in relationship with liquid nutrition as you would with a great friend. I invite you to use it as a ritual for wellness, as a sadhana.

Perhaps, at the beginning of each new habit, there are times of discomfort, times of inadequacy, times of doubt, of being too busy or even not motivated. Yet, persevere. The results are simply unimaginable to us right now. The results are none other than radiant health, none other than the pursuit of your heart's desires, none other than having the clarity of mind, of vision, of action to be your highest potential in this lifetime, here and now.

The ritual of liquid nutrition becomes sadhana, a spiritual practice to which you *gift the mightiness of your heart in complete reverence.*

SEASONAL QUALITIES OF LIQUID NUTRITION

I wonder if the snow loves the trees and fields, that it kisses them so gently? And then it covers them up snug, you know, with a white quilt; and perhaps it says, "Go to sleep, darlings, till the summer comes again."

—Lewis Carroll, Alice's Adventures in Wonderland & Through the Looking-Glass

---

We live on earth, *influenced by her rhythms and the seasons.* Every season has its own qualities and tastes that best bring us back to balance. From our perspective of using liquid nutrition, it's important that you pay attention to the taste of your nourishment and its heating or cooling qualities. In general, the tastes are balancing the opposite qualities inherent in the season.

SPRING

Seasonal qualities: cool, damp, moist, heavy.

- Season of birth, new beginnings, renewal, and growth. New life emerges all around in the natural world. Temperatures begin to warm up. Earthly time of rejuvenation, cleansing, detoxification. Lifestyle that invites a little extra lightness, sharpness, dryness, and heat into our lives.

Liquid nutrition qualities for wellness in spring:

- *Early spring:* drink slightly heating liquid nutrition. Balanced by pungent, astringent, bitter tastes.
- *Late spring:* drink slightly cooling liquid nutrition. Balanced by slightly sour and slightly sweet tastes.
- Avoid cold (frozen fruit), heavy, sticky drinks.

Juices: include bitter astringent greens in your juices (dandelion leaf, for example); green apples for their sour taste; ginger, turmeric, and slightly heating spices.

Smoothies and raw soups: keep them slightly sour, savoury. Include bitter astringent greens, sour fruit, slightly sweet (mid-glycemic fruit). No frozen fruit (thaw your fruit out the night before).

Nut mylks: slightly spiced, use seeds or soaked almonds.

Slightly fermented nut kefirs. Slightly sour bitter in taste.

Elixirs: drink slightly heating teas (early spring). Drink slightly cooling teas (late spring). Begin to ease up on the thick elixirs made with fats (nuts, seeds, nut mylks and butters, avocado, oils) and transition to lighter elixirs.

Brews: slightly sour kombucha, jun.

Best time to detoxify the body and liquid or juice feast, or even your Mighty detox! In general, it's a green juice, green sour smoothies, slightly heating elixirs kind of season.

SUMMER

Seasonal qualities: hot, dry, sharp, light.

- Season of strength, intensity, heat, passion. Time of expression, manifestation, showing our fullest potential. Life is busy, happening everywhere! Temperatures are warm or hot. Earthly time of growth, vibrancy, embracing the flow of abundance brought forth by the bounty of your gardens! Lifestyle that invites us to get outside, yet stay cool and calm.

Liquid nutrition qualities for wellness in summer:

- Drink cooling liquid nutrition. Use cooling veggies and fruits. Balanced by bitter, astringent, sweet tastes. Emphasize sweet taste.
- Drink extra water and lots of fluids.

Juices: use cooling veggies and fruits! Bring on your celery, cucumbers, mint, cilantro, apples, cooling sweet greens (spinach, collards, etc.), and lime.

Smoothies and raw soups: sweet, heavy, cooling higher-glycemic fruits, frozen fruits.

Nut mylks: sweet, use seeds or soaked almonds. Add them to your smoothies.

Elixirs: drink cooling teas such as mint. Elixirs are light in nature. Minimal use of fats (nuts, seeds, nut butters, avocado, oils).

Brews: sweet kombucha, coconut water kefir.

- In general it's a cooling smoothie, cooling juices, cold teas kind of season. Enjoy the bounty of your garden!!!

FALL

Seasonal qualities: light, dry, rough, hard, mobile, irregular, cool.

- Season of cooling down, winds blow, less sun, and the earth becomes dry, hard, rough. Time of gathering our personal bounty, savouring the fullness of Summer days and beginning to pause as we recalibrate for the dream of Winter. Temperatures begin to cool down. Earthly time of harvest, gathering, going within. Lifestyle that invites us to start slowing down, begin the journey of introspection.

Liquid nutrition qualities for wellness in fall:

- *Early Fall:* drink liquid nutrition that is slightly heating. Balanced by warming spices. Salty, slightly sweet taste.
- *Late Fall:* drink liquid nutrition that is heating. Balanced by warming spices. Sweet taste. Lower glycemic index.

Juices: slightly heating veggies, little fruit. Bring on your celery, root veggies, apples, fall fruit.

Smoothies and raw soups: slightly salty, slightly sweet warming smoothies and savoury soups. Use those ground veggies!

Nut mylks: spiced, use soaked nuts and seeds.

Elixirs: warming teas. Begin to thicken up your elixirs with fats (nuts, seeds, nut mylks and butters, avocado, oils).

Brews: Heating fermented drinks.

- In general, it's a warming juices, sweet soups, warming smoothies, and elixirs kind of season.

Enjoy the harvest of the garden!

WINTER

Seasonal qualities:

- *Early winter: cold, dry, windy, irregular, rough and vulnerable nature*
- *Late winter: dark, inert, wet.*

Season of withdrawing, going dormant, and embracing a long, dark season of slumber. Time of stillness, quiet. Cold temperatures. Life is slow. The natural world is in hibernation. Earthly time of harvest, gathering, slowing down, going within. Lifestyle that invites us to take time to rest, reflect, hold space, vision, hibernate, withdraw, stillness, quiet.

Liquid nutrition qualities for wellness in winter:

- *Winter is a time to build our physical, psychological and spiritual immunity. It is also a time to nourish and nurture our bodies deeply and build our vitality. Winter is a great time to bask in the love of herbal elixirs. Nutrition that builds our digestive fire. Avoid cold, frozen foods and drinks.*
- *Early Winter: focus on sweet, warming (use spices) and slightly drying qualities of your drinks. Drink liquid nutrition that is deeply nourishing, creates warmth and smoothness.*
- *Late Winter: Thicker and deeply nourishing drinks. Include bitter, astringent and pungent tastes that cut through the dark, inert and wet qualities of late winter.*

Juices: heating veggies, little fruit.

- Bring on your celery, root veggies, apples, ginger, turmeric, heating spices.

Smoothies and raw soups: warm, slightly sweet and savoury grounding smoothies and soups with a kick of spice. Use those ground veggies and heating spices! Use fats such as avocado, coconut or flax seed oil, nut butters.

Nut mylks: spiced. *Early winter:* seeds or soaked almonds. *Late winter:* soaked nuts.

Elixirs: warming immune building teas. Use cinnamon, ginger, clove, nutmeg, black pepper, turmeric, paprika, cayenne. Thicken elixirs with fats (nuts, seeds, nut mylks and butters, avocado, oils); that is, if your body is okay processing fats.

Brews: warming fermented drinks. Sour bitter.

- In general, it's a heating juice, warming soups, and elixirs kind of season.

LET YOUR INNER SHINE GLOW

As above, so below, as within, so without, as the universe, so the Soul.

—Hermes Trismegistus

You see, the journey ahead is full of possibilities. We live in exciting times. We have available to us the natural technologies that will enable you to deeply heal, turn on, and activate healthy gene expression, to be able to access higher levels of consciousness and allow for their expression to revolutionize not only your life, but also your impact on the world.

Health, to me, is the dynamic internal space of balance and harmony within all aspects of your self; physical, emotional, mental, and spiritual. Health is also a state of being fully present in the here and now in your life, embodying every inch of your skin.

Healing, to me, is the journey towards that state of balance and well being between the physical, emotional, mental, and spiritual bodies. It is the process of awakening to deeper states of conscious being, as much as the process of returning to the understanding of your connection to the spiritual world and the cycles of nature. It is a journey to rediscover, reconnect, and remember your true self, your true nature. It is a journey of growth and transformation, one that takes us back to inner peace with our body, mind, emotions and soul.

Radiant health, to me, is the knee-deep anchoring of your multi-dimensionality (body, mind, heart, and soul) into the earth, aware of your purpose, living from a place of truth and love, living an authentic ecologically responsible life. Radiant health is the effect of your healing, the gift of your transformation. It's the process of embodiment of the gift within, and the blossoming of your mightiness as it awakens to peace.

Medicine, to me, is a tool in the healing journey. I believe medicine is the wisdom that becomes one of the guides along the journey. Medicine does not need to be physical or chemical. Rather, medicine is any tool that facilitates or allows the inner energy to flow again. Medicine is energetic and flow promoting. It is sound, nature, love, and care. Medicine is creative, and brings you and me ever closer to our true self, and to embracing deeper awareness.

We have been trained to seek the expertise of others when it comes to our own body. Along the way, we have become strangers to ourselves, yet we know our own body best. So when did you forget, and let go of your sacredness in exchange for the magic pill? Because as you and I did, we began to forget that we are already magic; that alignment with all that is is at the root source of your health, and nobody else can do that for you.

As we forgot of our alignment with the earth, with the rhythms that make each and every one of our cells vibrate to the beat of our Mighty heart, we as a species have come into greater and greater disharmony, not only with our self and our multidimensional body, but also with our greater body: the Earth. Everything is interconnected and everything affects everything else. What we do and don't do have equal power in building our health or building our dis-harmony (dis-ease). Which road do you choose to journey on?

The time has come to empower yourself alive and *be your own revolution*. You can no longer afford to keep placing your life and your well being into the hands and authority of others without also empowering yourself with knowledge and wisdom. Educate yourself! Become the information you seek, but more importantly: **take action**. You know yourself best, and no one else can do the work for you.

The life beyond your dreams awaits one juice, one smoothie, one elixir at a time. You have access to your own inner power, to your own inner resources of strength, to your own ability to cope with change. You have access to activating your healthy gene expression. Your wonderful self can do it all, you only need to be willing—and to allow your revolution to be sparked from the inside out.

So I invite you to power up your health, to drink your medicine, to "*rawck*" it all, to dive within to be the very best you can, in service to yourself and the evolution of man on earth.

Liquid nutrition is a quest back to the self as soul, and to that space and consciousness of radiant health. It's a quest that will take you on, perhaps, the longest journey of your life—the 17 inches that separate your mind from your heart. It's a quest that will connect your heart back into your body, take you into your heart and through it, to the opening that will meet you as you follow your soul's guidance forward into your own emergence. This quest is a process of inquiry, one of diving within to allow your inner fire, your inner shine to glow. It is when you connect deeply to your own truth that you are able to stand more firmly upon your foundation, anchored knee-deep in the earth as you touch the sky.

Liquid nutrition has the power to spark your self alive. All the enzymes, its nutritional density, its ability to detox, clean, rebuild, repair, rejuvenate, and regenerate constitute the magic you've been searching for. It is life-force energy sealed with universal love straight into you, flooding your bloodstream and each and every one of your cells with its power. So come on, the time has come to step into your mightiness!

Allowing your inner shine to glow is as much a physical journey as it is an emotional, mental, and spiritual feast. Everything is interconnected and interrelated, and the one affects the whole, the whole affects the one. As you begin to align your physical body with greater health and radiance, the rest will follow. Your emotional, mental, and spiritual bodies will begin to shift, cleanse, detoxify, and rebuild. You will begin to upgrade your operating system and with that, your whole life opens up to a new dimension, to a ***brave new world.***

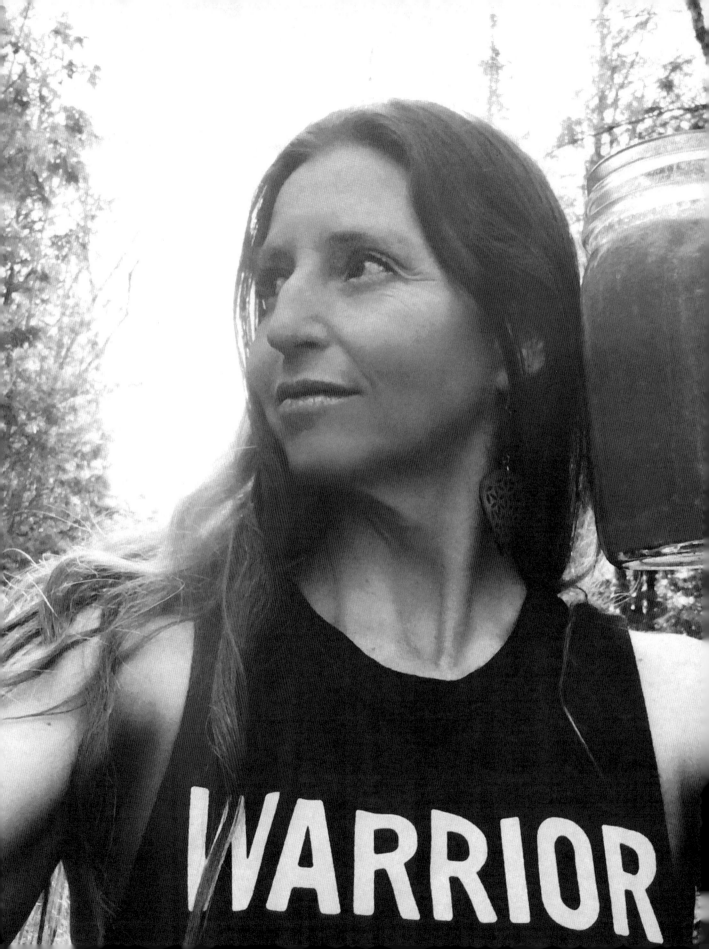

IV

108 LIQUID NUTRITION RECIPES TO POWER UP YOUR HEALTH

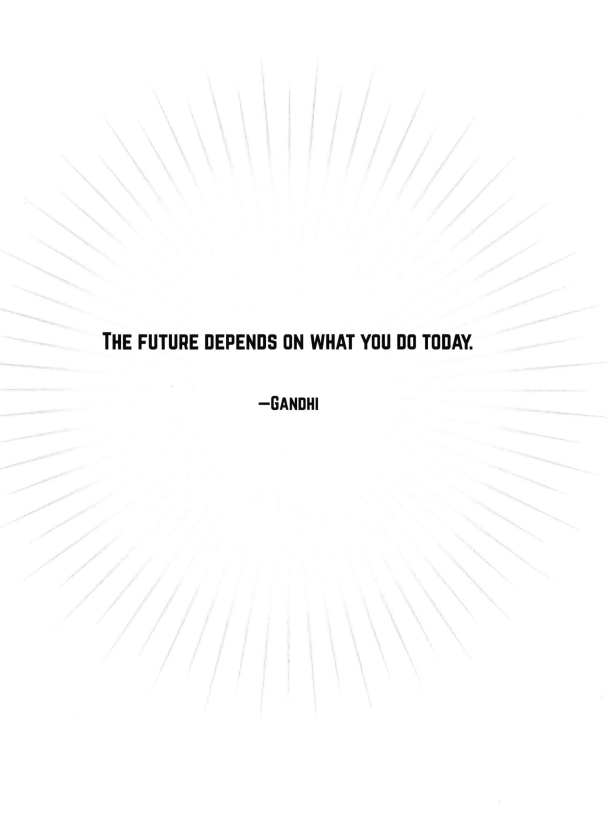

THE FUTURE DEPENDS ON WHAT YOU DO TODAY.

—GANDHI

TOOLS & TIPS OF THE TRADE

Life handed him a lemon,
As Life sometimes will do.
His friends looked on in pity,
Assuming he was through.
They came upon him later,
Reclining in the shade
In calm contentment, drinking
A glass of lemonade.

—Clarence Edwin Flynn

Tools of the Trade

For magic juice making you will need a juicer, yes you can do it in a blender and then strain it, but it's best to use a juicer to get the maximum power for the investment of time and money you have just committed to. What kind of juicer, you ask? The one you can afford, the one you will use, or the one you already have! If you are shopping for a juicer, consider the following prior to investing in one:

1. What is your price range? Search online for several options within that price range and read the reviews.

2. What kind of juices will you be making? Mainly green powerhouse juices? Will you be juicing grasses such as wheatgrass, barley grass, and so on? Will you be using more fruit than vegetables? Will you be juicing fruits that are hard or soft in nature?

3. Be honest: are you going to take the time to clean the juicer?

As you begin your journey, you may or may not know the answers to these questions. Only one thing is certain: things change. In time, your awareness, intentions, and conditions will change, and you may find yourself wanting to add wheatgrass to your juices! Who knew? Keeping your options open when buying a juicer is the way to go. Perhaps investing in one that meets your needs right now is best. Or, perhaps investing in one that allows for the possibility of adding grasses in the future is your best choice. Only you have the answer to your journey.

There are two kinds of juicers to consider: masticating juicers or centrifugal juicers.

Masticating juicers. These are the true cold pressed juicers. They work by gently masticating the fruits and veggies using non-sharp blades that rotate at low speeds to extract the juice. This results in a cold pressed juice, high in nutrient density and enzymes and richer in colour. The pulp that has been separated from the juice is dry, which is great because you want to be extracting as much liquid nutrition from your produce as possible. These juicers have minimal air exposure, so the resulting juice suffers minimal oxidization, also a great thing. These juicers are great for any and all veggies, grasses, and harder fruits. (Softer fruit is best saved for a smoothie.) These juicers generally come with a 5–10 year warranty, and last a long time. So they are a great investment in your well-being. There are a few options within masticating juicers.

Norwalk juicer. This is the hydraulic press juicer developed by Dr. Norman Walker, who became known as the leading expert in raw juice therapy when he opened the Norwalk Laboratories of Health Research in 1910. His research into the benefits of raw juices prompted him to begin production of a hydraulic press juicer. It was a revolutionary design at the time, for this juicer removes the fibres of the vegetables and fruits as it extracts the juice, with no loss of nutrients or enzymes. It is the ultimate cold press juicer.

Today's design has evolved from the original but stayed true to its mission. Norwalk juicers work by first passing the produce (veggies and fruit) through a triturating mechanism or grinder on one side of the machine, which transforms the produce into a wet pulp mixture that is then collected in a fine cloth bag, ready for pressing. It is then pressed in an electric hydraulic press on the other side of the machine, allowing you to enjoy the best cold pressed juice money can buy. This is the juicer used by The Gerson Institute, and the top juicer in the juice therapy industry. It is one of the most expensive juicers available on the market.

Twin blade or triturating juicers. These juicers were developed from the design of the Norwalk juicer. Through a dual blade system, the juicer finely crushes, grinds, or pounds the produce to extract the juice, nutrients, and enzymes. This system uses two blades that slowly rotate towards each other, grinding the produce into a fine pulp and extracting the juice, without producing any heat during the process, resulting in no loss of nutrients or enzymes. This action tears open the produce's cell membranes to release its deep-seated nutrients and enzymes, and, because of the low oxidization that happens in this process, you are able to enjoy a true cold pressed juice! This system also breaks up more of the phytochemical from the produce, resulting in a richly coloured juice which is also richer in nutrients and minerals, and leaving behind a drier pulp that is really just the fibre of the produce.

Twin blade or triturating juicers are powerful and popular because they produce large amounts of high-quality cold pressed juice, are simpler to use, faster to clean, and not as expensive. They are a mid-range juicer. Some brands of twin blade juicers (in no particular order) are: Champion, Kempo, Omega, Tribest Green Star, and Super Angel, amongst others.

Centrifugal juicers. These juicers work by using the power of centrifugal force created by a single, sharp-edged blade that cuts and pulps up the produce and separates the pulp from the juice simultaneously. The sharp-edged blade moves at a high speed, which lightly heats up the produce as it is being crushed into juice, causing oxidization of some of the nutrients and enzymes. The resulting pulp is wet in nature, as it still contains some juice.

Centrifugal juicers are faster to use, faster to clean (though that depends on the model), much less expensive, and more easily available. They only come with a 1–2 year warranty, and don't last as long as the masticating juicers. Some brands of centrifugal juicers (in no particular order) are: Omega J9000, Breville, Hamilton Beach Big Mouth, and Cuisinart amongst others.

For magic *smoothie* making, you will need a blender. Super power high-speed blenders are great for making smooth drinks and blending all the ingredients in a way that all you taste is goodness in a glass. Are they indispensable? No. You can still make delicious smoothies with the blender you have. When you are ready to invest in a higher-quality blender, I recommend you take a look at the following two powerhouses because they can be used for a whole lot more than just making smoothies. My Vitamix is my right-hand woman in the kitchen!

Two high-speed blender brands to consider are Vitamix and Blendtec. Due to popular demand, other companies now are coming up with their own versions of high-speed blenders. Both blenders are superpowers. Yes, you can actually blend your iPhone if you like, but I'd rather keep mine outside of my blender. Thank you very much!

To craft love making elixirs, you need a kettle (or boiled water), a blender, a glass Mason jar is always handy, a nut mylk bag (available at most health food stores), and some of the superfoods and super herbs you will get to know later in this book.

Tips of the Trade

Following are tips for making your journey into the Brave New World of liquid nutrition as smooth and easy a transition as possible, and best serve you as you power up your health:

Juices:

1. Wash and cut your produce to be juiced all at once, in handy pieces that fit through the mouth of your juicer.

2. Run the produce through the juicer by alternating the soft, the leafy, the hard, in no particular order, so your juicer doesn't get stuck with one type of produce. For example, celery and leafy greens are great juicer cleaners if your apples are getting stuck.

3. Drink your juice *right away*. This is when the nutrient content is most alive, most vibrant, and can do you the most good.

4. Light will oxidize the juice. If you plan to drink your goodness later, place it in a stainless steel container and cover it with a lid.

Smoothies:

Place the liquid contents first, then add all your superfoods, produce, and of course, magic to the mix. Blend. Serve. Enjoy.

Elixirs:

The best way to get to know medicinal herbs, mushrooms, wild edibles, and superfoods is to incorporate them slowly, one or a few at a time. We are all unique; they may love you or not or, rather, you may love them or not. They may facilitate a deeper healing, or create a healing crisis. Either way, if you approach it a little bit at a time, you will develop an intimate relationship with them and they will guide your way into radiant vibrant health! Sometimes you may need just ¼ tsp instead of a full tsp, or a tbsp of something else. Trust your body compass; it knows best.

COLD PRESSED FRESH LIVING JUICE RECIPES

The following recipes are for cold pressed fresh living juices made with a cold press juicer such as the centrifugal or masticating juicers mentioned in the previous section. (See page 134.) Wash your produce prior to use, cut them so they fit through the chute, and away you go! Be sure to mix the ingredients as you are juicing them to facilitate the process.

Celery Juice

1 full head of organic celery

Drink on empty stomach in the morning. Makes about half a litre of celery juice. Depending on the season and the celery, some contain more structured water, therefore yielding more juice.

Celery juice deserves the honour roll. It has been recently popularized thanks to the efforts of Anthony Williams, the Medical Medium. As he states:

> Celery is truly the saviour when it comes to chronic illness. I've seen thousands of people who suffer from chronic and mystery illness restore their health by drinking 16 ounces of celery juice daily on an empty stomach.[13]

Celery juice has the power to rebuild your digestive tract and system. It rebuilds the hydrochloric acid in your stomach, increases and strengthens the bile, and restores your central nervous system. It detoxifies and rebuilds the kidneys and liver from old poisons, toxins, heavy metals, and so on. It has been a super ally along my healing journey and I cannot stress it enough: "*Drink it up, drink it up, drink it up!*"

Celery juice can be made using a juicer, but it can also be easily made in the blender. Add chopped celery to blender. Add ¼ cup water. Blend till smooth. Strain through a nut mylk bag. Drink up.

The Rawlly Good Electromagnetic Green Juice Transfusion!

- 1 celery bunch
- 1 cucumber
- (5–6) green leaves such as kale, collards, chard, spinach, lettuce. Variety is key. (One day I use kale, the next a different green to ensure I get a variety of nutrients for me and for my family!)

---

13   Anthony William, "Celery Juice 101," Medical Medium Blog. Retrieved from: http://www.medicalmedium.com/blog/celery-juice-101

- 2 cups sprouts, such as sunflower, pea, buckwheat, alfalfa, clover, etc. (Again, variety is key.)
- 1 or 2 apples, cored
- 1 lemon, no rind
- ½-inch or 1-inch-long piece of ginger
- handful fresh mint leaves (optional)

Heavy Metals Be Gone

- 5 kale leaves
- 5 celery ribs
- 1 medium cucumber
- ½ bunch cilantro leaves
- ½ bunch parsley leaves
- 1 lime
- 1 inch ginger root
- 1 tsp chlorella (or a seaweed powder mix)
- 1–2 tsp chia seeds (to be mixed into the juice afterwards)

Chia seeds contain water-soluble fibre, which absorbs the toxins in your digestive tract, helping your body cleanse itself.

Digestive Aid Green Juice

- 1 whole fennel bulb, including stems, chopped
- 5 celery stalks
- 3 kale leaves
- 1 apple, cored
- 2 grapefruit, peeled

3 in 1: Beet Carrot Orange

- 6 carrots
- 2 beets
- 3 oranges, peeled
- Optional: 2 apples (cored), ½-inch–1-inch piece fresh ginger.

Electrolyte Me!

- 1 cucumber
- 2 celery stalks
- 2 apples, cored
- 2 limes, peeled
- Juice all together, and place in your blender. Add to the blender the following:
- 2 cups coconut water
- 1 tbsp spirulina or seaweed powder
- 1–2 oz wheatgrass juice
- pinch Himalayan salt

Blend all ingredients. Serve. Bliss out.

Ginger Ale Mojito Kombucha

- 3 green apples, cored
- 1 inch ginger root
- 1 lime, peeled
- Juice it all up!
- 1 cup kombucha

Add the juice to the kombucha. Sit back and relax!

Ginger Lemonade

- 3 apples
- 2 lemons, peeled
- 1-inch-long piece of ginger root

In a blender, place:

- 1 L water
- 1–2 tbsp xylitol or sweetener of choice

Add juice and blend. (Add 1 cup of raspberries and blend all together for Raspberry Ginger Lemonade.) Drink it straight up, or strain for a more smooth lemonade.

Post Workout Regenerator

- 3 apples, cored
- 3 carrots
- 3 celery ribs

August Garden Harvest

- 3 broccoli florets
- 1 garlic clove, peeled
- 4 carrots
- 2 stalks celery
- ½ green pepper, stem and seeds removed

Garden's Delight

- 3 cups spinach or any combination of dark green leaves (kale/chard/collards)
- ½ cup parsley
- 4 celery ribs
- 1 broccoli floret
- ½ red pepper, stem and seeds removed
- 3 medium carrots
- 2 tomatoes
- 1 cucumber

Liquid Sunshine

- 2 cups buckwheat sprouts
- 1 cup sunflower sprouts
- 1 cup pea sprouts
- 1 cucumber
- 5 celery ribs
- 1 lemon, peeled
- 1 green apple, cored

Sprouts are the ultimate activators and regenerators, as they contain all the information they need to become mature plants that have the ability to thrive and survive in the elements. When you include them in your diet and in your juices, you are ingesting the essence of that information. Pure liquid sunshine goodness for greatness on earth.

Tropical Paradise

- 2 cups pineapple, cored and peeled
- 2 apples, cored
- 1 kiwi, peeled
- 1 orange, peeled
- 1 lemon, peeled
- 1 lime, peeled

Golden Times

- 2 apples, cored
- 2 pears, seeded
- 2 carrots
- 4 celery ribs
- 1 lemon, peeled
- 1 inch ginger root
- 1 inch fresh turmeric root (or ½–1 tsp ground turmeric root, added to the juice)

Digestive Tonic

- ¼ pineapple, with skin on
- 1 apple, cored
- ¼-inch slice ginger root

Kidney Glory

- 5 celery ribs
- 2 apples, cored
- 2 oranges, peeled
- 1 lemon, peeled

Iron Power

- 6 carrots
- 1 beet
- ½ cup fresh parsley

Adrenal Power

- 4 carrots
- 4 celery ribs
- 2 apples, cored
- ¼ broccoli head
- 5 asparagus spears
- ½ cup parsley

Immune Power

- 4 carrots
- 2 apples, cored
- ½ cup parsley
- 1/2 inch ginger root
- 1/2 inch turmeric root
- 1 garlic clove, peeled
- pinch cayenne (optional)

Liver Lover

- 1 cup green leaves (spinach, kale, Swiss chard)
- 1 cucumber
- 8 dandelion leaves
- 1 large pear or apple, cored
- 1 lemon, peeled

Awaken your Brain Power

- 8 romaine leaves
- 1 cup spinach
- 1 pear, seeded
- 1½ cups grapes
- ½ lime, peeled

WELLNESS SHOTS RECIPES

The following are recipes charged with superpowers. These foods will aid in your healing and, because of their potency, a little goes a long way.

The Queen of Grasses

- 1 oz wheatgrass juice (or more!)

Works best first thing in the morning on an empty stomach. Unleash the force of the queen!

Good Morning Power Shot

- 1–2-inch slice ginger root juiced
- 1 lemon, juiced
- ½ cup water
- 1 tsp raw honey (optional–added afterwards)
- Pinch cayenne (optional–great when facing the alMighty winter cold season)
- A few drops of oregano oil (optional–cold and flu defence and speedy recovery)

Anti-inflammatory Wake-Up Call Shot

- 1–2-inch slice ginger root, juiced
- 4-inch piece fresh turmeric, juiced (or 1/4 – 1 tsp of ground turmeric)
- 1 lemon, juiced
- ½ cup water (or straight up!)
- 1 tsp raw honey (optional, added afterwards)

Aloe Vera

- 1 inch fillet of the inner leaf of the aloe vera plant
- 2 oz water
- Blend together and enjoy!

Aloe vera increases nutrient absorption, aids in removal of toxins, supports digestion and immunity, and acts as an anti-inflammatory.

E3 LIVE

- ½ tsp or 1 oz of liquid blue green algae to boost energy, improve mental focus, and balance blood sugar
- ½ lemon, juiced
- ½ inch fresh ginger root, juiced
- dash sea salt
- 1/2 cup water

Pineapple Turmeric Gut Shot

- ½ cup fresh pineapple juice
- 1–2 tsp apple cider vinegar
- 1–2 inches fresh turmeric root, juiced
- dash sea salt

Popeye Shots

- 3 cups of spinach, juiced
- ¼ lemon, juiced
- 1 green apple, juiced

Apple Cider Vinegar Elixir

- 1–2 tsp apple cider vinegar
- 1 apple, juiced
- ½ inch fresh ginger root, juiced
- ⅛ tsp cinnamon powder
- 1 tsp raw honey
- 8 oz of water

Wellness Shot

- 3 stalks celery, juiced
- 1 Granny Smith apple, juiced
- 1 lemon, juiced
- 1–2 inch fresh ginger root, juiced
- Dash cayenne pepper

Glow Shot

- 2 medium beets, chopped, juiced
- 1 medium cucumber, juiced
- 1 inch fresh ginger root, juiced
- 1 lemon, juiced

SWEET AND GREEN SMOOTHIE RECIPES

The following are recipes for all types of smoothies, easy 1–2–3 all ingredients go in the blender. Blend until smooth. Enjoy!

Smoothie to Heaven!

- 1 banana, peeled
- 1 cup blueberries or strawberries
- 1 tbsp flax or hemp seed oil
- 1 tbsp hemp seeds or nut butter
- 1 cup of almond milk (homemade is best, see page 155 for recipe), or water
- ½ – 1 tsp green powder (best if fermented)
- 1 scoop vegan protein powder
- pinch of sea salt

Note: Most green powders contain sea vegetables. They can have a detoxifying effect, so start with a little bit and observe how your body does. Once your body has adjusted to them, you can increase the amount.

Optional:

- ½–1 tsp sea vegetable powder (chlorella, spirulina, E3Live, Blue Majik, or any combination).
- 1 tbsp bee pollen
- 1 tbsp raw cacao powder or carob
- 1 tbsp raw cacao nibs

Mango Kale Green Smoothie

My kids' first love! Simple, yet so good and satisfying.

- 1 mango
- 1 cup kale
- 1 cup water or coconut water for added sweetness
- 1 banana, peeled, for a sweeter smoothie (optional)

If you wish to make this smoothie into a heavy metal detox, add the following:

- 1 cup cilantro
- 1 cup parsley
- 1 date
- 1 tsp chlorella

Matcha Pear Green Protein Smoothie

- 1 cup almond mylk (homemade is best, see page 155 for recipe)
- 1 cup spinach
- 1 pear, cored
- 1 scoop protein powder
- ½ tsp matcha tea powder

Chocolate Banana Shake

- 2 cups almond mylk
- 1 banana, peeled
- 1 cup frozen cherries or raspberries
- ½ fresh avocado
- 1½ cups fresh spinach
- 2–4 medjool dates or 1 tbsp sweetener of choice (raw honey, xylitol, stevia)
- 2 tbsp cacao powder
- 1 tbsp maca powder (optional)
- 1 tbsp cacao nibs, sprinkled on top (optional)

Mint Lemon Green Smoothie

- 1 cup fresh mint
- 1 avocado, peeled and seeded
- 2 apples, cored
- ½ lemon
- 4 cups water

Energy Pick-Me Up

- 2 green apples
- ½ avocado, peeled and seeded
- 3 kiwis, peeled
- 2 cups spinach
- 1 cup water

Green Peach Delight

- 1 bunch cilantro
- 3 ripe peaches, quartered and pits removed
- 2 mangoes, peeled and chopped
- 1 cup fresh apple juice
- 2 cups water

Beauty Smoothie

- 1 head romaine lettuce, chopped
- 3–4 stalks celery
- 2 apples, cored and chopped
- 1 banana, peeled
- ⅓ bunch cilantro
- ⅓ bunch parsley
- 1 lemon, juiced
- 1½ cups water

Velvet Blue Margarita

- 1 frozen banana
- 1½ cup pineapple
- ½ mango, peeled and pit removed (optional)
- 2 limes, peeled
- ½ tsp blue-green algae (E3Live or Blue Majik)
- dash cayenne
- pinch sea salt
- 1 cup ice
- ½ cup water

Oh—Green—Oh!

- 2 handfuls spinach
- 2 cups fresh orange juice
- 1 grapefruit, seeds removed, peeled and chopped
- 1 mango, peeled and chopped

The Regenerator Smoothie

- 2 cups fresh kale
- 1 orange, peeled
- 1 cup pineapple, peeled and chopped
- 1 cup blueberries
- 1 cup coconut water or water
- 2 tbsp chia seed

Summer Loving

- 1 cup strawberries
- 1 mango, peeled and chopped
- ¼ medium watermelon, chopped
- handful fresh mint
- 2 cups lettuce or spinach

Liquid Gold Smoothie

- ½ cup golden beets, chopped
- ¾ cup red grapes
- 1-inch piece fresh turmeric root, juiced
- 1 lemon, juiced
- 1 tbsp pumpkin seeds
- 1 cup water

Kiwi Double Up

- 2 kiwis, peeled and chopped
- ½ cup mesclun lettuce mix, or spinach
- 1 pear, cored
- 1 tbsp chia seeds
- 3 tbsp cashews
- 1 cup water

Superfood Oatmeal Smoothie

- 1 zucchini, peeled and chopped
- 1 banana, peeled and chopped
- 3 tbsp rolled oats
- 1 tbsp pumpkin seeds
- 1 tsp lucuma powder
- 1 tsp cinnamon powder

Pink Coconut

- 1 frozen banana, peeled
- ¾ cup frozen strawberries
- ¼ cup zucchini
- 1 red medium beet
- 1 cup coconut milk
- 1 tsp lemon juice (optional)
- 1–2 scoops vegan protein powder
- water, as needed

RAW SOUPS / SAVOURY RECIPES

Raw soups or blended foods are easier for your body to digest. Since that step has already been done, there's no need for your body to spend a lot of energy breaking down and digesting what you've eaten. In general, when making raw soups it's best to use water that's at room temperature, or warm water (towards hot), especially if you live in a cold climate. Embarking on your revolution is not about eating cold foods. Raw foods can be eaten warm by adding warm water to the recipe, by using the dehydrator to heat your food, and by adding warming spices to bring heat into your body.

Cucumber Dill Savoury Smoothie – A Soup Evolution!

- 2 medium cucumbers, chopped
- 1 avocado, peeled and seeded
- 5 leaves dinosaur kale, stems removed
- 2 stalks celery
- 2 tbsp fresh lime juice
- 1 clove garlic
- ½ cup water

Mango Cucumber Soup

- 2 mangoes, peeled and cut
- 2 cucumbers
- ¼ cup water or coconut water
- ¼ cup fresh mint leaves
- 2 tbsp fresh lemon juice
- 2 tbsp olive oil
- ¼ tsp sea salt

So long Heavy Metals… So long!

- 1 avocado, peeled and seeded
- 1 red pepper, stem and seeds removed
- 1 ripe tomato
- 1 lemon, seeds removed
- 1 bunch cilantro

Blend all ingredients until smooth. To serve, add the following:

- ½ bunch cilantro, chopped
- 1 ripe tomato, chopped
- 1 carrot, grated
- 1 handful dulse (seaweed) leaves, chopped
- 1 handful sunflower sprouts, chopped

Green Pea Mint Soup

- 2 cups green peas
- 2 cups spinach
- ½ avocado or ¼ cup raw cashews
- 1 garlic clove
- 1 cup mint
- 2 tbsp fresh lemon juice
- 2 tbsp nutritional yeast
- 2 tbsp gluten free tamari
- 2 cups water or nut mylk of choice

Naty's Gazpacho

- 3 large ripe tomatoes (about 3 cups)
- 1 cup chopped cucumber
- 1 red pepper or green pepper, stem and seeds removed
- 2 Tbsp fresh lime juice
- ¼ red onion
- 1 cup of basil
- 1–2 garlic cloves
- ½ tsp sea salt
- 1 Tbsp olive oil
- ½ cup water or more, until desired consistency has been reached.

To make a chunky soup, blend all ingredients on low speed, or faster to create a smoother, more creamy gazpacho. If you prefer it even chunkier, add some more veggies to your bowl along with the blended soup. In this case, because it is a gazpacho, add more chopped tomatoes, cucumber, red or green pepper, a slash of olive oil for decoration, and you have created a master gazpacho!

Savoury Coconut Soup

- 2–3 cups mixed greens (kale, chard, parsley, cilantro are good)
- 1 celery rib
- 3–4 whole tomatoes
- 2 tbsp fresh lemon juice
- ½ avocado, peeled and seeded
- 1 tbsp miso paste (I prefer chickpea miso as it doesn't affect *Candida* issues)
- 1 tbsp gluten-free tamari
- 1 cup warm to hot water
- 1 cup homemade coconut mylk or 1 small can of organic coconut mylk (see recipe page 156)

Separately:

- ½–1 leek, finely sliced
- 1 garlic clove, finely sliced
- 1 lemon juiced and drizzled over the leek and garlic mix

Blend the first set of ingredients. Add to serving bowl. Add leek and garlic.

Cream of Celery

- 1 head of celery
- 1 avocado, peeled and seeded
- 1 tomato or 1 red pepper, stem and seeds removed
- 2 cups water
- 2 Tbsp fresh lemon juice, about 1 lemon
- 2 tbsp nutritional yeast or more (It gives it that cheese taste without the consequences!)
- 1 tsp gluten-free tamari sauce
- ½ tsp sea salt

Blend all ingredients together in a high-speed blender. Serve. Or, add additional veggies like red pepper, zucchini, or kelp noodles for serving. Enjoy!

Curry Carrot Soup

- 3 cups of carrots
- 1 cup chopped celery
- 2 cups water
- 1 avocado, peeled and seeded
- 1 clove garlic, peeled
- 1 inch of fresh ginger
- 1 tbsp fresh lemon juice
- 1 tsp curry powder
- ½ tsp cumin powder
- ½ tsp Celtic or Himalayan salt
- ¼ tsp cayenne powder
- ¼ tsp fresh ground pepper

Process all ingredients in a blender until smooth and creamy.

Watercress Power

- 3 medium cucumbers, peeled
- 1 cup watercress, large stems removed
- ¼ cup onion
- 2 tbsp fresh lemon juice
- 2 tbsp gluten-free tamari
- 2 tbsp flax seed oil (olive oil works as well)
- ½ cup water

Blend all ingredients until smooth and power up!

NUT MYLK RECIPES

The truth is out. If you don't believe me, do your research. Check it out. Conventional dairy products from milk—pasteurized, full of antibiotics, chemically enriched, and containing a whole lot more sugar than it used to—are one of the leading causes of osteoporosis, acidity, and mucus in the body, amongst other things. These are just three truths, and they are pretty big ones. The business of dairy has changed the quality of dairy products. Dairy is not building us up as much as we think it is.

Wait, what? Isn't milk supposed to be good for my bones? What about calcium? What about all those years of advertising telling me I have to drink my milk to grow strong and healthy? Yes— note the key word there—*advertising*. And it worked pretty well. It's a complicated story that like most, has little or nothing to do with your health, and a lot more to do with the evolution of the dairy industry as a business in today's world. Yikes, did I say that out loud?

But hold on … raw milk, ethically sourced from grazing cows that have not been inundated with antibiotics and growth hormones, and are not fed corn or soy? What about them? Well, there is your source for the healthy dairy industry that sustained previous generations.

If you are going to include dairy in your life, please invest in organic dairy. Do your research and support companies that raise cows with as little antibiotic and hormone usage as possible, so there is less of it in the milk you love.

But … if you are looking to change your habits and your sources for calcium, and the milk you want to nourish your body, you have great options! Leafy greens have greatness for calcium in there—yes! Add them to your juices and smoothies. Raw nuts and seeds are also power calcium, magnesium, and selenium-rich foods.

So, let's make *mylk* (raw nut mylk) to improve your intake and absorption of calcium, magnesium, and selenium! *Raw nut mylks* are also a great base for thicker smoothies, salad dressings, and kefir.

Step 1: Soaking and sprouting (activating nuts and seeds). To be able to fully enjoy the benefits and powers of homemade raw nut and seed mylks, it is important they be activated through soaking for at least four hours, or even overnight. Soaking them releases the enzyme inhibitors that keeps them dormant until the right forces and conditions are in place for them to release their power and begin to grow and thrive. This is nature's way of preserving itself. This is our way of awakening their mightiness!

Soaking the raw nuts and seeds activates the food's full nutritional potential, along with your ability to better digest and get the most from them.

Upon activation, their enzymatic powers for growth and survival rise to exponential levels, exactly what you want to bring into your body! This is an exponential-level enzymatic power that you can then assimilate, and allow to function through you. You can also take the extra step of allowing nuts and seeds to begin to sprout, again allowing all that enzymatic growth to happen.

Step 2: Blend with water. Strain using a nut mylk bag, and use the liquid as your nut / seed mylk. Use the pulp to make all sorts of raw pulp crackers, cookies, wafers, and so on!

Fresh Nut or Seed Mylk – Almond Mylk

- 1 cup raw nuts or seeds (such as almonds, cashews, walnuts, or brazil nuts), soaked and, if possible, sprouted
- 4 cups water
- 4 medjool dates, soaked, if possible. (For those with sugar sensitivities, use other sweetener such as Lakanto monk-fruit sweetener, stevia, or birch-derived xylitol. Substitution is 1:1. 1 tbsp sweetener = 1 date)
- pinch sea salt

Soak the nuts overnight, leave on the counter to sprout for a day. If you are pressed for time, soaking them is the most important part. Sometimes I soak nuts and seeds in batches, dehydrate them, and have them already pre-activated to make mylk on my busy days.

Blend all ingredients together in a high-speed blender for 30–60 seconds. Pour into a nut mylk bag and "milk it" to get the mylk out. You will be left with the pulp of the nuts in the bag. This pulp can be used for all sorts of wonderful recipes—from croutons to cookies and toast. Your imagination and creativity are the limit!

Fresh Nut Chocolate Mylk

(I like using almonds for this recipe)

- Add 1 tbsp raw cacao powder to the fresh nut/seed mylk recipe above.

Fresh Nut Vanilla Mylk

(I like using almonds for this recipe)

- Add 1 tsp raw vanilla powder to the fresh nut/seed mylk recipe above.

Fresh Golden Mylk

- 2 cups of mylk fresh nut/seed mylk (warm or hot)
- 1 tsp turmeric
- ¾ tsp fresh ginger (chopped)
- ½ tsp cinnamon powder
- pinch black pepper
- 1 tsp – 1 tbsp raw honey

Blend all. Enjoy your liquid gold!

Fresh Live Homemade Coconut Mylk

- 1 cup shredded coconut
- 4 cups water
- 2 medjool dates or 2 tbsp xylitol (or sweetener of choice)
- pinch sea salt

Blend all ingredients in a high-speed blender until the coconut has been pulverized, about 1 minute. Pour through a nut mylk bag to strain any reminder of shredded coconut.

Almond Mylk Kefir

- 1 recipe of fresh almond mylk (made with warm water is best)
- two vegan probiotic capsules
- 1 Mason jar (sterilized)
- cheesecloth

Place 4 cups of fresh almond mylk in blender. Open two vegan probiotic capsules. Blend all together. Transfer to Mason jar and cover the mouth of the jar with the cheesecloth. Leave on the counter for a day or two (at room temperature) until it ferments. Drink an espresso shot every day! Almond mylk kefir is a great probiotic for your gut health.

FERMENTED RECIPES

Fermented liquid foods are very high in enzymatic powers. Natural probiotics, they help your system maintain gut health and overall systemic health. In order for your immune system to be at its best, the balance of good and bad bacteria in your system needs to remain stable with more of the beneficial bacteria ruling the kingdom.

Our gut has become known as our "second brain." The health of your gut system is a key factor in your overall health and, yes, there is a lot you can do about it! Fermented liquid foods are a wonderful addition to your new lifestyle. The life that brews within these fermented liquid powerhouses is rich in micro-organisms that cannot be reproduced in a lab. They get pretty close, but these are the real deal!

Water Kefir (Fermented Electrolytes)

(I double this recipe every time I make it—it is that good. It just doesn't last)

Supplies Needed:

- a 2-litre, or two 1-litre glass jars
- cheesecloth and rubber band
- water kefir grains (from Cultures for Health)

Ingredients (per glass jar):

- ¼ cup hydrated water kefir grains
- ¼ cup Sucanat, rapadura sugar, or organic cane sugar (do not use honey)
- 1 litre water

Add sugar to the glass jar. Add water, and stir until the sugar is thoroughly dissolved. Add the kefir grains to the sweetened water. Cover the mouth of the jar with the cheesecloth and secure it with a rubber band. Let it sit at room temperature to ferment for 24 – 48 hours. Once the water kefir has reached your taste buds' level of satisfaction, strain through a nonreactive (plastic or wood, avoid metal) strainer or nut mylk bag.

If you prefer a strong fizz and more flavour, you can do a secondary fermentation. Wash the grains with clean water. Freeze them for later use, or if you are ready to make another batch, they are ready to be used again! I like to keep a few grains in my kefir, they are just so tasty.

Secondary Fermentation:

Add ½ cup fruit juice, a small piece of ginger root, 1 lemon (halved), ½ cup of fruit or 1 tbsp organic sugar to a 1-litre glass bottle (with a lid).

Add your water kefir to it, leaving about an inch of empty space at the top. Place the lid on it in order for it to develop natural fizz. Place on the counter for 2–3 days. Then, into the fridge it goes! It is ready to serve! Be mindful that when you open it, the extra fizz might just be bursting to come out, so be standing by the sink. Note: if you used lemon in your second fermentation, take the halved lemon pieces out before placing your Mighty kefir in the fridge.

Spirulina Lime Water Kefir

Follow instructions for your initial fermentation of water kefir (page 157)

Secondary Fermentation:

To your initial water kefir, add:

- 1 tbsp spirulina
- 2 tbsp fresh lime juice (1 lime juiced)
- 1 tsp Sucanat, rapadura sugar, or organic cane sugar (do not use honey)

Add all the ingredients to a 1-litre glass jar along with your water kefir, leaving about an inch of empty space at the top. Place the lid on it in order for it to develop natural fizz. Place on the counter for 2–3 days. Then, into the fridge it goes! It is ready to serve! Be mindful that when you open it, the extra fizz might just be bursting to come out, so be standing by the sink.

Wheatgrass Coconut Lime Water Kefir

Follow instructions for your initial fermentation of water kefir, but use coconut water instead of water to make the initial water kefir. (page 157)

Secondary Fermentation:

To your initial water kefir, add:

- 1 tbsp wheatgrass powder
- 2 tbsp of fresh lime juice (1 lime juiced)
- 1 tsp Sucanat, rapadura sugar, or organic cane sugar (it will become extra carbonation)

Add all the ingredients to a 1-litre glass jar along with your water kefir, leaving about an inch of empty space at the top. Place the lid on it in order for it to develop natural fizz. Place on the counter for 2–3 days. Then, into the fridge it goes! It is ready to serve! Be mindful that when you open it, the extra fizz might just be bursting to come out, so be standing by the sink.

Rejuvelac

Rejuvelac is fermented wheat berry water, but it can also be made with any grain or seed, like kamut, rye, or quinoa. This very powerful probiotic does take a few days to make.

Day 1: Combine the wheat berries and rye berries in a 24-ounce jar with a vented lid (or use cheesecloth to cover the top). Add 3 cups water. Place the jar in a warm spot, and let it sit at room temperature for the day.

Day 2: Discard the liquid. Transfer the berries to a nut mylk bag and put the bag in a bowl. (I hang mine).

Day 3 to 4: Rinse the berries under cool running water three to five times a day. (I only do it morning and night for sure. If I remember to do it at other times, I do).

Day 5: When the berries have tiny tails, it means they have sprouted! Rinse the sprouted berries once more. Put the berries in a one-gallon glass jar with a lid. Fill the jar completely with spring (filtered) water and let sit overnight in a warm spot.

Day 6: Strain and discard the berries, but save the liquid. The sprouted berries will produce 1 gallon of fermented liquid called rejuvelac. It will be pale yellow and cloudy, with quite a pungent smell. Refrigerate for up to one month. The same berries can be used up to three times.

Rejuvelac can be drunk on its own, or used instead of water in a variety of recipes, such as nut mylks, raw nut cheeses, and others.

Kombucha

This fermented drink, traditionally made with black tea and sugar, uses the Mighty power of a kombucha scoby, a symbiotic culture of bacteria and yeast, to alchemically ferment the drink. You can also use green tea, white tea, oolong tea, or even mix them up. Always include a few bags of black tea to ensure your scoby is getting all the nutrients it needs. Avoid flavoured teas or teas that contain oils.

Supplies Needed:

- glass jar with a wide mouth to allow enough oxygen to interact with your brew
- kitchen towel or large piece of cheese cloth to cover the wide mouth
- kombucha scoby (the magical being who will be fermenting your kombucha)—you can find one online, or ask your friends. You never know where a scoby might be waiting to be found!

Ingredients:

- 8 cups water
- ½ cup organic (preferably) cane sugar or raw coconut sugar (it gets "eaten" as part of the fermentation process)
- 4 bags tea (at least 2 bags black tea, and 2 other bags of your choice)
- 1 cup of pre-made kombucha (generally the kombucha your scoby was patiently awaiting its next brew on)
- 1 kombucha scoby

Bring water to a boil. Add sugar and tea bags. Let the sugar dissolve. Turn it off. Allow the tea to steep for about 10 minutes.

Remove the tea bags. Allow the brew to cool. Transfer it to a large glass jar with a wide mouth (or several wide-mouth Mason jars). Stir in 1 cup of pre-made kombucha and drop in scoby in on top.

Cover with a kitchen towel. Place it in a quiet spot. Your Kombucha will need 7–10 days to ferment. Taste and delight.

When your brewed kombucha is ready, remove the scoby, the bottle it in a glass jar with enough brewed kombucha to cover it, and place it in the fridge until you are ready to make your next batch. Brewed kombucha should be bottled in glass jars and placed in the fridge.

Sacred Kombucha

- 4 cups strained ancient wisdom tea (recipe under Tea Decoctions, page 175)
- 4 cups water
- 1-inch stick palo santo wood
- 6 tbsp tulsi (holy basil)
- 3 teabags yerba mate
- 3 tea bags rooibos red tea
- ½ cup organic (preferably) cane sugar or raw coconut sugar (it gets "eaten" as part of the fermentation process)

Bring water to boil. Cover and simmer for 20 minutes. Stir in sugar until it dissolves. Turn it off and allow to cool down. Strain using a plastic strainer.

- 1 cup pre-made kombucha (generally the kombucha your scoby was patiently awaiting its next brew on)
- 1 kombucha scoby

Allow the brew to cool. Transfer it to a large glass jar with a wide mouth (or several wide-mouth Mason jars). Stir in 1 cup of pre-made kombucha and drop in scoby in on top.

Cover with a kitchen towel. Place it in a quiet spot. Your Kombucha will need 7–10 days to ferment. Taste and delight.

When your brewed kombucha is ready, remove the scoby, the bottle it in a glass jar with enough brewed kombucha to cover it, and place it in the fridge until you are ready to make your next batch. Brewed kombucha should be bottled in glass jars and placed in the fridge.

Jun Tea (Kombucha's Cousin)

Jun tea is a fermented drink traditionally made with loose green tea leaves and honey. It is alchemically fermented by the one and only Mighty jun culture (like a scoby). Jun is an ancient Tibetan drink, but newer to us here in the Western world than kombucha.

Supplies needed:

- glass jar with a wide mouth to allow enough oxygen to interact with your brew
- kitchen towel or large piece of cloth to cover the wide mouth
- jun culture and jun tea starter (available at Kombucha Kamp)

Ingredients:

- 8 cups water
- 1 cup raw organic (preferably) honey
- 4 tsp loose green tea, preferably organic
- 1 jun culture
- 1 cup jun tea Starter

Heat up the water, but do not boil. Remove pot from heat. Place 4 tsp loose tea in a stainless steel tea mesh and hook to the side of the pot. Let steep for 2 minutes. Remove tea mesh and pour the hot tea into the glass jar. Stir in honey and let mixture come to room temperature.

Stir in jun starter. Place jun culture on top. Cover with a clean white tea towel or cheese cloth and secure with a large rubber band. Place in a quiet room. Leave undisturbed to ferment for 3–6 days. Harvest after 3 days. If you wish to bottle and add more fizz to this Mighty power, bottle and cap for 3 more days, then place it back in the quiet room. Or leave your brew for a full 6-day fermentation.

Remove the jun culture from the jun fermented tea. Place in a glass jar, cover with enough brewed jun tea, and place in the fridge until you are ready to make your next batch. Brewed jun tea should be bottled in clear glass jars and placed in the fridge.

POWERHOUSE WITH SUPERFOODS

These foods contain within them incredible amounts of power that are considered beneficial to your health. Depending on the food, it can contain very high amounts of protein, antioxidants, nutrients, minerals, and so on. They can be added to any recipe; I like to add them to smoothies, juices, salads, desserts, and make deep, nourishing teas out of them (goji berry, chaga tea). You name it!

Superfoods have become very popular as a dense vehicle to increase our nutrition. They are the ultimate superpowers, and can supply your body with much-needed nutritional support. Just remember that for some of us, a little can go a long way. Now, having said that, a lot of superfoods in the marketplace are exotic, expensive, and come from faraway lands. Some are indeed powerful and have a place in your healing and well-being, yet the most powerful superfoods you will ever find are the weeds growing in your backyard! They are local, perennial, have really long taproot systems, and appear seasonally just in time to provide your body with what it needs when it needs it.

Some options we have available that can turn your super juices and smoothies into nutritional powerhouses are: spirulina, chlorella, E3Live, or Blue Majik, marine phytoplankton, sea vegetables (kelp, dulse, nori, hijiki, bladderwrack, Irish moss), hemp seed, flax seed, chia seed, maca, lucuma, mesquite, raw cacao, goji berries, golden berries, bee pollen, green powders (wheatgrass, barley grass, alfalfa, brown rice protein, pea protein, etc.), medicinal mushrooms (chaga, reishi, lion's mane, turkey tail, cordyceps, maitake), coconut (meat and water), triphala, ashwagandha, camu camu berry, MSM (methyl sulfonyl methane), noni juice, mangosteen juice … and, oh, don't forget your local superweeds! Yes! Add your dandelion leaf and root, burdock root, and nettles to the mix, AND—add your maple sap and birch sap too.

There are even products in the market today that combine a few of these superfoods into one, for your convenience. How thoughtful, but *please* read the fine print. Avoid consuming products that have extra fillers, preservatives, natural or artificial flavours, and artificial colours. What good is it to get all the way here, and then continue to damage your body with these harmful additives? Choose clean products for a clean healthy body. It's that simple.

Throughout this recipe part of the book, you have already seen many a superfood included in the recipes. I am adding a few more to the collection, but know that they are meant to be included in the synergy of the magic you are creating. Spark your body into action and ease your way into radiance by creating new practices and protocols that support your intention to live in Radiant Health.

Morning Liver Tonic

- 1 cup warm/hot water—spring water is best
- 1 inch fresh ginger, juiced
- 1 inch fresh turmeric, juiced
- ½ lemon, juiced
- 1 tsp raw honey or xylitol
- pinch cayenne (optional)

Add juiced ingredients to your cup of warm/hot spring water. Add cayenne and sweetener of choice. Drink first thing in the morning while still warm/hot. Like its name says, it is a powerful liver tonic.

If you are considering doing a liquid feast for a couple of days, or if you are ready to include more superfoods and their powers into your life, I recommend you start the day with your *Morning Liver Tonic* and follow it with the *Deluxe Detox Lemonade*. I have integrated this practice into my daily rituals and as part of my daily self-care protocol.

Deluxe Detox Lemonade

- 1 litre water
- juice of ½ lemon
- ½ –1 tsp MSM powder (plant-derived). See below.
- ½–1 tsp buffered vitamin C powder or Camu Camu berry powder
- 1 tbsp raw honey or xylitol (birch tree derived) or stevia if needed.

Mix all the ingredients together in a 1-litre glass Mason jar. Slowly sip through the morning.

The combination of *water and lemon* is a natural alkalizer for the body.

MSM (methyl sulfonyl methane) powder or crystals is an organic sulphur compound naturally derived during the earth's rain cycle. This compound is a powerful supplement for longevity, and a key anti-inflammatory protocol for health. Most of us are dealing with some sort of inflammatory condition in combination with other conditions. MSM is a key protocol because it detoxifies the body by making the cells more permeable.

MSM is also a calcium phosphate dissolver (dissolves bad calcium deposits that are at the root of degenerative diseases), it improves joint flexibility, it improves skin health and complexion, it strengthens nails and hair and accelerates healing. It is most powerful as an anti-inflammatory because it allows metabolic waste to be removed from cells. Note: beware of synthetic by-products found in most MSM supplements. Look for and demand "organic plant-derived MSM" powder or crystals.

MSM powder or crystals in combination with buffered vitamin C or camu camu berry powder or lemon juice is just pure synergy. We live in an age where our allies are becoming well-known. When you combine them, you can increase the inherent power of a superfood, super herb or supplement like MSM. Specific to MSM is vitamin C.

Vitamin C is a free radical scavenger, and when you combine that power with MSM's inherent power to detoxify and decalcify (bad calcium), your detoxification process will be deeper and more effective. When these two super supplements are taken together, they also help reduce scar tissue, bring more elasticity to your skin, and assist each other in helping your nails and hair grow faster and stronger.

Optional Add-ons:

- fulvic acid (a dropper)
- 1 tsp zeolite
- black mica extract (a dropper)
- 2 oz. aloe vera juice (highly recommended to soothe internal inflammation)
- 2 oz. noni or mangosteen juice

Fulvic acid is a humid compound made largely of organic matter. It aids in the biochemical processes of the body, and optimizes its functions. Considered to be one of the most chemically active compounds in the soil, fulvic acid contains a wide variety of beneficial nutrients, such as hormones, fatty acids, ketones, flavonoids, vitamins, and minerals. It promotes cell life, helps boost energy, improves circulation, stimulates metabolism, remineralizes the body, controls inflammation, regulates hormone production, boosts the immune system, and promotes brain function.

Zeolites are natural volcanic minerals mined in certain parts of the world. They are natural chelators of heavy metals with no side effects, and they help balance the body's pH to healthy alkalinity. In today's world of abundant heavy metal toxicity, including zeolites in your morning lemonade detox is great, safe preventive idea.

Black mica extract is extracted from black mica volcanic rock, and has long been used to clean and purify water. Since our body is mostly water, it's an incredible tool for cleaning and purifying our whole-body system. Black mica has the ability to reduce or remove bacteria, viruses, parasites, heavy metals, petrochemicals, and pharmaceuticals from our water—and our bloodstream. It also oxygenates water, and can restructure and charge water molecules. It has the ability to decalcify bad calcium deposits in the body, as well as remove candida overgrowth.

Aloe vera is a powerful anti-inflammatory superfood known as the "Essene and Egyptian secret of immortality." It is high in antimicrobial properties, dissolves mucus in the body, has a lubricating effect on the joints, brain, skin, and nervous system, and supports the immune system to fight back against chance viral, nanobacteria, and fungal infections. It is a tonic adaptogen that supports our kidneys. Topically, it absorbs quickly through all seven dermal layers into the muscle, and when used on a burn or other injury, its proteolytic enzyme action promotes healing and cell reproduction at twice the normal rate, from the bottom up, reducing and minimizing scar tissue.

Noni juice (organic) is made from whole noni, a tart superfruit that grows along the rocky beaches and sandy shores of the South Pacific. It supports detoxification and digestion, assists in the healthy functioning of the liver, is beneficial to skin and scalp conditions, is anti-cancerous, antibacterial, antiviral, and antifungal, and boosts the immune system. It is also a natural antidepressant as it stimulates serotonin and melatonin production.

Mangosteen juice (organic) comes from the tropical evergreen mangosteen tree, and is another powerful anti-inflammatory superfruit. It is extremely high in antioxidants and vitamin C, is antifungal and antibacterial, and is an immune system booster. It has anticancer properties, helps maintain healthy skin, regulates blood pressure and heart rate, improves digestion, contains antihistamine properties, and assists the body in maintaining healthy weight.

Mangosteen Aloe Anti-Inflammatory Power Boost

- Juice 2 grapefruits
- Add 2 oz mangosteen juice
- Add 2 oz aloe juice or fillet your own aloe leaf

Add all the ingredients to your blender. Blend for a few seconds. Serve. Drink. Feel the power.

If you are dealing with inflammation in your body, this power boost will become a great tool along your healing journey. Mangosteen is the greatest anti-inflammatory super fruit! And working in synergy with aloe vera, well, that inflammation will all soon be history.

Hydration with Determination

- 1 L spring water
- ½ tsp Sea Salt (good quality)

Good-quality sea salt (not the common health-hazard known as table salt) has the power to balance the electrolyte, mineral levels and fluids in your body. It gently cleanses your body by forcing out toxins from your gut and bowel, it clears up your digestive systems, lowers pain in inflamed muscles, clears fluid retention, establishes normal pH balance, provides trace minerals, and facilities metabolic processes.

There are many more superfoods that can be included in your diet to upgrade your body's current operating system, and almost just as many books about them. Get curious, start by adding one (well, two) superfoods, such as MSM and Vitamin C together. Carve your own road to wellness, and your own education about superfoods by safely experimenting to discover what works or doesn't work for you.

ELIXIR RECIPES: TEA INFUSIONS, OVERNIGHT INFUSIONS AND DECOCTIONS

I have put together a ***sadhana of tea*** recipes in alignment with a cycle of seven days that follows the body's seven chakra energy centres, which will further help you align your body, mind, and spirit.

Energy is subtle and it seeks alignment in subtle ways. Please know that you really can drink any of the following tea recipes at any time, but if you wish to further align the subtle expressions of you being, then please follow the sadhana of tea roadmap recipes below.

To keep this busy life of mine flowing, I usually prep seven jars filled with plant ally wisdom at the beginning of every month. Then voila! It all flows!

To make a ***tea infusion,*** simply add a handful of plant wisdom into a 500 ml jar, fill it with boiling water, then let it steep and cool down a bit. I drink it slowly throughout the day. Or if you prefer to have a cup of wisdom a day, great! Add 1 tbsp of plant wisdom to your favourite cup, add boiled water, steep, drink, and self-nourish.

Tea infusions are a wonderful addition to your detox. They can be used as the base for your smoothies or savoury soups! If so, keep them light (only ½ cup or less of leaf mix per 1 L water). The key is to "play"; get to know yourself, get to know what strength a tea infusion is just right for you.

To make an ***overnight infusion,*** place ½ to 1 cup of plant wisdom into a 1-litre glass Mason jar, add boiling water, cover, and let it steep overnight. In the morning, you can strain the leaves, or leave them in the jar and drink the stronger tea infusion throughout the day.

Tea decoctions are stronger teas, usually using roots, berries, medicinal mushrooms, and barks that require longer steeping time, and sometimes gentle simmering, as well. To make a tea decoction, bring herbs to a boil and simmer gently for 20 minutes. Strain what you will drink. This tea is great as it can be reheated and more medicinal properties will come out of your ingredients!

As time has passed, I've added a few more jars to my collection that I use for times like the new and full moon, as well as more specific teas for times of need such as colds and, in particular, tonics. Please know that I too have been, and continue to be, in process, but I'd rather give you a lot of recipes from which you can choose and build your own foundation according to your current needs.

If you don't have the time to prep the loose-leaf teas, I strongly encourage you to seek pre-mixed loose-leaf teas that are beneficial to the different systems, and enjoy the benefits of drinking the plant wisdom. Here in Canada, my friends Simon and Ellery offer a great variety of loose-leaf teas through their business www.simonsteeps.com. We always have options.

The following recipes can be steeped as short infusions, overnight infusions or decoctions, unless otherwise noted.

. . . .

Day: Sunday

1st Chakra: Root Chakra
Location: Base of the spine, perineum
Element: Earth
Glands: Adrenals
Other body parts: Legs, feet, bones, large intestine
Relates to: Safety, survival, security, and stability. Self-preservation. Will to live.

When imbalanced: Issues with the legs, feet, bones, rectum, and immunity. Feeling all over the place, feeling anger or even depression. Living on survival mode, eating disorders.

Sunday Bone Density Tea Recipe

- Equal parts horsetail, oat straw, stinging nettle, red clover, alfalfa, hyssop, violet leaf, raspberry leaf, and comfrey leaf.

Sunday Deep Nourishment Tea Recipe

- Equal parts nettle leaf, raspberry leaf, red clover blossoms, alfalfa leaf, and horsetail

Sunday Root Chakra Tea Recipe

- 1 tbsp raspberry leaf
- 1 tsp ginger root
- 1 tsp dandelion root
- 1 tsp red clover
- 1 ½ tsp elderberries
- pinch valerian root

....

Day: Monday

2nd Chakra: Sacral Chakra
Location: Sacrum
Element: Water
Glands: Gonads
Other body parts: Womb, genitals, kidney, bladder, low back
Relates to: Emotions and sexual energy.

When imbalanced: Urinary tract infections, eating disorders, reproductive imbalances.

Monday Reproductive System Tea Recipe:

- Equal parts rose buds and raspberry leaf

Monday Kidney Tonic Tea Recipe:

- Equal parts parsley root and hydrangea root. Simmer for 10 min. Strain. Drink.

Monday Urinary System Tea Recipe:

- 2 tbsp each dried dandelion leaves, calendula flowers, and yarrow
- 1 tbsp dried marshmallow root

Monday Sacral Chakra Tea Recipe:

- Equal parts calendula flowers and hibiscus tea

. . . .

Day: Tuesday

3rd Chakra: Solar Plexus Chakra
Location: Solar plexus
Element: Fire
Glands: Adrenals, pancreas
Other body parts: Digestive system, liver, gallbladder
Relates to: Personal power, will and self-esteem.

When imbalanced: Person may feel depressed, anxious, and low self-esteem. Issues in the liver, kidneys, or digestive system.

Ayurvedic Digestive CCF Tea Recipe:

- Equal parts coriander seed, cumin seed, and fennel seed

Note: This is a great recipe to drink a cup of every day.

Tuesday Digestive Tea Recipe:

- Equal parts catnip, spearmint, lemongrass, calendula, skullcap, rosemary, sage, and fennel seed

Tuesday Solar Plexus Chakra Tea Recipe:

- Equal parts rosemary, fennel root, cinnamon tea
- Equal parts lemon, ginger tea
- Equal parts lemon, ginger, turmeric tea
- Equal parts lemon, ginger, fennel tea
- Equal parts lemon balm tea
- Equal parts lemon balm, mint tea
- Mint tea

Day: Wednesday

4th Chakra: Heart Chakra
Location: Sternum
Element: Air
Glands: Thymus
Other body parts: Heart, lungs, circulatory system, arms, hands
Relates to: Expression of love, forgiveness, and compassion.

When imbalanced: Feeling disconnected from others, issues with loving others or yourself, poor circulation, lack of motivation, lack of empathy, and inability to heal.

Wednesday Lymph-Moving Tea Recipe

- 4 parts cleavers
- 2 parts red clover
- 1 part ginger
- ½ part calendula flower

Wednesday Heart Tonic Tea Recipe

- 2 parts each of hawthorn flowers or berries, peppermint, ginkgo leaves
- 1 part motherwort leaves
- ¼ part yarrow leaves

Wednesday Heart Chakra Tea Recipe

- Hawthorn berry tea
- Tulsi (holi basil) tea
- Nettle tea
- Green tea

. . . .

Day: Thursday

5th Chakra: Throat Chakra
Location: Throat
Element: Sound (a quality of Ether)
Glands: Thyroid, parathyroid glands
Other body parts: Throat, ears, mouth, shoulders, neck
Relates to: Self-expression, speech, communication and creativity.

When imbalanced: Inability to speak one's truth or thoughts, lack of confidence, codependency, and issues with thyroid.

Thursday Thyroid Tea Recipe

- 2 parts gotu kola
- 1 part red clover blossoms
- 1/5 part liquorice root

Thursday Healthy Hormones Tea Recipe

- 2 parts each of nettle, red raspberry leaf, chamomile, lemon balm, and oat straw
- 1 part lavender

Thursday Throat Chakra Tea

- Equal parts rosemary, thyme, sage

. . . .

Day: Friday

6th Chakra: Third Eye Chakra
Location: Brow
Element: Light (associated with Ether)
Glands: Pituitary gland
Other body parts: Eyes, brow, base of skull
Relates to: Intuition, clairvoyance, imagination and seat of consciousness, the pineal gland.

When imbalanced: Issues with lack of imagination, inability to connect with our intuition, weakness in the ears and eyes, migraines, insomnia, and nightmares.

Friday Visionary Tea Recipe

- 1-3 tsp of Mugwort leafs per cup of water. Infusion.

Note: Caution should be observed when consuming large amounts of mugwort tea or drinking it over a prolonged period, due to its content of thujone,[14] which can be toxic at high doses. So enjoy it, but don't drink it daily.

Friday Ancient Wisdom Tea Recipe

- Equal parts white pine, sweetgrass, and sage

Friday Third Eye Chakra Tea Recipe

- 1-2 tsp of Blue Lotus flower per 1 cup of water. Infusion.

. . . .

Day: Saturday

7th Chakra: Crown Chakra
Location: Top of the head
Element: Thought (in relationship with Ether, the sacred space that contains all thought)
Glands: Pineal gland
Other body parts: Central Nervous System, cerebral cortex
Relates to: Knowledge, personal connection to the universal or source. Responsible for wisdom and enlightenment.

When imbalanced: Feeling disconnected spiritually, lack of purpose and direction, nervous system disorders, migraines, learning disabilities, and mental illnesses.

---

14   "Thujone is a fragrant, oily substance, naturally found in a variety of common plants and flowers. Thujone is perhaps best known in connection with absinthe, the drink that inspired a generation of nineteenth-century artists, writers and thinkers." "Thujone," Absinthe Fever (2006). Retrieved from: https://www.absinthefever.com/thujone

Nervous System Tea Recipe

- 1 part milky oat tops
- 1 part nettle leaf
- 1 part lemon balm leaf
- 1 part ashwagandha root
- ½ part rose hips
- ½ part lavender flowers

Happy Day Tea Recipe

- 3 parts lemon balm
- 2 parts chamomile flowers
- 2 parts nettle leaf
- 2 parts eleuthero (Siberian ginseng) root
- 1 part St. John's wort
- 1 part oatstraw

Saturday Crown Chakra Tea Recipe

- Equal parts gotu kola, tulsi, american ginseng, lavender

OTHER MOON MAGIC AND WELLNESS WARRIOR ELIXIRS:

New Moon Nourishing Herbal Tea

- Equal parts calendula flowers, red clover, skullcap, chamomile flowers, lavender flowers, lemon balm, catnip, oatstraw, lemon peel

My method is to mix equal parts of these herbs (except the lemon peel) into a large jar and label it New Moon Nourishing Herbal Tea. Then it's always at hand. I add the lemon peel fresh when I'm steeping the tea.

Bring your water to boil. Add ingredients. Let it infuse for about 5 minutes. Drink up. Feel the magic!

Drink on the new moon, or during days before and after.

Magical Full Moon Herbal Tea

- 2 bags organic tulsi and rose tea, or 2 tbsp loose-leaf tulsi tea and 1 tbsp rose petals
- 1/2 tsp true cinnamon chips or cinnamon powder
- 1/2 tsp hibiscus flower
- 1 cardamom pod
- ½ tsp ground ginger root

Bring your water to boil. Add ingredients. Let it infuse for about 5 minutes. Drink up.

Feel the magic!

Ginger Goji Berry Chaga Tea

- 2 inches fresh ginger, sliced
- 2 inches fresh turmeric, sliced
- 2 tbsp goji berries
- 2 tbsp chaga mushroom powder or chunks
- 8 cups water
- sweetener of choice, optional

Bring to a boil and simmer gently for 20 minutes. Strain what you will drink. This tea is great as it can be reheated and more medicinal properties will come out of your ingredients! Goji berries and chaga mushrooms can be reused for multiple brews.

Ancient Wisdom Tea

- 1 tbsp pau d'arco bark (antiviral, anti-*Candida*)
- 1 tbsp cat's claw bark (antiviral, anti-*Candida*)
- 2 tbsp reishi mushrooms (or 2 dried strips)
- 1 tbsp chaga mushroom powder or chunks
- 1 tbsp horsetail
- 2 tbsp goji berries
- 1 tbsp red ginseng
- 8 cups water
- 1 tbsp ginger root, dried and ground (optional)

- 1 tbsp cinnamon (optional)
- ½ nutmeg nut, grated or ground nutmeg (optional)

Cover all ingredients with water. Bring to a boil. Lower temperature and allow to simmer for at least 20 minutes. Allow to cool down a bit. I reuse this recipe all week long; just keep adding water to the mix as you drink the tea, then re-boil. And keep on drinking! Enjoy it on its own, or add a little raw honey, allow to cool down completely, and give your kids the best-ever iced tea!

Lover's Chai Tea

- 4 cups nut mylk of your choice (see page 155), made with warm/boiled water
- 1 inch fresh or 1 tbsp ground ginger
- 2 tsp ground cinnamon
- ¼ tsp nutmeg
- ½ tsp cardamom
- ¼ tsp cloves
- ¼ tsp black pepper or 4 black peppercorns
- 1 tsp raw vanilla powder

This wonderful chai recipe can be made on the stove or in your high-speed blender. Combine mylk and the rest of ingredients in a pot. Bring to a boil, then simmer for 10 minutes. Strain. Delight in its healing aroma, or place all ingredients in a blender and blend on high for 1 minute. Strain. Drink up.

THE ULTIMATE ELIXIRS: BREWS

The art of making elixirs is complete herbal synergy at play. I love learning about natural allies, and how we can maximize the benefits of their friendship. They are immunity builders, and build a reservoir of vitality in our body.

To Make:

Combine your tea infusion or decoction with power foods and other herbal superpowers in the form of powders, seeds, berries, and bee pollen, and sip up. They can be combined in the pot or blender, depending on the recipe.

Mayan Heart Power

- 3 cups warm/hot Ancient Wisdom Tea (recipe page 175)
- 2 tbsp sweetener of choice
- 2 tbsp unrefined coconut oil, or splash of nut mylk of choice
- 1 tbsp raw cacao powder
- 2 tsp–1 tbsp maca powder
- 2 tsp–1 tbsp lucuma powder
- 2 tsp–1 tbsp mesquite powder
- 1 tsp goji berries
- 1 tsp bee pollen
- pinch cayenne

Blend all ingredients together and share it!

Aloe Cool Power

- 2 inch inner filet of aloe plant, or use ½ cup inner leaf aloe juice
- 1½ cups of water (room temperature)
- 2 tbsp of fresh lemon juice
- 1 tbsp chopped mint
- 1 tsp chia seeds
- 1 tbsp raw honey (optional)

Burdock Shilajit Latte

- 1 cup burdock root tea (1-2 tbsp of cut and sifted burdock root + 3 cups of water. Simmer for 30 min. Turn stove off, and let it sit for another 20 min. or make the night before.)
- 1/8 tsp Shilajit powder or a nip spoon (250mg) Pure Himalayan Shilajit Signature Blend (www.purehimalayanshilajit.com/?ref=401)
- 1 cup hot almond mylk (see page 155)
- 1 tbsp maple syrup

Ashwagandha Sleep Tonic

- 1 cup + 2 tbsp hot water
- 2 heaping tbsp macadamia nuts (or soaked almonds)

- 1 medjool date or 1 tsp raw honey
- ¼–½ tsp cinnamon powder
- ¼ tsp nutmeg powder
- ¼ tsp clove powder
- ½ tsp vanilla powder or ⅓–½ vanilla bean
- ½ tsp ashwagandha root powder
- pinch sea salt

BROTH RECIPES

Some people really enjoy having broths during their feasts. I must say I am not one of them, but on cold days you might just find me making one batch!

Preparation for either recipe: Place all the ingredients in a pot and bring to a gentle boil. Reduce heat to low and simmer for about an hour. Strain and sip for a mineral-rich, healing and restorative broth.

Healing Broth, by Anthony Williams[15]

- 4 carrots, chopped, or 1 sweet potato, cubed
- 2 stalks celery, roughly chopped
- 2 onions, sliced
- 1 cup parsley, finely chopped
- 1 cup of shiitake mushrooms, fresh or dried (optional)
- 2 tomatoes, chopped (optional)
- 1 bulb garlic (about 6–8 cloves), minced
- 1 inch fresh ginger root
- 1 inch fresh turmeric root
- 8 cups water

Vegan Gut Healing Broth

- 12 cups (2¾ L) filtered water
- 1 red onion, quartered (with skins)
- 1 garlic bulb, smashed
- 1 thumb-sized piece ginger, roughly chopped (with skin)

---

15   Anthony William, "Healing Broth," Medical Medium (2016). Retrieved from: http://www.medicalmedium.com/blog/healing-broth

- 1 cup greens, such as kale or spinach
- 3–4 cups mixed chopped vegetables and peelings (I used carrot peelings, red cabbage, fresh mushrooms, leeks, and celery)
- ½ cup dried shiitake mushrooms
- 30 g dried wakame seaweed
- 1 tbsp peppercorns
- 2 tbsp ground turmeric

RAW CRACKERS RECIPES

You've got that new juicer going, and now what are you gonna do with all that pulp? I know you've been asking yourself that question throughout these pages.

PULP CRACKERS. PULP COOKIES. PULP WAFERS. PULP SOUP STOCK. PULP YOU NAME IT.
PULP = Potentially Unlimited Loving Power

The following are pulp cracker recipes for your delight. Your imagination is the limit.

Savoury Pulp Crackers

- 2 heaping cups of juice pulp
- 1 heaping tbsp chia seeds
- ½ cup flax meal or flaxseeds
- 3 tbsp tamari or coconut aminos
- 1 tsp dried chopped parsley
- ½ tsp turmeric
- 1 tsp dried chopped oregano
- black pepper, to taste
- ¼ cup water

Blend all ingredients except water in a food processor. Add just enough water to the mix to create a dough-like consistency that isn't too watery.

Dehydrator: Roll out mixture onto one or two sheets and spread evenly. Cut into squares with a knife. Dehydrate at 118F for 4 hrs, flip, then dehydrate for another 4 hours or until crispy.

Oven:

Option 1: Preheat oven to 320F. Thinly spread the mixture on a parchment-paper-lined baking sheet. Cut into squares. Place in the oven and bake 40–50min. Flip half way.

Option 2: Preheat oven to its lowest temperature (150F or 170F). This option will minimize nutrient and enzyme loss. Thinly spread the mixture on a parchment-paper-lined baking sheet. Cut into squares. Place in the oven and bake 1 hour. Flip. Bake for another hour or until crackers are crisp, checking every ½ hour, or turn the oven off after 2 hours, don't open the oven door, and leave the crackers in the oven overnight to crisp up.

Store the crackers in an airtight container.

Mexican Flare

- 1 cup celery and carrot veggie pulp left over from juicing
- 1 cup golden flaxseeds
- ½ cup chia seeds
- ½ cup raw sunflower seeds
- ½ cup raw pumpkin seeds
- ¼ yellow onion, diced
- ¼ red pepper, diced
- 1 small garlic clove
- 1½ tsp chipotle powder
- 1 tsp sea salt
- ½ tsp cayenne pepper

Place flax, chia, sunflower seeds, and pumpkin seeds in separate bowls. Fill each bowl with just enough water to cover the seeds, and soak for 6 hours or overnight.

Place onion, red pepper, and garlic in food processor. Process well.

Drain sunflower and pumpkin seeds and place in a large bowl. Add flax and chia gel. Add the rest of the ingredients. Mix well.

Dehydrator: Scoop 2 cups of mix per dehydrator tray, lined with a non-stick dehydrator sheet. Spread thinly. Score into squares. Dehydrate at 115F for 6 hours. Peel, flip crackers onto mesh screens. Dehydrate again for 6 hours or until crispy.

Oven: Follow above oven instructions for making pulp crackers.

Note: Dehydrating time will vary with each batch as there are many factors at play: how much moisture is in your vegetable pulp, how efficient your food dehydrator is, how low your oven will go, and how humid the air is where you live, to name just a few. So please stay curious, play, exercise your patience, take some notes, and next time you make them you will be a pro!

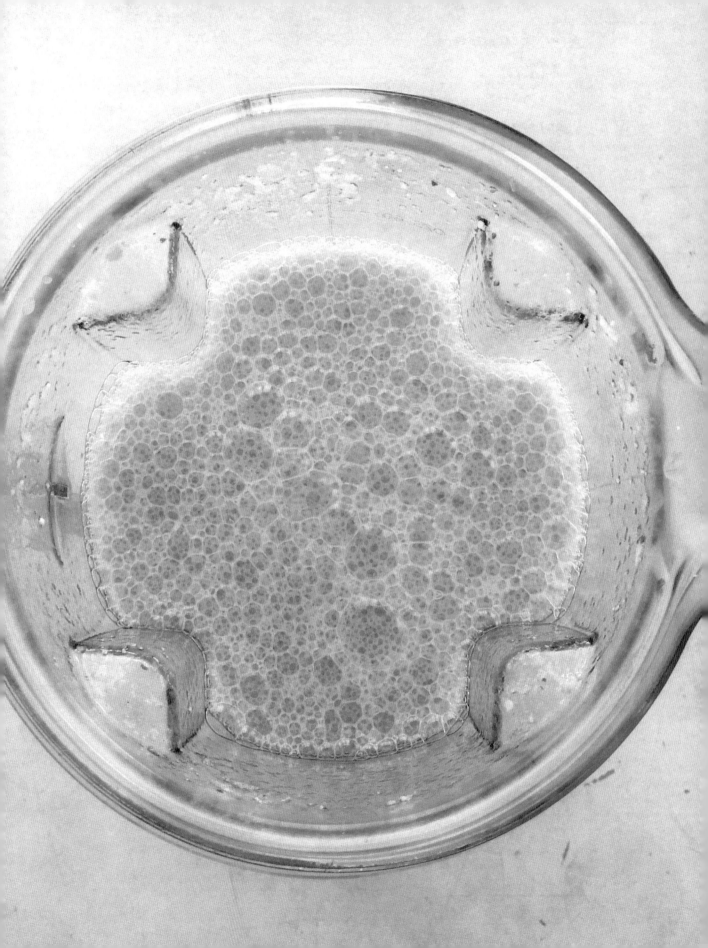

V

THE RITUAL OF DETOX

IT IS NEVER TOO LATE TO BE WHAT YOU MIGHT
HAVE BEEN.

-GEORGE ELLIOT

THE RITUAL OF DETOX

Everyone can perform magic, everyone can reach his goals, if he is able to think, if he is able to wait, if he is able to fast.

—*Hermann Hesse, Siddhartha*

All spiritual paths hold rituals for detoxification of the body temple to bring coherence back into the body, and to bring coherent and congruent thought and action into our lives. In our modern secular world, we have lost touch with the art of the ritual of detox to bring us back to the inner space of source, home, and reconnection with self and with that which is beyond the self.

Over the last couple of centuries, the ancient lineages that understood the need for these practices were greatly affected by occupation, war, and displacement. These lineages also understood that we live in relationship with—not ownership of—the ALL, with our self, with one another, with the earth and with spirit.

In our efforts at being and living "in relationship," we begin to reclaim ourselves, our roots, our heritage, and our need to be on the spiritual path. We begin to reconnect with and remember the wisdom of the ancient ones. We begin to remember the power of ritual to anchor our lives into sacredness and the need for the ritual of detox as a practice for deep healing.

Every fibre of your being is made of ritual, and it is through ritual that you can re-embody every fibre of your being.

We begin to remember the ritual of detox is more than just the detox of our physical bodies; it is a detox of our emotional and mental bodies as we begin to deeply nourish our souls, gain support for our emotional and mental clarity, reconnect with practices of self-care and daily rituals for health, connect deeply with the space of radiant health, reclaiming our health and therefore our wholeness through our process.

Our bodies will only detoxify in as much as they are being nourished. As we begin to heal the fragmented pieces of our selves, we reclaim our power and wholeness. The veil of our disconnection then begins to lift as we embrace our healing journey, our bodies begin to trust us again, and we deepen our connection to the inner space of sacredness within our hearts.

Like any other habit, the ritual of detox must be created and instilled with *Blisscipline!* Yes! Even the tools and practices with the potential of opening your inner doors of perception towards bliss need to be carved into your very being with discipline. It's a great muscle to develop; it allows you to access your will and your resilience, and it will serve you well on those days halfway through a detox when you must find your resolve to persevere, where you must engage in battle with your demons and the deepest of your shadows, and surrender to their teachings, as you become aware of your power to choose to no longer need to be defined by "your story."

The ritual of detox enables us to build our foundation with consciousness, brings great coherence into our lives, leads us to act with awareness and authenticity, and facilitates our engagement with the world from a place of peace, trust, unity, and love—both for self, and others.

TO JUICE FAST OR FEAST? THAT IS THE QUESTION

What the eyes are for the outer world, fasts are for the inner.

—Ghandi

The art of juice fasting is the action of only drinking freshly made juices for one or more days in a row to allow your digestive system to rest, thus allowing your body to use this now-available energy to detoxify, repair, rebuild, rejuvenate, and regenerate itself. During a fast, you usually consume a limited number of juices (between four and five) that contain all you need to thrive, yet because you are totally infusing your body with this magical liquid source of nutrition, it has a more detoxifying effect on your body. You may also feel more tired, and feel a deeper need to slow down in all aspects of your life.

The art of juice feasting is the action of juicing for one or more days in a row, just like during a juice fast. The difference is you are infusing your body with larger amounts of nutrient-dense fresh raw living juice. I will usually drink up to 3 litres of fresh raw living juice, 5 ounces of wheatgrass diluted in 1 litre of water, 1 litre of deluxe detox lemonade (find recipe on page 164), and tea infusions each day of my feast.

There is a lot going in, and a lot flushing out, but I don't feel as tired as I otherwise might. I find I am better able to cope with my worldly responsibilities, while still facilitating the cleansing action of a juice fast. Although I still recommend you slow down and support yourself through this time, for those of us who must continue to engage with the world, this might be a better option. We are all different, and you must respect and get to know your body, and support your journey at the moment.

The digestive process is one of our body's most energy consuming processes, so when you juice fast or feast, because your nutrition and sustenance are coming into you through a liquid form, your body is able to take the much-needed digestive break, and overall physical rest. Juicing can be done one day per week, or for three days, seven days, ten days, or really as many days as you wish.

It's always a good idea to juice fast one day per week, or once per month—perhaps with the change of seasons, on new and full moons, and/or with the solstices and equinoxes—to allow your body an opportunity to rest, to slowly detox, rebuild, and rejuvenate in alignment with the earthly rhythms. I see it as insurance, prevention, and the opportunity to recalibrate my heart compass seasonally. I am sure you've heard these words before: ***Prevention is really the only true cure.***

This day is like pressing the reset button on your phone and allowing it to restore and clear any corruption in its code. It is an opportunity to pause, feel, and reset as you ignite your Mighty inner healer, restore, and heal. Juice fasting or feasting allows you to re-centre yourself, to ground, focus, and reconnect with your true self, reconnect with your intuition, and build a more solid foundation. The process of juice fasting or feasting is one of coring in, of rooting down in order to rise anew.

Juice fasting or feasting also allows you and I to make sense of our world, with some "processing and integration" time and inquiry time, and then return to our lives with more balance, *oomph*, energy, passion, trust, and belief in our own abilities to make our dreams happen.

If you are new to the idea of a juice fast or feast and it simply sounds just too far-out for you right now, not to worry; start by adding juices to your daily life. Create and integrate the new juicing habit first into your life, and soon enough you'll find yourself ready. Your body will guide you, trust your intuition.

It is a good idea to also consider slowing down your everyday busyness, turning off your electronic devices or using them less, and becoming aware of your everyday wear and tear when you are choosing to do a juice fast or feast. For some it is possible to fully slow down. But for most of us it's not that simple. But wouldn't you want to disconnect from all your earthly responsibilities and greet heaven on earth at its door step for a day or two?

Can you think of a way you can slow down your life, as you gift yourself with a juice fast or feast?

When you juice fast or feast, you also begin the process of quieting your mind, of connecting in greater clarity with your heart, and so begin to hear your truth. You can also begin to recognize those places within you where you still hold onto your traumas and your emotional wounds. It is a completely normal experience to re-visit some of these places within as you quiet down and reconnect. So please find compassion for yourself and those who may have hurt you or whom you may have hurt, and create your sacred space where you can process and release all that no longer serves you, be it physical, emotional, mental, or spiritual.

Get out your journal, write those density releasing letters that no one else will read—but the writing of them allows that stuck energy to free itself. Then afterward, burn them (safely) in a small ritual of compassion and forgiveness. (More on the Hucha Ceremony on page 307.) Give yourself the space and the time to dive in and create room for the dream you want to build. Clean house. Reach out if you need to. Recalibrate. Trust. Accept. It is the death of that which no longer serves you, in order to reclaim your self alive. It is what in shamanism is called dying while still being alive, or the dark night of the soul; it is a necessary process in your revolution.

SMOOTHIE CLEANSE

You're in pretty good shape for the shape you are in.

—*Dr. Seuss*

A smoothie cleanse is the ritual of committing to drinking smoothies—green, purple, polka dotted if you wish, during a specified amount of time. It could be for a day, a week, twenty-one days, a month, and so on.

A *smoothie cleanse* is a similar process to doing a juice fast or feast in that you are committing to nourishing your body with liquid nutrition, but because the fibre is still present in the smoothies, your digestive system does not fully go to rest in the same way it does during a juice fast or feast.

A smoothie cleanse also has the power to rebuild your system because, along with the fibre, you are putting in a vast amount of nutrient dense food for which, once the fibre has done its job, your cells will be extremely thankful.

You will feel fuller during a smoothie cleanse; you will feel more grounded just because of the thickness of the liquid powers you are consuming. You will feel a deep sense of satisfaction and deep nourishment from the nutrients now within the boundaries of your body. You will feel their cleansing action as well, and that might just send you to the loo for a few extra trips, which is a great thing. You want to move all that toxicity out! It will still provide you with physical, mental, emotional and spiritual clarity, and connect you to the life-force energy in all.

One easy way to build up both your immunity *and* your bodily reserves is to include wild edible foods into your smoothies, in particular when doing a smoothie cleanse. Always remember the power of synergy and alchemy. Use them, they will be glad to help. Some wild edible plants you can include into your smoothies are: dandelion (leaves and flowers), wild spinach or lamb's quarters, purslane, chicory (leaves and flowers), clover, malva, miner's lettuce, plantain, sorrel, and wild strawberry leaves. There are many books available about wild edible greens for you to dive into.

You can also add tea infusions made from our wild edible friends as the liquid part of your smoothie, or simply drink tea infusions while you are doing a smoothie cleanse.

In my experience, doing a smoothie cleanse differs from a juice fast or feast in the subtle experience of the energy and the mental body. There is (for me) a subtle difference of experience in the quality of my quietness, and in the quality and depth of my meditation and movement practices. But as with juicing, when we drink smoothies, we begin or perhaps accelerate the process of deeper alignment that is an aspect of our Mighty revolution.

FOUNDATIONS FOR A SUCCESSFUL DETOX

Discovery consists of seeing what everybody has seen and thinking what nobody has thought.

—*Albert Szent-Györgyi*

Whether you choose to do a juice fast or feast or a smoothie cleanse, or choose to combine all liquid nutrition into a Mighty detox, here are a few key steps that will help create a stronger foundation for your journey.

Plan for success. First make a feast plan and map, and then stick with it. Food planning has its place in your busy life. Plan and map your detox so you feel supported along your process. You may of course switch recipes around to serve the taste you desire, but get organized and plan and map your days ahead. Invest the time to build your food shopping guide or download mine from: www.natyhoward.com/food-shopping-list

Clear your schedule. You got it. Clear your schedule as much as possible to create space for deep healing. Ask for support around you, if you need to get your kids to here and there and everywhere. Choose a time that you can turn into "quiet time," one that will support your process. Feasting on the busiest weeks of your personal schedule will only add more stress to the equation.

Speak your intentions out loud. Speaking your intentions is a two-step process. First you must slow down enough to listen to your heart and create your personal intentions for doing a feast. Write them down. Don't think this is just a fluffy new age concept. It's not. This is a key step in your process, for your intentions begin to recalibrate your heart. Once you have written them down, speak them out loud. When you speak your intentions aloud, all aspects of your being get on board with the plan. Your intentions will help keep you true, and support you on those days that may be difficult. They will anchor your journey and provide you with resilience.

When you speak your intentions out loud to others, it allows them to know where you're at. They will know that for the next three days while you are detoxifying, you might be grumpy, emotional, and not as available to them. They will understand that you might actually need them to fill in for you for those few days, while you take care of yourself. And … they might just be so inspired by your commitment to your own revolution they may choose to join you.

Focus on adding in recipes, veggies, and fruits that inspire you and build you up. When we focus on adding in, the habits and foods that do not support our process will naturally fade away. But if we focus on what we are missing, on what we are denying ourselves and not having now, we will be miserable. So do your best to focus on the positive, on the new recipes and actions you are taking that are going to build a new state of wellness for yourself.

Make synergy your BFF. Through this book I have spoken of and will continue to speak of other practices you can begin to add synergy to your detox. Please remember to consciously move your body (a walk in nature or do gentle yoga), to anchor your mind (with meditation and deep breathing exercises), and to look within as you are able, to best serve your process. Please remember to align your detox with your lifestyle and the seasons.

LEVELS OF DETOX

We are what we repeatedly do.

—Aristotle

As I guide people through their journey in doing a detox, I come across people at all different levels of their journey. Some have never done a liquid detox before, some have never had a fresh pressed juice before, but they're heard the call and they're ready. For some, liquid nutrition is already a part of their life: juicing daily, consuming smoothies, elixirs and liquid delights are part of their every day.

Through leading the *Mighty detox online program,* I have found that everyone is unique and dealing with a unique set of life circumstances. You may have already been juicing, you may have been smoothing, or perhaps you are new to the whole adventure and may only have a blender at hand!

To assist you along your process of *becoming,* I've created a guide to levels of detox. Please know that each person is *unique*, and no level is better than the other. It's all a process of evolution, and being honest is key in determining if you should be doing a juice feast, a smoothie cleanse or all of the above — and for how long.

You may be fortunate enough to be able to take time off work and dive in deep. Or, you may have the opportunity to continue to work through the detox, and find ways to stay supported and grounded during the process.

Stay clear on the intention you made prior to beginning your detox, and commit to *staying true to it*. You might currently only have access to a blender, but go ahead with your detox and blend away! Speak your intention out loud to yourself, a*nd stay true to it. The universe is watching for your highest self to become your true expression.*

Beware, Beware! Your old Self (Ego) will trick you. You might, just might, develop cravings, thoughts, emotions and behaviours that send you for a loop. Breathe into it. You are transforming, and shedding your old skin. Know that as you detox— as you cleanse, as you get hungry, as you begin and continue to release your physical/emotional/ mental/ heart/ and spiritual blockages—you **will** be challenged. But also know this: you **are** being supported by your higher self, the unseen world holds your heart—and most importantly know that you do have the power to do it. Don't give in or give up. I fully trust in your mightiness to **do** this, to answer the call of recalibrating of your heart compass, and release some of the blockages that have been keeping you bound.

THE THREE LEVELS OF DETOX

Level 1: Level I consists of drinking water followed by celery juice, lemonade detox in the early morning, smoothies, raw soups, and tea infusions for mid-morning, lunch, afternoon, and evening, and perhaps a few fresh pressed juices. This level of detox is for those of you who are perhaps new to the whole concept of liquid nutrition altogether, are new to detox, only have access to a blender at this time, or for whom life is simply too busy.

In Level 1 we are consuming liquid nutrition with fibre in it to begin the process of *brooming*—of stirring and cleansing our digestive track with fibre power!

. . . .

Level 2: Level 2 strives to include more fresh pressed juices than smoothies or raw soups. It also includes elixirs, and begins the process of including more superfoods, super herbs that take the detox to another level and assist in further upgrading your operating system. They allow you and I to address with more awareness our unique physical-emotional-mental-heart-spiritual blockages, as all food, superfoods, and super herbs have subtle energetic qualities we can use to our advantage.

In Level 2 we strive to consume liquid nutrition with less fibre in it, moving towards more fresh pressed juices than smoothies and raw soups, but still including both. We begin to add some superfoods like seaweed powders, goji berries, and bee pollen to our liquid nutrition. Be sure to include celery juice to start your day, and to help maintain mineral balance throughout your day, have a celery, cucumber, apple juice blend after midday.

Note: Some of the recipes for elixirs I've included here may need more ingredients than you have at this time. No worries. Perhaps there's one elixir recipe calling your name, for which you can invest in the ingredients (in particular the superfoods). Yes, this is an investment because once you buy them you will have them for a while, as you continue to build up your pantry of nutrient dense superfoods and functional foods to serve your liquid nutrition revolution!

. . . .

Level 3: Level 3 consists of mainly water, celery juice, morning lemonade detox, fresh pressed juices, and tea infusions (fibre-less elixirs). Here we are using superfoods and super herbs in our liquid nutrition.

In Level 3 we strive to consume fibre-less liquid nutrition and no fats (no nuts, nut mylks, or elixirs made with nut butters). By doing so, we are able to fully shut down our digestive system, completely freeing the energy normally used for digestion to be available now to detox, repair, rebuild, regenerate, and rejuvenate our body at deeper levels. Have a juice made out of celery, cucumber, apple in the afternoon to continue to support your mineral balance.

Note: Drinking water to start your day and during the day is key to continuing to flush your system and dilute the toxicity being released through your feast. You want to be urinating often, as in hourly. If your urine is cloudy and dark, support your detoxification process by drinking more water. You want your urine to be light; this way you know your kidneys are not being taxed nor overwhelmed by the process, and you will also know that the toxicity is not sitting on your kidneys.

Dear Mighty healer, as with any great leap you're about to take, it's good—perhaps wise—to see it as a transition rather than an end onto itself. If you are going to detox for three or more days, it's important to transition yourself into and out of your detox to best support your body. Transitioning into it with plant-based foods and then raw foods as you begin will support your inner organs and your mind, and get you ready for your process. At the end, it works well to break your detox with a raw plant-based meal (no oils), followed by heavier plant-based meals until you finally reintegrate yourself into your normal diet.

Are you interested in doing a detox together?

Well, the universe has conspired and you are at the right place at the right time. How amazing is that? You might just find the guidance, support, and empowerment you are seeking through my online program Mighty Detox. It is an opportunity to reclaim your strength, your health, and your radiance as you detox with me, as I guide you through the power of liquid nutrition, the ritual of detox, the art of mindfulness practices and the alchemy of inner questing. This book actually started as the manual for this program. Full details are available at www.natyhoward.com.

1 DAY MIGHTY DETOX

This is a one day Mighty detox for you, broken down by level. You have everything you need to do it. You got this. Always allow at least 30 minutes in between consuming your liquid golds.

	Level 1	Level 2	Level 3
Upon arising	Morning Liver Tonic (one cup) (recipe page 163)	Morning Liver Tonic (one cup) (recipe page 163)	Morning Liver Tonic (one cup) (recipe page 163)
Early morning	Water 1 L Celery juice, 16 to 32 oz. (recipe page 137)	Water 1 L Celery juice, 16 to 32 oz. (recipe page 137)	Water 1 L Celery juice, 16 to 32 oz. (recipe page 137)

	Level 1	Level 2	Level 3
Mid-morning snack: wheatgrass! **(if needed, but best to try and wait until early lunch)**	Deluxe Detox Lemonade (recipe page 164) or 1 to 2 oz wheatgrass as a shot or in water. (Optional) Sweet/ green smoothie (1 serving up to 1 L) (recipes page 145)	Deluxe Detox Lemonade (recipe page 164) or 1 to 2 oz wheatgrass as a shot or in water. (Optional) Sweet/ green smoothie (recipes page 145) or fresh pressed sweet or green juice (recipes page 137) (1 serving up to 1 L)	Deluxe Detox Lemonade (recipe page 164) or 1 to 2 oz wheatgrass as a shot or in water. (Optional) Fresh pressed sweet or green juice (recipes page 137) (1 serving up to 1 L)
Lunch	Smoothie (recipes page 145), Savoury Raw Soup (recipes page 150), or fresh pressed juice (recipes page 137) 1 L	Fresh pressed juice (recipes page 137) 1 L	Fresh pressed juice (recipes page 137) 1 L
Afternoon	Tea infusion (recipes page 167)	Warm tea infusion or elixir (nut free) (recipes pg. 167)/ Wellness shots (recipes pg. 143)	Warm tea infusion or elixir (nut free) (recipes pg. 167)/ Wellness shots (recipes pg. 143)
Early evening	Savoury Raw Soup. Sit down and enjoy them as a meal (recipes page 150) 1 L	Savoury Raw Soup. Sit down and enjoy them as a meal (recipes page 150) 1 L	Fresh pressed green juice (recipes page 137) 1 L
Evening (after sunset)	Warm tea infusion with nut/seed mylk (spiced) (recipes page 176)	Warm tea infusion or elixir with nut/ seed mylk (spiced) (recipes page 176)	Warm tea infusion (nut / mylk free) (recipes page 167)
Personal notes	An additional 1 L of water (spring water is best) should be drunk during the day	An additional 1 L of water (spring water is best) should be drunk during the day	An additional 1 L of water (spring water is best) should be drunk during the day

7 TOOLS TO IGNITE YOUR MIGHTY INNER HEALER

If you're always trying to be normal you will never know how amazing you can be.

—*Maya Angelou*

Along my journey, I've learned that detoxification is an art well worth getting to know. Here are seven tools to ignite your Mighty inner healer, engage in radical self-care, and detox your body.

1. *Dry Skin Brushing*

   Have you tried dry brushing your skin to awaken your lymphatic system? Oh, it just feels so good to brush away; it's the best alarm clock ever. This invigorating practice is great for exfoliation, increases circulation, reduces cellulite, calms the mind, relieves stress, and has the potential of improving digestion and kidney function. Using a specific dry skin brush, you start at your feet and begin brushing in a circular motion all the way up towards your heart. Brush every part of your body, thoroughly and lovingly. Then brush from your hands up to your shoulders, neck, chest, and back towards your heart again, in small circles. It feels like having a massage!

2. *Neti Pot (Nasal Rinse Cup)*

   This ancient Ayurvedic art of rinsing your nasal passages with warm saline solution is done using a Neti Pot. The warm saline solution is easily made with warm water and a teaspoon of sea salt or Himalayan salt. It naturally refreshes cleanses, prevents, protects, and keeps your nasal passages moist, thus enhancing your health. It removes excess mucus naturally. For best results, it should be done daily.

3. *Tongue Scraping*

   Tongue scarping is the ancient Ayurvedic art of scraping your tongue to remove the coating that builds up on it daily, and which is more visible as you detoxify. Your tongue holds within its structure the map of your organ systems, along with vital information about their health and how they are functioning. It is through the tongue, pulse, and constitutional diagnosis that Ayurveda is able to get to the root cause of disease.

Tongue scraping is done in the morning upon rising, before brushing your teeth, and again at night before brushing your teeth to remove any toxicity that has accumulated. It feels like a massage—and it is a massage to your internal organs.

Some benefits of tongue scrapping are: it cleans toxins and bacteria from your mouth, removes any coating on your tongue that may lead to bad breath, enhances your sense of taste, gently stimulates your digestive system and internal organs, and increases your awareness of your state of health. Tongue scrapers are available at most health food stores. For best results, it should be done daily.

4.   *Oil Pulling*

Oil pulling is an ancient Ayurvedic technique of pulling toxins from within your body by swishing one tablespoon of raw sesame oil in your mouth, optimally for twenty minutes, but for a minimum of five. As you do this, draw it through your teeth and "chew" it to mix it with your saliva, and activate the enzymes in the oil that will draw the toxins out. Oil pulling cleanses bacteria, viruses, and toxins, pulling out all uninvited and unwanted guests from within us.

After five to twenty minutes, remove the oil from your mouth. Do not swallow it, as it's become a toxic time bomb. Discard it. Afterwards, make sure to rinse your mouth thoroughly several times with a cup of water to which you've added a ½ teaspoon of sea salt and a ½ teaspoon of baking soda. They will assist in further removing and neutralizing any residual toxicity that may be left in your mouth.

It is also recommended to scrape your tongue and brush your teeth, gums, and tongue using the combination of sea salt and baking soda. Gargle afterwards with the same water/sea salt/baking soda combination.

Some benefits of oil pulling are: it aids your immune system, reduces internal inflammation, detoxifies your body, increases energy, whitens teeth, and promotes oral hygiene—amongst many others. For best results, it should be done daily.

5.   *Sesame Oil Skin Massage (Self-Abhyanga)*

Abhyanga is another wonderful and powerful ancient Ayurvedic art—this time of self-massaging your body with sesame oil. Sesame oil is naturally antibacterial and powerfully healing, often infused with herbs and usually warm. You lovingly massage the oil over your entire body. It provides the feeling of being deeply grounded, stable, supported, comforted, and warm. Sesame oil, in particular, is able to penetrate into your body's deep tissue layers.

Abhyanga benefits the skin, calms the nervous system, nourishes the body, and decreases the effects of aging, thus increasing longevity; it increases circulation and stimulates your internal organs, among others. To do it, first gently warm the oil in a double boiler. Sit or stand in a warm room and, using a small circular motion, begin to lovingly massage your body from the extremities towards your core. Take your time. Massage for five to twenty minutes. Give attention to your joints, scalp, ears, and feet. When you are done, have a warm shower or bath. For best results, this should be done at least once a week.

I like to first dry skin brush and then deeply nourish my body with Abhyanga self-massage at least two times a week. If you are dealing with anxiety, feeling ungrounded, or experiencing any disturbance of the mind, do Abhyanga daily.

6. *Bath Soaks*

Pure delight. Being in warm water sends us back to the primordial cellular memory of being in the womb, safe, protected, and encapsulated by the rich viscosity of life. When we have a warm bath, our body, at the cellular level, is reliving that experience. We may or may not be conscious of it, but our nervous system begins to calm, and our muscles, joints, and whole body begin to relax deeply. Yes, the warm/hot water has a lot to do with it, but there is much more at play when we soak in a warm bath.

A bath soak is a conscious effort on our behalf to detoxify, and deeply nourish our body at the same time. So softly play your favourite tunes, light your candle and/or your incense, and just like we created a sacred meditation space earlier, create your sacred bath soak ritual.

Add 1 cup of Epsom salts to your bath (the great detoxifier), 1 cup of baking soda (the great alkalizer) and ½ cup of sea salt or pink Himalayan salt (the great re-mineralizer). Then add a few drops of essential oil—lavender is one of my favourites.

7. *Colon Hydrotherapy*

Colon hydrotherapy (known as a colonic) is an alternative way to cleanse the toxic residue from the colon and the large intestine, as well as flush the liver. It is also a Mighty tool to assist the body when deeply detoxifying, in order to flush out all that toxicity, and not have it be re-absorbed into the blood stream.

During a colonic session, a disposable proctoscope (nozzle) with tubes attached is inserted gently into the rectum. One of the tubes is connected to a clean water system; the other will carry the fecal matter out and away from your body. Approximately 50 litres of water will pass through your system, flushing the colon and saturating the impacted waste throughout the length of your colon. The water pressure on the colon stimulates it into peristalsis, helping to tone and support a weakened colon. This safe practice has the potential to speed up your recovery into health, as well as release the current levels of toxicity in your body during a detox, or as a regular protocol for longevity every couple of months.

DEEP NOURISHMENT AS RADICAL SELF-CARE

If the foot of the trees were not tied to the earth, they would be pursuing me. For I have blossomed so much, I am the envy of the gardens.

—Rumi

Deep nourishment means truly nourishing your whole-body system from the inside out. It is the art of nourishing your physical body with the whole foods and liquid nutrition that will build, repair, rejuvenate, and regenerate the life-force energy within you. It is the art of nourishing your heart by engaging in heart-filling activities, be it mindfulness, or something you deeply love and find nurturing, and which brings you joy.

Deep nourishment is the art of nourishing the mind; grounding your chatter and elevating your consciousness. It is the art of nourishing your spirit through the art of devotion, through being in relationship with the world around you. It is the art of falling in love with life again; of opening your heart to appreciate the beauty, and allowing life to fill you up again. Deep nourishment is soul food. Deep nourishment is radical self-care.

Igniting your Mighty inner healer will require you to commit to some radical self-care. Today is the day to nourish yourself like never before. Today is the day to love yourself like never before. Claim your sacred womb for healing and reconnection. You might just awaken into your mightiness.

The time of detox is just for ***you***. As you create the space you need to detox, you must also tap into what nourishes you deeply. I know a lot of us find deep nourishment in food, but away from food, what nourishes you deeply? What activities, books, and practices serve you in slowing down, in connecting, in calming your nervous system, and helping you feel rejuvenated?

Some suggestions are: surrounding yourself with your favourite books, practising conscious movement, meditating, walking in nature, listening to talks by inspirational and motivational teachers and speakers, journaling, practising creative expression, engaging in vocal practices such as singing and chanting, keeping warm, or sipping your favourite tea while reading your favourite book might be what nourishes you.

During your detox, I highly encourage you to slow down, to take time away from your social media and electronics. Give yourself the gift of silence. Even if it's only for five or ten minutes. Be by yourself in silence. You could do this as your meditation, or while you walk in nature, or while you have a bath! Notice your senses, and the clarity and sharpening that begins to appear as you spend more time soothed and embraced in and by silence.

A detox is a great time to notice yourself. Take the time to notice the quality of your mind, the quality of your heart, the quality of your breath. Notice what feeds you, supports you, inspires you, and sustains you. Notice how you feel when you radically self-care. Notice how you feel when you deeply nourish yourself. Can you make that depth of nourishment an integral part of your foundation for life?

Also, *notice what is noticing.*

DO YOU, TOO, HOWL AT THE MOON?

Generally speaking, a howling wilderness does not howl: it is the imagination of the traveller that does the howling.

—*Henry David Thoreau*

The moon, with all her beauty, controls the movements of the waters on our planet with her gravitational pull, and has a profound effect on our psyche, and our feelings, emotions, and desires, both conscious and subconscious. Depending on the planetary alignment during new and full moons, there are specific energies at play at these times that greatly influence our behaviours.

The *rhythms of the moon* offer us an opportunity to come into a deeper space of stillness within us. They provide an opportunity to align and anchor into our true nature, as we pause and feel, tap into our heart, and recalibrate with our own rhythms, on a monthly basis.

The *new moon* is a symbolic portal for new beginnings, a time for planting the seeds of that which you want to bring forth into your life and into the world. It's a womb time of time, of darkness and stillness, of slow movement, of self-inquiry, and of dropping deeply within. What is it you wish to bring forth? What kind of physical, mental, emotional, and spiritual seeds are you planting? What kind of radiant health do you want to experience?

The new moon is also a time of deep release and letting go of what is not serving us that has become density in our body systems, by giving them space outside of your body (through the ritual of the Hucha Ceremony, on page 307), so as to create the fertile ground for the conscious seeds we are now planting in our inner garden. Are there habits and behaviours you need to let go of in order to access that deeper space and state of radiant health? What new tools are you developing to upgrade the operating system of your whole body complex?

Can you connect with the subtle energies of the new moon to fine tune the process of recalibrating your heart compass? Can you commit to your vision? Can you open yourself to receiving the guidance, healing, and support from the spirit world that is always near you? New moons are a time to voice your dreams out loud.

The *full moon* is a symbolic portal for completely letting go of the densities (Hucha) that was first seen and given space outside of our bodies in the new moon. The full moon is also a time of taking action and celebrating the growth of your choices. It is a time of "harvesting" that which you planted with the new moon, a time of releasing the dream into the world, of being out in the world, of bold actions, of becoming, of radiance and illumination. As you tune into the moon's cycles, just like the full moon shines her beauty and states her presence, you and I are asked to step into our own light.

The quest for lunar alignment can be enhanced by doing a detox on the days of the new and full moons, for one day, or for a three- or seven-day detox, keeping the actual day of the new or full moon as mid-point of your detox.

ALIGNMENT WITH THE EQUINOXES AND SOLSTICES

In the depth of winter, I finally learned that within me there lay an invincible summer.

—Albert Camus

The equinoxes and solstices mark the movement of the earth around the sun, in a yearly cycle. The equinoxes occur in spring and fall. The solstices occur in summer and winter.

The equinoxes and solstices are energetic solar portals of alignment with the cosmos, and with celestial and earth rhythms. On these days, the portals between worlds are thinnest, allowing you and I greater access to the wisdom beyond the veils of our illusion.

Equinoxes and solstices provide you and me with a point of magnetism in the recalibrating of our heart compass, a deepening of our experience on earth, our connection to the celestial world, our reception of the cosmic forces, and our awareness and expansion of consciousness of our inner sun. The equinoxes and solstices define our seasons and the changes in earth rhythms. They provide the wisdom of when to plant, when to harvest, when to stay put, and when to travel.

For our ancient peoples, they were times of sacred ceremony with the cosmic and celestial realms. Many of the sacred sites around the world, from Stonehenge to the Egyptian pyramids and Karnak Temple Complex at El-Karnak, to Chichén Itzá in Mexico, Machu Pichu in Peru, and so on, have been built in perfect alignment with the position of the sun at equinoxes and solstices.

The word *solstice* means sun standing still. It is a day to stand still, bear witness, pause and feel. Feel deeply into our hearts, and consciously recalibrate our way forward.

The word *equinox* means equal night, referring to the roughly 12-hour day and 12-hour night that occurs only on the two equinox days of the year. It is a day to honour both our light and our darkness equally.

The **Spring Equinox** around March 21 is a time when light starts to increase after the dark winter. It is a time of new birth, new beginnings, sowing seeds and creating new paths into fertile grounds. A time of renewal, purification, and cleansing. Life begins to bloom gloriously again, and we begin to step into the excitement of spring, light, growth, new energy, and inspiration.

It's also a time when nature will offer you plants to detoxify your system after winter. It's a time of rebirth, of activating your potential and the perfect time to do an extended detox.

The *Summer Solstice* around June 21 is the day of the year where the sun is at the highest point over the equator. There is a positive energetic opening up to our celestial potential. It is a time of new creations, growth, intensity, high energy, light, and warmth. A time of connecting with pure life force energy and stepping fully into our light. A time of bursting gardens and bursting into our Mighty power.

The *Fall Equinox* around September 21 is a time when light begins to diminish. The days begin to shorten as the nights get longer. It is harvest time, a time to reap the seeds we sowed in the spring and nurtured in the summer. A time to begin to face our darkness (shadow), as we head towards the darkness of winter. It is a time of inner reflection as we rebalance and recalibrate, and harvest the fullness of our mightiness.

The *Winter Solstice* around December 21 is the darkest day of the year; the sun is at its lowest point over the equator. This is a time of physical and spiritual hibernation. A time of contemplation, reflection, quietude, and *going within*. It is a time to root down into our own light, a time to "dream" into our own vision of ourselves for the year to come.

The shifts in nature provide clues to the shifts that are happening within us. It's important to pause and feel, recalibrate, and come back into alignment with the rhythms of nature.

Why are the equinoxes and solstices important for radiant health, you might ask?

Well, as much as radiant health is the process of allowing your inner shine to glow, your inner beauty to be your outer expression, it is also the process of anchoring or embodying your mightiness with the subtle forces of the sun, the moon, and the cosmos, in both the seen and unseen worlds.

The more you are able to align and deeply anchor your soul with the laws of nature, the more you will be able to consciously evolution yourself alive. And though these words may sound catchy, they are not.

By now you know me as a firm believer in synergy. I am also a firm believer in being the alchemist of my heart, and being the magician in transforming the density of our personalities into the gold of our spirit. I invite you to seek your own philosopher's stone, and to become the hope activist in your own life.

Introducing a detox on the days of the equinoxes and solstices has the power to consciously spark your heart and recalibrate your heart compass to unimaginable depths. You are simply combining two well-known technologies for the developing and anchoring of your Mighty true nature, in synergy and alchemy with each other.

RECALIBRATING YOUR HEART COMPASS

Our bodies are our gardens – our wills are our gardeners.

—*William Shakespeare*

Can you hear the thump within your chest? Can you hear the rhythm of its song? Can you feel its desire to express itself?

Your heart: the thumps that keep you going, the vibration that keeps everything else in resonance, the rhythm that pulsates creating your sacred body, one thump at a time. So tender, once open, with the potential to lead into a world of freedom and equality.

Our Heart: still beating as it gets broken. We spend a lifetime inside our stories, coping and guarding our heart—trying to keep it safe. Yet while trying to keep it safe, we miss so much; we miss ourselves, our soul expression of ourselves. We miss our spontaneity, our youthful perspectives and boldness, courage, desire, joy, peace, and aliveness.

Our Heart: our body-soul compass. It's always guiding us in the right direction—towards growth, evolution, learning, and inspiration, towards love. But so often we get in the way and allow our mind to take over. We live then from our mind, and close off our heart.

How do we begin to re-connect with our body/soul compass? How do we begin to feel our way through life, rather than just thinking our way through? How do we begin to crack ourselves open to bare our heart, and allow ourselves to shine? How do we begin to actually live our life, rather than allowing our life to live us?

You and I begin by considering our best possibilities and true potential. Then, in order to connect with the best version of yourself, you must turn your gaze inwards. You must make time to sit quietly, in inquiry, and allow yourself the opportunity to sort yourself out. Who else will give us the opportunity of this gift, if not us?

You and I give ourselves the opportunity to surrender to our heart. First, you must listen to it, and then hear it—to know what it is you are yearning for. To feel what must be felt and honoured, and then release it. Feeling is a good thing, but most of us are afraid to really feel that which is within our heart. We have lost the intimate connection with our soul centre, and have often taken years of wonder in order to find our true ourselves again.

Once you give yourself the opportunity to find your true north, you will begin to walk, breathe, move, and act in a way more congruent with your Mighty heart and your highest self into the world.

Above all, you give yourself the opportunity to return home to the space within that is whole, sacred, and truly yours. This is your opportunity to move beyond that which keeps you bound, stuck, and unable to move forward to living the life your heart desires. It's your opportunity to reconnect with grace; to surrender your Ego and allow your essential self to shine, glow, lead, and change the world.

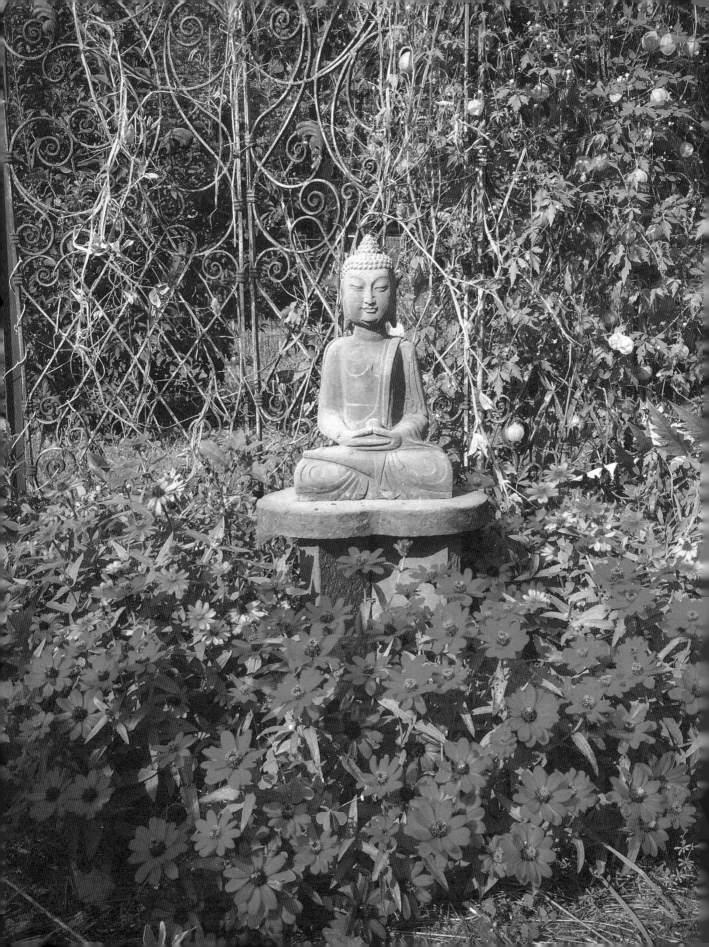

VI

THE ART OF MINDFULNESS

You cannot see the Seer of seeing.
You cannot hear the Hearer of hearing.
You cannot think the Thinker of thinking.
You cannot understand the Understander
or understanding.
He is your Self, which is everything.

—Yajnavalkya, Brihad-Aranyaka Upanishad three.4.2

STAYING IN YOUR SHIT

Only in the darkness can you see the light.

—Martin Luther King Jr.

Let's face it, *most of us are as happy as pigs in shit.* Not knowing we are standing in it, and not really knowing we are really *not* that happy, either. Many of us are currently sitting in park in a place of complacency with life. We have become resigned to the way things are, and to our suffering. We have given our power away so many times, there is very little left. We have come to accept the current state of affairs as a matter of fact. We have given up—and not given our choice for change a second chance.

In Eastern philosophies, people strive to move beyond the state of their suffering into happier states of being. It is understood that our human minds play a big role in the state of our suffering, and that happiness or liberation from suffering is an inner journey that requires *us* to change. It is a journey that requires you and I to **PAUSE (Pay Attention Use Sensory Experience)** as we shift away from our *stories* and living in the past, to being present—here and now—and feel. This journey requires us to slow down so we can develop the awareness and the skills to embody our inner warrior.

The recognition that we are indeed ***standing in our shit*** can be quite a brutal awakening. But it can also open your life to a brave new world of possibilities and potential that will indeed challenge you to change your thoughts, perspectives, attitudes, beliefs, words, patterns, habits, and behaviours. But it will also gift you with the philosopher's stone: happiness.

The quest for the philosopher's stone is the journey of transformation of mercury, lead, or heavy metals into gold. It is the alchemical process of transforming the densities you and I stand on (the shit) into light, love, life; a golden light awareness of our being that is infused by love.

Each of us carries within us the *karmic seeds*—the conditions and causes of our life circumstances, relationships, and our very being—that we need to open (for they will open themselves anyway). You and I must come to understand them at their root for us to transcend them. This is the process of awakening to our potential. This is the healing journey, the path towards wholeness that will require us to change, to look within, to develop mindfulness and remember our inner voice and inner wisdom. It's a path that requires courage, discipline, patience, self-care, generosity, kindness, compassion, and self-compassion.

The very awareness that we are standing in our shit begins to crack our hearts open. It begins to let the light in, begins to open us to those karmic seeds and demand that we transcend the *coping mechanisms* we've been using. No longer in park, you begin developing the inner skills and tools for your forward journey. This journey will ask you to listen deeply, beyond your personality and your Ego, to the silence within, the inner sanctuary where sacredness and grace reside. It will ask you to look at the root causes of your wounding, for your psychology will always become your biology. It is a process that will demand you take responsibility for your part, that you awaken the adult within. In order for you to learn to manifest your potential, your gifts into the world, you must begin with the question *What cracks my heart open?*

WHO DO WE THINK WE ARE?

It's hard to be humble when you are as great as I am.

—Muhammad Ali

As we journey on into deeper levels of healing, we come to greet the higher mind, the source of illumination and the seat of our mental realm. Our mental realm is but an antenna (whether in tune or not) to perceive the universal wisdom of the mind.

Our mental realm or **Mind (uppercase M)** is composed of three constituents:

1. Our **mind (lowercase m),** responsible for processing our thoughts and lived experiences through the senses. It stores these into our memory bank which then begins to weave the fabric of our mind.

2. Our **Ego,** the shape of the little self, the identifier, the I-shape that creates distinction between our self and others.

3. Our **intelligence,** wisdom, our true self—the source of our discernment and decision maker.

These are three distinct aspects of our Mind, for as we begin to bring awareness to our process, we can begin to understand that we are not just our mind, not just our Ego, but rather have the capacity to go beyond the senses, beyond the memory, beyond the "story," beyond the Ego, into engaging with our self and the world from a place of intelligence (wisdom), in tune with the greater universal intelligence.

Without the awareness of the three aspects of the Mind, most of us tend to define ourselves through *the seat of our Ego.* The Ego is a very necessary tool in our own evolution, but one that can sometimes trick us into believing we are something or someone we are not. But if we over-identify with our belief system, we will become so rigid we won't be able to flow with life. If we over-identify with our Ego, we won't be present to the here and now.

A healthy amount of Ego is necessary for us to awaken to self-compassion and kindness, to self-love through self-care. Yet we don't live in isolation; we must equally take care of others. The art of living in sacred reciprocity is an evolution of our Ego; it's that spot in our awareness of the fine balance between our individuality and our inter-connectedness.

For a lot of us, the Ego mind rules the show. It's a world built with the Ego mind as ultimate governor, with no acknowledgement that there are a few other *minds* involved in this thing called *World,* let alone the worlds that exist beyond the veil of the senses.

For most people, the Ego mind becomes the blueprint that governs their whole experience. It is where the core beliefs (often limiting) that we inherited and adopted from our parents and ancestral lines become our own, along with the belief systems (BS) that we ourselves have created. It is the space that shapes your life, for what you "think" of your story, creates strong emotional reactions and attachments within the boundaries of your own skin.

Your Mind is a personal, human element of your true self or soul (seed of eternal consciousness); it's just one of the tools soul uses in order to have a human experience.

Your Mind contains your thoughts and beliefs, your concepts, attitudes, strategies, thought patterns, emotional reactions, and automated behaviours. It contains your Ego and also contains the seat of your wisdom. These are all key elements in how you interact with other people and the world around you, yet they can also be quite limiting, and a top contributor to your suffering.

The quality of your thoughts, beliefs, concepts, attitudes, strategies, patterns, emotions, and so on, along with your ability to move beyond the seat of your Ego into the seat of your wisdom, will lead to a certain quality of body, quality of mind, quality of heart, and ultimately quality of reality and quality of life.

Committing to our happiness is a spiritual responsibility. Perhaps spending time inquiring about the question **Who do we think we are?** is a worthwhile exercise for bringing awareness to the quality of life you are creating for yourself. Honesty and transparency will be key in your process if you are truly seeking to change the quality of your life.

THE ROLE OF THE EGO IN OUR EGO-LUTION. ME? NEVER.

The mind has a mind of its own.

—Old saying

The Ego is the small sense of self. It is also our false sense of self, false personality. It is a necessary tool in our evolution, yet one that can be at the root cause of our suffering if we don't realize that all systems need an upgrade once in a while.

The Ego is formed in early childhood, highly influenced by the thoughts, concepts, beliefs, attitudes, strategies, patterns, emotional reflections, and automated behaviours of our parents and our ancestry.

Yet this Ego is not who we truly are; it is formed by the inevitable reactions to the people and events in our most intimate environment. The Ego has shaped our self image, our worldview, and how we approach the world and our world vision.

The Ego begins to "solidify" at a very young age. As a baby, our personal consciousness was undeveloped and inexperienced, and we had no understanding of the world outside of us.

The Ego begins to solidify after we experience our first psychological wound, our first "trauma," the very first time our newly formed false-self felt hurt. That instant became the frame for our "glasses"—the lenses through which, going forward, we will view the world around us. These lenses will shape our core beliefs, thoughts, and attitudes, creating a "filter" through which we will interpret all the events in our life and the world. This interpretation will determine our reactions and responses to that world and the people in it, all to suit our false-self sense of righteousness and survival.

There is a reason we ALL develop the Ego ... it's called ***Ego-lution!*** All right, it's called ***Evolution!***

I like to call the EGO the place of Evolution Going On. What do you think?

The Ego allows us to interact with the world and to form our own "limited" identity, a crucial step in our evolution. Whoever you and I finally identify our self to be is first a process of identifying who we are not. This step is crucial in your personal development from infancy to adulthood. It allows you to shape who you want to be, hopefully more and more in alignment with your true nature—your soul. It allows you the choice in how you give expression to your mightiness while here on earth, and that is a great thing.

The danger here is actually believing that the illusionary mirage the Ego presents us is the ultimate reality. When we come to believe that our thoughts, attitudes, concepts, values, and beliefs, and the resulting reactionary behaviours they create—is who we truly are, then by definition we're saying that other people's thoughts, attitudes, concepts, values, and beliefs are not true or valid—in fact—***wrong.*** And as we all know, great and multiple wars have been fought over that illusion.

The very role of the Ego is to keep us *separate* enough from the world to allow us the opportunity to define ourselves and form our own character. But if we don't allow for the process of evolution, it will *always* keep us separate from everyone else, and from all of life.

Remaining separate from everything and everyone only creates further suffering. In our illusionary separateness, we must protect and defend ourselves, our beliefs, our thoughts, our attitudes, and our values at all costs, for our very survival appears to depend on it.

(Please read that again.)

Is it true? Does any other being in the world actually live in separation from all else? What actually happens when we feel we must protect and defend ourselves, our beliefs, our thoughts, and our values at all costs for our survival?

The answer? Great suffering on both the personal and global levels of our existence is what happens.

We cannot develop our compassion muscle if we believe we exist separately from the world and everyone else in it. We cannot take care of each other or the earth if we believe our actions don't affect anything or anyone else. Ultimately, we cannot access our hearts. We cannot access universal love, not for ourselves, and not for Mother Earth or humankind.

As we begin to access the inner space of using the Ego as a tool, it no longer holds us bound on our earth walk. It will no longer limit your health or the possibility of healing. It will no longer limit your mind to the possibility of hope. It will no longer limit your heart to the possibility of feeling intimacy (*into me you see*). It will no longer limit you and I, for we truly are limitless radiant beings of light.

If your Ego is no longer serving you; if your attitudes, beliefs, values and thought patterns are old and need *upgrading*, if they are limiting your healing, and limiting your living from a place of your highest potential, then surely it's time for an upgrade!

So, thank you, Ego, for bringing us to this point in time and space. Thank you for your lessons. Thank you for anchoring us into the physical plane, as without you, our souls would not get the opportunity to have a human experience. How liberating is that?

A HEALTHY RELATIONSHIP WITH OUR EGO

When ego is lost, limit is lost. You become infinite, kind, beautiful.

—*Yogi Bhajan*

It's time to come into a healthier relationship with our Ego. We cannot erase it; we cannot use a magic spell and make it disappear, though sometimes that might be nice. *We can call a truce and begin to live in a healthier more conscious relationship with it, instead of allowing it to continue running the show—usually to our detriment.*

The first step is to begin to recognize the judgmental thoughts and shaming—towards both ourselves and others—that perhaps we naturally do. Then, as we begin to recognize our programming, patterns, and reactions to life and to others, we can begin the process of rewiring our brains as adults, and leave behind the negative ego reactions of the child we once were. We can begin reprogramming our minds, our ego, our operating systems and our personalities—a process that will allow us to live a life of beauty and peace, and let go of the need for extra drama and suffering in our lives.

Challenges and obstacles will always come, but when you realize they are not a part of who you are, but rather a part of the *story* you are living, of the tools you've developed, or need to develop as your life lessons, everything changes. Knowing this, you can now find greater inner courage, resilience, strength and love to deal with them, and both seek and allow the solutions to come to you.

The Ego or false-self thrives on drama and dictatorship. So as you begin to take charge of your life as co-creator, just know that Ego will do anything and everything it can to stay in power and continue running the show. This is simply part of our human journey, and will be unique to each of us. But also know that as you're able to reduce the inner noise, it will be easier to tap into your true self—soul—more consciously and at will. The more you do that, the more you begin to develop your inner voice muscle.

This inner voice is truly your map—and your compass—to guide you in your choices and actions while here in this world. You learn to recognize the presence of the Ego. You acknowledge it, yet you act according to your higher truth; your inner wisdom, as spoken by your inner voice, as guided by your Inner heart compass, as an expression of your true self: *your soul.*

FULL OF MIND

Many people are alive but don't touch the miracle of being alive.

—Thích Nhất Hạnh

As you become ever more mindful, what are you filling yourself with? Are you filling yourself up with the cosmic consciousness—the universal mind? Or are you filling yourself with Ego?

There is a large difference in my opinion, between becoming *full of mind* and becoming *mindful.*

The third aspect of our individual mind is the seat of our wisdom, our intelligence, our true self directly connected to, influenced by, and inspired by the universal mind. How often do you connect with your own wisdom? How often does it guide your thoughts, your actions?

> The u**niversal mind** refers to the consciousness that exists outside of us that created everything; the life force energy that infuses all life to carry on, to evolution, to be, to be love. This single, intelligent consciousness animates the entire universe. It is all-present, all-knowing, all-powerful, and all-creative. It is present everywhere, and in everything at the same time. It is present in you, and me, and yes—them too. In the Star Wars movies, it was called the Force, the energy field that surrounds us, penetrates us, moves through us and binds the entire universe together.

The universal mind is that which inspires our own intelligence, wisdom, and inner fires; that which is the source of our inspiration and illumination. It is your inner space of source, your ultimate home. By connecting with it more deeply, by purifying your body, heart, and mind, you begin to become all-present (omnipresent), all-knowing (omniscient), all-powerful (omnipotent), and all-creative (omnificent), which is the nature of the universal mind. Our healing journeys are really to become one with the nature of the universal mind—that which created us.

As you ignite your Mighty inner healer, as we travel through our healing journeys and connect more deeply with our true self, we begin to align with the five Elements, which are the building blocks for our external and internal realities, the seen and unseen worlds. Our process is one of remembering the seed of our own potential, of coming into *right relationship* with the Earth we live on, and with the great mystery to which we will return.

MINDFULLY MOVING INTO STILLNESS

"What day is it?" asked Pooh. "It's today," squeaked Piglet. "My favourite day," said Pooh.

—AA Milne

Mindfulness is the art of becoming aware of one's self, of witnessing yourself in the moment. It is the art of getting to know ourselves so intimately, that ultimately we hold our relationship to our self as sacred, for now you know intimacy is another word for ***into me you see.***

You engage in mindfulness by paying attention to the here and now, and by grounding yourself through the five senses. Engage in it by pausing (remember, PAUSE = Pay Attention Use Sensory Experience) yet knowing that beyond the senses lays your true self, the master of the senses and the wisdom that will guide your actions.

While mindfulness may seem to be the newest new-age thing, it is not. The roots of mindfulness are anchored deeply in the ancient systems that first developed in this world.

We live in an era of distraction and of mindless movement. We are moving faster than ever before, yet often forgetting to root down, to feel our heats, to feel the depth of our breaths. Part of our healing journey is to come back to focus, back to mindful movement, and back to stillness from where we can more easily PAUSE and feel, use our senses to ground, recalibrate our heart compass, and act from a place of wisdom (our true self).

Mindfully moving into stillness is the art of being more conscious and aware of our movements, both the ways in which *we act* in the world, and the ways in which *we are moved* by the world. They both require awareness on our behalf. Are we being moved in ways we no longer wish to be? Are our actions in alignment with our beliefs? Are we engaging in actions that are damaging others? Have we grown into a place where our old beliefs are holding us back from greater conscious action?

Stillness is the inner space between breaths, the *stillpoint*, the spaces in between our thoughts, our heartbeats, and our movements that brings us to connect deeply with our inner source. Stillness does not mean empty space, but rather it is a space so full we can deeply feel the power of our very own heartbeats.

There are many ancient mindfulness rituals and practices, such as yoga, meditation, Qi Gong, and Tai Chi, among others. I invite you to explore them. I invite you to build layers of conscious deep nourishment, by mindfully moving into stillness.

Mindfulness is the foundation for awareness, grounding, and compassion. Mindfulness practices allow you to anchor your mind in your body, connect your mind with your heart, and then connect with that which is the witness: your soul, your sense of source, your true home. They allow you to cultivate your innate potential for being present in and for your life.

Mindfulness practices allow you to face the inner constructions of your illusions and, in doing so, you begin to awaken. You awaken to the knowing that all movement begins in the spaces within your mind, and in order to shift the excessive movement currently expressing itself as dis-ease into coherence and harmony, a conscious effort is needed to still the current fluctuations of your mind, to still your mindless movements.

Mindfulness practices allow you to move beyond your current state of movement or reactivity, beyond your current coping mechanisms into developing focused attention, receptive awareness, kindness, true empathy (inner and outer), and mindful and compassionate listening. Ultimately, they open the gateway of self-compassion, and the capacity to find compassion towards your own humanity. Mindfulness allows you to access the stillpoint, the space between the breaths, where you can just be.

Reverend Andrew Blake, a Buddhist chaplain who trained under Roshi Joan Halifax PhD, and co-founder of Sarana Institute, describes five facets of mindfulness practice as taught by Roshi Halifax:

1. Concentration and focus (coming back to the present moment awareness)
2. Observation (noticing)
3. Discerning awareness (describing or labelling our thought/experience)
4. Non-judgement (letting go of attachments to our thought/experience)
5. Non-reactivity (not engaging with a thought/experience, allowing it to pass)

Mindfulness creates stability in our lives; it grounds the way we experience ourselves and the world around us. It opens us up to acceptance of what is, and develops our non-judgemental muscle, which further develops intimacy, kindness, empathy, compassion towards self and others, and interconnectedness. It creates the necessary conditions within to develop our inner trust and inner faith, which brings further healing to our experience of separation into wholeness.

Ultimately the practice of mindfulness extends well beyond our mat or cushion into mindful living. Mindfulness allows you to create the inner space needed for you to journey safely through your healing, as you activate your Mighty inner healer, in the process of remembering and reconnecting with your true nature, your wisdom.

Remember, our bodies are 9.9999999999996% empty space and about 0.000000000004% matter. How you choose to connect to the space that is you has the power to transform your whole being.

MONKEY MIND

When meditation is mastered, the mind is unwavering like the flame of a candle in a windless place.

—Bhagavad Gita

As we approach beginning a mindfulness practice, most of us are under the illusion we will be striving towards having *no thought*. I used to think that too, and it's always the first question I get asked in my classes.

The goal of your mindfulness practice is to create *more space in between your thoughts, to access the spaces in between thought, in between breaths, in between actions.* It's in these spaces in between that you find the opportunity to bear witness to yourself in process. This process of witnessing, and of noticing what and who is noticing, allows your mind to ground within your body, and access the inner space of stillness, what the yogis call the ***stillpoint.***

We live in fast times, in fear and stress, under the constant threat of attack from the shadow of the tiger. As a result, we spend most of our days acting or, rather, reacting with our sympathetic nervous system, our fight or flight response. Yet our bodies are not intended to remain in the fight/flight response, or to be constantly stressed, for as we know stress is one of the key players in the manifestation of dis-ease. Rather, our bodies are intended to shift into the parasympathetic nervous system in order to repair, restore, and heal.

Monkey mind is the accepted description for the nature of our human mind. It is said we think 1,000 thoughts per blink of the eye. Only one of those thoughts is grasped by our conscious mind and, if we get attached to its story, we will travel along with it until the end of times. The other 999 thoughts get passed into our subconscious mind. So, clearly, most of our Mind is actually composed of the subconscious, and most of us are carrying quite a heavy load there, which results in making our subconscious truly the director of the show. Most of us spend 95% of our day controlled by the unconscious thoughts, beliefs, and emotional drivers that burden our subconscious.

As we begin to quiet the mind, we begin to empty the subconscious mind and, through the life-force energy we bring into our body via the breath, we actually begin to reorganize and bring coherence into our subconscious. This greatly affects and brings coherence into our conscious mind. We also come to realize, neither our mind nor our body is who we truly are.

Our mind is always seeking to be engaged. It needs to be busy. So what are you feeding it? What are you choosing to engage it with? Are you building the field of coherence in your mind—the one that manifests in your body? Or do you continue to feed the chaos or incoherence that has taken a hold of you, and controls you?

The great news is our monkey mind can be trained. Through your mindfulness practice, you can develop skills to work *with* your mind, not *against* it, in order to create a conscious life.

STILLPOINT AWARENESS

At the still point of the turning world. Neither flesh nor fleshless;
Neither from nor towards; at the still point, there the dance is,
But neither arrest nor movement. And do not call it fixity,
Where past and future are gathered. Neither movement from nor towards,
Neither ascent nor decline. Except for the point, the still point,
There would be no dance, and there is only the dance.

—*T.S. Elliot*

Do you think that if you are always scattered in thought, which leads you to be scattered in action, you will ever find the ever-escaping present moment? Do you think you will ever find the depth of the healing you seek? Do you think you will ever find happiness?

Stillpoint awareness is the deep awareness and acceptance of the present moment. We access stillpoint through the spaces in between thought, in between breaths, in between actions, in the thin spaces between the veils of our illusions, where wisdom resides. *Stillpoint* is also the place of simply being, here and now.

Being present to your breath, to your mind, to your actions, and to the world outside yourself is truly an art. This art of living fully present and embodied demands that through your senses, you pay attention to what is happening right ***now.*** Not yesterday or tomorrow, because that is a part of your *story.*

Stillpoint is also the inner space where your personal power resides; you know, the one you've been giving away all these years. Reclaiming your personal power is part of your journey in and through your stillpoint, towards wholeness.

The nature of our mind as monkey mind was given to you and I to help us to discover who and what we are not. It is for you to discover and exercise your free will in the shaping of who you choose to be, and the remembering of who you are. The wild garden of life is always blooming and luring our senses into many directions. But as you begin to access the space of stillness within, you become your own master; you begin to consciously choose your path and the ways you wish to bloom yourself into the world.

The nature of your being is stillpoint; the great field of coherence, the great web of which you are a part. *Reconnecting with the inner space of stillpoint reconnects us with the inner space of stillness, which is the portal to the universe.* **Stillpoint awareness** is the journey back from our individual mind (from form) to higher consciousness or source. It allows us to now expand our own awareness, our own consciousness into the great originating mystery.

Mighty inner healer, in the stillness of the pauses in between your heart beat, the universe has your back.

BEARING WITNESS

Feel the feeling but don't become the emotion. Witness it. Allow it. Release it.

—*Crystal Andrus*

Bearing witness is the process through which we actually begin to see and know ourself. In order to bear witness, we must create a sacred space within to be become aware, and to be present to our thoughts, emotions, beliefs systems (BS), patterns and circumstances. Bearing witness is part of the path of accessing stillpoint awareness.

Moving into bearing witness to ourselves rather than remaining in a state of autopilot where we don't actually feel our emotions, and are unable to recognize our thought patterns or habitual belief systems, is a process that brings us into greater intimacy with our story and our personal narrative or conditioned thinking, without becoming attached to it, getting triggered by it or going into shame over it. We begin to move away from judging ourself, which allows us to begin seeing the roots, causes and conditions of our own suffering, the suffering of others and the suffering of the world. It's a process of awakening to our true self.

As we move into bearing witness we create a safe space within where our intellectual inner adult learns to process our thoughts and emotions with honesty, as we hold and support our emotional inner child from a place of sacredness, trust, peace, self acceptance and self love.

As we learn to embrace our own humanity in our practice, we connect with the space within of empathy, acceptance, stillness and receptivity. We learn to cultivate an open heart and mind for self, other and the world.

As we find the courage to face ourself in this way, we begin to awaken and develop fierce self-compassion. In facing what-cracks-our-heart-open, we learn to bring the self-compassion, self acceptance, empathy, stillness and receptivity with us into the world.

The more we awaken and move into bearing witness, the more we are able to step into a sense of interconnectedness and interrelationship with all life. Bearing witness connects us to the greater web that runs through all life and binds it together, and to a new and very personal realization of the wholeness of life. It allows us to weave together the fragmented aspects of ourself as we come back to feeling whole and centered again. We are One, even if we have forgotten.

Just as our mindfulness practice gifts us with the possibility of accessing and anchoring into stillpoint awareness, it also gifts us with the tool of bearing witness or witness awareness. Both of these, if we are consistent with our practice, can rapidly transform the mind, allow us to make peace with our ego, facilitate making peace with our emotions, re-connect us with our inner knowing of our wisdom and our truth, and shift the body from the sympathetic to parasympathetic nervous system, among other benefits.

When you gift yourself the opportunity to create the sacred space within to bear witness to yourself, you become accountable and responsible for your thoughts, emotions, words and actions. You come to understand that while your thoughts and emotions are yours, they are not actually you, but rather reactions to the world around you as you process them through your own filters. You come to understand there is great power in choosing your response, rather than your unconscious reaction. You become accountable for teaching Love by the way you choose to live. You become a vessel for new ideas, options and congruent paths of effective action to emerge from deep within you. This process and the practice awaken your own need to serve, your need to remediate not only your own suffering but the suffering of others and the suffering of the world, and it asks the question, how can I serve?

As you access new pathways for deep healing and begin to engage in new, perhaps different actions to power up your health, you begin to serve yourself and those around you. You realize your light is needed to brighten up the world, and your gifts, your talents and dreams have a purpose in the weaving of each other's lives. As you awaken into a greater relationship with yourself, you will also come to be more authentic in your relationship with those around you, and in your relationship with Mother Earth.

Truly bearing witness to yourself is not always an easy task. But it is necessary if you are to begin changing your habits, power up your health, ignite your transformation, and spark your revolution. As you awaken, you begin to reclaim yourself away from the thoughts, emotions and patterns that have kept you on autopilot.

FEAR

/fir/[16]

noun

1. *an unpleasant emotion caused by the belief that someone or something is dangerous, likely to cause pain, or a threat.*

verb

1. *be afraid of (someone or something) as likely to be dangerous, painful, or threatening.*

Fear has the power to cause a change in the metabolic and organ functions of our body, and ultimately a change in our behaviour, for it keeps us in the sympathetic nervous system, in the fight or flight response, 24/7. Emotions have the power to dramatically change our physiology. Do you think we, as a society, are living from a place of fear or a place of love?

Do you think fear keeps you in your past, in your future, or in the present moment? Fear keeps us so far from the present moment that most of us have never even heard of stillpoint. It is fear that

---

16   "Fear", Merriam-Webster Dictionary

keeps us so far away from feeling our hearts and the depth of our emotions; quite simply, we are afraid that if we were to feel them, we might just not survive them.

And it's true. If you and I were to feel the depth of the array of our emotions, we actually might not survive them. We haven't been taught *how* to feel them. We haven't been taught to create space both within and around ourselves to ***feel***. As children, we were connected to our feeling bodies. But, as children, we used to feel so much that the traumas of our experiences began to shut down our hearts, for the depth of the array of our feelings was simply too much to bear.

The tear in the fabric of our ancestral wisdom doesn't just break our lineages; it breaks our hearts. It breaks down the passing of the supportive web and practices that held us together in love, in sacredness, in respect, and in dignity.

But what if you and I were to gift ourselves and our children mindfulness practices to anchor our experience into the present moment awareness; practices to anchor our emotions (energy in motion) into a supportive field that holds us as we go through our shit? What if we gifted ourselves the opportunity to move the energies in motion that have gotten stuck within our very cell structures? For here is what most people don't know: ***all*** of our experiences have been recorded into the memory of our cells.

The emotions you and I do not allow to move and flow become stagnant energy within us. The trauma, sadness, grief, anger, fear, guilt, and shame you carry in your cells become blockages along the energy currents of your body. They become distortions in the field of your coherence and dis-ease in the field of your harmony, to the point that chronic headaches set it, cancer sets in, heart disease sets in, autoimmune disease sets in—the list is endless. As you can see, a big component of the root cause of disease lies in our emotional body.

What are you still holding onto that's creating an interference field and incoherence in your field? The cellular memory of your fears and of your deepest emotions. Can I perhaps offer you a different approach to ***FEAR? Face Everything And Rise.***

BREATHE DEEP INTO HEALTH

When you own your breath, nobody can steal your peace.

—Author Unknown

Let's just pause for a sec. Take a deep breath. Actually close your eyes, and take five deep breaths. How do you feel now?

Breath is defined as *"a noun that refers to the process of taking in and expelling air during breathing."*[17] Breath is the vehicle for breathing life.

Prana is the intelligent life-force energy of the world/heaven/spirit. With each breath you are being in-spirited or inspired. It is the vehicle through which pure consciousness journeys into form.

Breathing is the process through which pure consciousness enters our bodies. It is the process through which you are being breathed in and out by the power of life itself.

Did you know that the surface area of a pair of lungs is equal to that of a tennis court? Did you know that our estimated lung capacity is 180–200 cubic inches? Did you also know that through our regular, normal breathing cycles, we are only accessing about 30 cubic inches of our potential?

And lastly, did you know … deep breathing exercises allow you to access up to 100 cubic inches of your lung capacity? The length and the depth of each breath increases your lung capacity. When you breathe deeply you oxygenate your blood, which causes your brain to release endorphins—the feel-good hormones. These endorphins then help reduce stress, anxiety, and pain in your body.

Both Prana and the Mind are the main activators of our whole-body system. It is here where movement within your body is initiated. Prana is the spark that ignites your Mind into action. The deeper the breathing, the more Prana you accumulate in your lungs to ignite your whole-body system into patterns of greater coherence, which results in better health, clarity, and yes, more coherence.

---

17   "Breath", Vocabulary.com

From the smallest expression of the proton into the largest expression of life on earth, life communicates and expresses itself through patterns. What is the pattern of your breath? Is this pattern helping you? Is it building you up? Or, is its shallowness leaving you feeling like you're on empty all the time? Is its shallowness depriving your body of the precious oxygen and life-force energy it needs to thrive?

Deep breathing exercises also increase your vitality. Yes, we know there's an increase in our levels of oxygen intake, but most of us don't realize our vitality is linked directly to the state of coherence and harmony within our body system. As you breathe deeply, you increase this field of coherence and harmony in your own body through the depth of the flow of the life-force energy you're taking in along with the oxygen.

Deep breathing exercises also draw the senses within, purifying them and quieting the noise or chatter in our minds. And you already know about the power of cleansing the senses, right? (See page 253.)

Deep breathing exercises are by nature a mindfulness practice. They allow both hemispheres of your brain to synchronize, and change the structure of your brain by facilitating it to enter the lower brain wave frequencies that restore health to the body system.

It's been scientifically proven that deep breathing increases the alpha, theta, and delta brain waves. What does this mean to you? Well, well … ready?

The **beta state** is our regular state of being. Our brain waves have a frequency of 14–40 Hz (per second). We are attentive, actively thinking, and alert. Our state of being ranges from actively calm, to stressed out. Beta state is our walking consciousness and reasoning wave.

We experience **alpha waves** when the frequency of our brain waves lowers to the range 7.5–14 Hz. We are relaxed and reflective, and our experience of stress is significantly reduced as compared to the beta state. The alpha state has been widely recognized as an optimal state for learning; it reduces depression and boosts creative thinking. It is the state we access when meditating or daydreaming. Alpha is our deep relaxation wave.

We experience **theta waves** when the frequency of our brain waves lowers to the range 4-7.5 Hz when we are sleeping. We are even more relaxed, and are extremely receptive and open in this state. Theta waves also occur in the deepest stages of Zen meditation, and they are our meditation and sleeping waves.

We experience **delta waves** when the frequency of our brain waves lowers to the range 0.5-4 Hz. This is an extremely relaxed state mostly associated with deep dreamless sleep. Delta waves are our deep sleep waves.

Lowering the frequency of your brain waves increases the frequency of your energy field, and your overall state of being along the spectrum of conscious awareness. Remember, everything in the universe is vibrating at a particular frequency. The quality of this vibration has been studied and paired with the depth of our emotions. *The higher the frequency of your energy or vibration, the lighter you feel in your physical, emotional, and mental bodies. The more you will experience greater personal power, clarity, peace, love, and joy.*

According to the scale of human consciousness, the lowest emotional vibrations are those of shame and guilt. They are the most-contracted forms of human emotional consciousness. As we begin to raise the frequency of our emotional vibration through deep breathing and expansion of consciousness, we move through apathy, shame, guilt, grief ,and fear into desire, anger, and pride, into courage, neutrality, and willingness. From there we move into acceptance, reason, love, joy, peace, and ultimately enlightenment.

So my dear friend, will you *breathe deeply into health*? The journey sure seems promising.

BENEFITS OF MINDFULNESS PRACTICES AND DEEP BREATHING EXERCISES

If you want to conquer the anxiety of life, live in the moment, live in the breath.

—*Amit Ray, Om Chanting and Meditation.*

In this era of distraction, it is no wonder so many of us have turned to mindfulness practices to anchor into our centre, to find our true north, to reconnect with our purpose, and to heal our bodies from disease and pain. But the above are just a few of the benefits you may experience as you make your practice a daily non-negotiable. I invite you to bask in the benefits of these powerful practices, I invite you to become the magnet that attracts this long list of benefits into your life. You got this.

Physical:

- Change the inner terrain of your body
- Oxygenate the body. Purify blood, lower blood pressure. Dual-action aid in remineralization of body, in detox, and lowering of inner toxicity
- Fast alkalizer
- Strengthen your immune system
- Reduce heart disease
- Cleanse your sense organs
- Reduce stress, anxiety, and pain in your body
- Enhance brain functioning
- Lower brainwave frequency
- Improve memory retention
- Decrease depressive symptoms
- Increase overall vitality
- Improve digestion and absorption of nutrients
- Create overall feeling of whole-body wellness
- Aid in deep cellular nourishment, the building block for whole-body radiant health
- Aid in the repair, rebuilding and regeneration of our DNA
- Full of life-force energy from the world of spirit
- Build our pranic body; reorganize the life-force energy within
- Reconnect you to your awareness of your senses
- Reorganize your entire system into coherence
- Enhance your ability to deal with illness
- Facilitate your recovery from dis-ease
- Ignite your Mighty inner healer

Emotional:

- Facilitate emotional clarity and greater flow of emotions, both current and past
- Facilitate your feeling of connectedness to self, to others, to the world at large
- Deepen emotional intimacy to self and emotional availability to others
- *Improve clarity of purpose that is rooted in self, world, and ecological and spiritual responsibility*

Mental:

- Improve mental discipline and clarity of thought
- Create awareness of your thought patterns, habits, and addictions
- Facilitate the process of quieting the mind
- Facilitate the emergence of the witness awareness
- Facilitate access to ***stillpoint awareness***—the *spaces in between* and the world of the unseen
- Facilitate entering lower states of brainwave vibration
- *PAUSE TIME IN MOTION. Anchor the mind in the body. (One of the root causes of disease.)*

Energetic:

- Enhance awareness of your energetic body
- Enhance, rebuild, repair your energetic circuitry, your energy body—your biofield
- Enhance awareness of the sacred within, and the sacred within all
- Enhance awareness of your interconnectedness
- Enhance awareness of the understanding that we're a part of the universe, the earth, and life beyond your bodies
- Enhancer of the understanding of life-force as your ultimate source of spiritual nutrition
- Tool for evolutionary consciousness transformation

Spiritual:

- Reconnect with your soul
- Enhancer of the understanding of life-force as your ultimate source of spiritual nutrition
- Spiritual enhancer of your connection with grace and the god of your own understanding
- Tool for evolutionary consciousness transformation
- Activator of your spiritual and karmic evolution
- Serve as portal into the realm of quantum healing
- Gatekeepers into the inner space of deep nourishment and deep healing, where you can spark your own revolution and ignite your inner healer
- Anchors the mind into the body
- Ignites your mind into action

- Reconnect you to your own wisdom
- Ignite your remembering of your primordial nature
- Awakens your mightiness

Do any of these benefits seem familiar to you? I hope so. Mindfulness practices, deep breathing exercises, and liquid nutrition share a lot of the same benefits. And now that you're familiar with the alchemy of synergy, are you ready to double-up on happiness?

If you remember, the root cause of the root causes of dis-ease is the forgetting of our primordial nature. Nice to know we have a tool available to assist us in remembering … assist us in the *remembering of our primordial nature*. The very word **remember** stems from two words: re-member, and the action of re-membering, re-assembling ourselves anew.

Mindfulness practices and deep breathing exercises are to be done with great respect for the process, and for the force that will begin to move through you once you've cleared the pathway, which is simply this vehicle, your body. Deep breathing exercises are by nature mindfulness practices that will ground your experience of this alMighty force, practices that allow you first to root down in order to rise.

What happens when a balloon (the body) is filled with air (life force) and is not grounded or held by a string? It flies off into thin air where it eventually pops—and then its pieces come crashing down, back to earth. So, please, ground your body (the balloon) before you fill it with activated intelligent life force energy (air) so that you can root down and be held by the string of grace throughout your body, before you rise up into the thin air of expansive consciousness.

17 INCHES

To discover new oceans, one must have the courage to lose sight of the shore.

—*Don Oscar Miro-Quesada*

The longest journey of all is perhaps *17 inches long*. It begins in your mind, and takes you into the depths of your Heart (capital H, for the totality of our heart space, not only the physical heart). As you further the journey along your path of becoming, you perhaps realize this is not the first time you have walked this path, and likely not the last time either. Yet you viscerally know this is the path of your truth; the path of your awakening.

Surrendering to the journey, surrendering to the awareness that there's more going on than meets the eye is so important. And though you would very much like to be in control, *this ship is being piloted by the masterful spirit. We—you and I—are but cosmic travellers,* and though we are very much in control of our intentions and choices (for free will choice is our spiritual birthright), we know there is just so much we don't know, and won't know about our journey, about our life lessons, about the characters of our story. So, can we trust the path of these 17 inches that may take lifetimes to travel? Can we trust that you are actively choosing and engaging with soul to awaken?

If so, you are answering the call of soul to heal yourself and each other, and the deep inner yearning to become whole. Perhaps, deep down, you already trust this crazy journey you're on. But can you bring that level of trust up into your Mind, and let go of the Ego and the barriers you've created that have kept you safe, but bound at the same time? Can you open up to the risk of the journey? I'm not suggesting you leave it all behind. But I am asking, can you get out of your comfort zones and take that leap of faith into making your soul dream your reality?

We first break the cycle of being *in our head* by diligently recognizing that we *are* in it. Sometimes we have a breakthrough, and can begin to find the space of our hearts. Tools such as mindfulness and meditation practices are great allies in getting out of our head and into our Heart; they provide tools to begin to recognize and silence the chatter, the patterns, and the Ego.

But mindfulness and meditation practices alone won't get us out of our head. What happens on the cushion or mat is one thing: what happens when we leave it is very different. But we must begin somewhere, and for many it works to begin with practices that calm the mind, anchor the nervous system, and reduce stress; little do we know they are a portal to the journey into the Heart. We must spark our journey; we must leap forward. We have feared this moment all our lives. Well, here we are.

Mindfulness and/or meditation are not the only methods one can use. Any practice that gets your brain to access a lower brainwave pattern will open the gates to heaven. Okay, maybe not quite that fast. Try this: any practice that gets your brain to access a lower brainwave pattern will open the gateway into your Heart. For some people, that practice may be running. Or it may be yoga, or their workout, or canoeing, or skating, or doing art, or spending time in nature, or sitting by a sacred fire, or listening to classical music. Whatever works for you. But whatever it is, work it. Work it good.

PAUSE AND FEEL

Energy cannot be created or destroyed, it can only be transformed.

—Albert Einstein

Here is a quick question for you: What is more important—what you feed your body, or what you feed your mind?

Pause and feel. Pause and feel.

Come back to the ***stillpoint,*** present moment awareness. Come back to the breath. Come back to your centre, your inner source.

The ability to pause and feel is truly the alchemical process of transformation of your *stories and attachments* into the here and now moment, which brings forth great compassion (to self and other), kindness, connectedness, and wholeness.

What do you feel when you pause? What do you feel when you connect with the feeling body?

You feel your heart beat. You feel alive. You feel each and every one of your senses engaged with the world.

What do you feel when you've been running around so much you can't even recognize the beat of your own heart?

*The ability to pause and feel allows you to transform the energy in motion (e-motion) that is currently in your life, allows you to become the witness, to become aware that you are aware, allows you to simply **become.***

Becoming the witness is the process by which we access stillpoint, the process through which we can expand our emotional resiliency and move up the emotional chart of consciousness into the higher frequencies of courage, neutrality, willingness into acceptance, reason, love, joy, peace, and ultimately the awakening of our mightiness.

The tipping point of our health journeys, of our journeys to ignite your Mighty inner healer as we anchor into our inner source, is the point *when the resonance of the higher emotions become a force greater than all the other forces.* That resonance begins to shape shift every single cell in your body, from its nucleus containing your genetic material to the outer expression of your body.

When you pause and feel, you become the still lake waiting for the stone to be thrown; the stone that will shift and elevate the resonance of the whole system into greater coherence and health. *The stone, in this case, is your mindfulness practice.*

THE ECHOES OF SILENCE

Let silence take you to the core of life.

—Rumi

Is silence really the absence of sound or perhaps the absence of man-made sounds? Does nature exist in silence? Is silence empty or full?

Nature does not exist in silence. *Nature exists in the echoes of the subtleties of sound that are coherent, and which bring great coherence to all that experience it.* To me, silence is quite full. It's full of vibrating energy and frequencies that promote great healing in our body system.

Silence is full only when we've given ourselves the opportunity to just be, to be still. Silence offers an opportunity to tap into the vastness of our inner reality and the echoes of our soul.

Silence is full of energy vibration, full of coherence, and full of patterns of sound waves inaudible to the human ear. The beauty of silence is that it simply "is." It is the vehicle through which life echoes and ripples.

Silence gifts us the opportunity to cleanse our sense organs, to reorganize our body systems, to recalibrate our Heart. It gifts us the ability to listen to our inner guidance, our inner wisdom, the ability to create space in our mind for what needs to emerge and the ability to remember our mightiness.

Silence is truly a gift in this modern world—in this era of noise and distraction where most of us feel uncomfortable being in silence, or simply being silent. We are so used to always being on the go and to experiencing the constant hyper-stimulation of man-made noise that we have forgotten the importance of being still for our health.

The soul speaks in silence. How can we hear our soul if we are constantly busy, constantly creating or engaged with noise, constantly outside our body?

In this brave new world, you and I must create silence—as much as that may sound absurd. We must create *space* for silence. We must create a daily practice of basking in silence to allow for a time of processing and integration of our life experiences; a time for decompressing, a time for deep listening, a time for reconnection with our hearts, a time for anchoring the mind, a time for conscious travel of the 17 inches, a time to commune with soul, a time to just simply *be*.

BEING

/ be·ing /'bēiNG/[18]

noun

1. *existence.*
2. *the nature or essence of a person.*

verb

1. *present participle of be.*

When was the last time you spent a day just ***being?*** Mmmh, perhaps an hour just being? I mean being; as in away from your phone, your gotta-do list, your book, your family life, your work life, your kids' hockey lives? Being, as in just you and your breath and the nature that surrounds you?

For most of us, being is not something that happens often enough. Being with ourselves just as we are. Being away from the distractions of our worldly affairs and the demands of our everyday living is not something we have the luxury of? Right? Life here in this world is busy, or so we

---

18   "Being", Oxford English Dictionary.

think. But what if being was the state of existence we actually need the most? If so, is it then a luxury? Or is it a human necessity for health and deep healing?

And no, being doesn't mean doing nothing on your couch, watching TV, and zoning out. Being means *being fully present with all your senses in direct relationship with the elements and the natural world that surrounds you.*

I had a chance to be up close and personal with the concept of being during the summer of 2016. Under the guidance of Grandmother Dianne Ottereyes-Reed, I did my first four-day vision quest. Dry fast (no food, no water), no phone, no books, no journals; nothing but me, myself, and I … well and a tent in the hills of Labelle, Quebec, Canada.

Being is an art. A quality of living in the present moment, engaged with the world around us. My four days in the bush taught me a lot about my mind, about my body, about fear and trust, about the echoes of nature and the ripples of my inner nature, about my senses and about how I relate and engage with the world around me. It taught me a lot about the noise I carry within, my ancestral wound, my shit, my BS, and the many layers of the depth of the healing that I was seeking.

Beingness takes us away from mindlessness, into more mindful states of existence. Being allows us to tap into *stillpoint awareness* more often and, as we begin to learn how to be with ourselves more often, away from all the inner and outer distractions, the more we'll be able to truly engage mindfully from a place of deep peace and stillness through our movements into the world.

Being brings you closer to both your light, and your shadow. For without your awareness of both, there would be no opportunity to exercise your free will. Yes, your free will. Do you choose to stay in your shit and your BS? Or, do you choose to release, transform, surrender, and integrate it in order to rise to the power of living life through your best potential? Can you quiet your mind enough to listen to your soul speak? Can you tune into the power of the ancestral wisdom that moves through you?

THE ART OF CREATING SACRED SPACE

Your sacred space is where you can find yourself again and again.

—Joseph Campbell

As we surrender into being, we will come to feel there are sacred spaces that hold us more than others. We will come to yearn to claim a sacred space of our own, one that will nurture us into wellness. This sacred space will become a womb-like space of refuge, safety, and deep nourishment and it will begin to root you into the inner space of sacredness.

Choose a space in your home to become your sacred space. It can be a corner in your bedroom or a room onto itself; it can also be a place in nature you always return to. But right now you are making a conscious choice to create a space in your home that will hold you in your practices. Before creating sacred space, first close your eyes, take a few deep breaths, and connect with the inner space of sacredness that you desire. Then, and only then, begin to create that quality of sacredness in your outer space.

Through resonance, the creative expression of your outer sacred space will further activate, ignite, spark, and heal the space of sacredness within you. Everything is always in relationship and, as we build each other up, we also build our own innate power for creation and healing.

Ritual is a powerful portal to open up sacred space. You and I have been creating sacred space all along during our time together. The following are rituals generally used by many ancient traditions to open up sacred space prior to beginning mindfulness practices:

1. ***Smudge*** yourself and the space around you with incense or dried sage to clear and purify both self and space from the densities of the day. Then, remind your whole-body system you are entering into sacredness.

2. ***Set your intention*** for being in this space.

3. ***Sanctify*** the space with corn/sage/tobacco/cedar by placing a pinch of either one of them in your space. This further honours the space itself as a sacred vessel that will hold and support you. You can also do this by lighting a candle.

4. Do your **breathwork,** a deep steady breath to the count of five (inhale for five seconds, hold for five, exhale for five). This ignites your body, calms the mind, integrates them both, activates the space, and lets your soul know you are getting ready for your mindfulness practice. See pages 253 for more complete descriptions of breathwork.

5. Use the space you just created for **meditation/mindfulness practices,** or any other tools for self inquiry.

SHADOW WORK

One must have chaos in oneself in order to give birth to a dancing star.

—*Friedrich Nietzsche*

Psychologist Carl Jung stated the shadow to be the unknown dark side of the personality, which the conscious Ego does not identify in itself, or the entire unconscious (everything a person is not fully conscious of).

Our shadow is made up of the wounds that have us believing we're flawed, unlovable, unworthy, undeserving people. These wounds are often created in childhood, yet they are also inherited through our social, cultural, and religious systems. When these wounds are left unattended, we come to live life from a place of deficiency, contraction, and victimhood. When we begin to engage in our shadow work, we begin to walk the path towards a more authentic and fulfilling life.

Shadow work is the journey of alignment, healing, and growth we are all on, whether you and I admit it or not. Along the journey, we stop interpreting the actions of others from the place of the wounded self, and begin to understand that most things in life we choose to be hurt or triggered by are not about us; instead, they are the unconscious actions, reactions, and expressions of others from their own place of unhealed wounded-ness. As Ronald D. Siegel (2010) wrote:

> *By illuminating how we construct our identity, Mindfulness practice helps us recognize and accept our shadow moment by moment. Every desirable and undesirable feeling, thought, and image eventually arises in meditation, and we practice noticing and accepting them all. We see our anger, greed, lust and fear along with our love,*

generosity, care, and courage. Seeing all these contents, we gradually stop identifying with one particular set and rejecting the other. We eventually see that we have a great deal in common with everyone else – including those we are tempted to judge harshly. We see for ourselves why people in glass houses shouldn't throw stones.[19]

As you begin to quiet your mind through mindfulness practices, you also begin to bear witness to the noise and static that has always been within you. You begin to notice the content of your mind, even of your subconscious and unconscious minds, which are really the structure of your personality. The conscious mind is only 10% of our mind; our subconscious is 50% and our unconscious mind is the remaining 40%. So you see, if you do not consistently "empty" the contents of your subconscious and unconscious minds, they will continue to drive your life more than your conscious mind ever will.

Mindfulness practices assist us in bringing to light parts of our subconscious and unconscious minds—they also allow us to *sit*, and to *be present* to our shadow self. To be present to all the difficult emotions—the hidden traumas, wild desires, obsessions, complexes, negative thought patterns, shame, guilt, regret, aggressiveness, violence, resentment, anger, rage, and vindictiveness we have felt yet denied expression to.

According to Jungian analyst Aniela Jaffé, the shadow is the "*sum of all personal and collective psychic elements which, because of their incompatibility with the chosen conscious attitude, are denied expression in life.*"[20]

Yet, as you already know, every experience you have ever had, and every emotion you have ever felt lives in the subtle field of your cells; your entire psychology becomes your biology. So your shadow self lives within you. It is the denser aspect of your self, but the more light and awareness you bring to it, the more you will begin to shift the densities that lie within into spaces of greater harmony.

Disease is the accumulation of density in the body, of incoherence in the bio-field. The seed of consciousness of our shadow self is passed down along with our unique seed of consciousness from one lifetime into the next. Mindfulness practices such as yoga, deep breathing (pranayama), and meditation allow you and I to shine a light on our shadow self.

> *"In Indian and Yogic philosophy, Samaskaras are the mental impressions left by all thoughts, actions and intents that an individual has ever experienced. They can be*

---

19   R. D. Siegel, R.D. The Mindfulness Solution: Everyday Practices for Everyday Problems. (New York, NY: The Guilford Press, 2010.)

20   "Anger, Madness, and the Daimonic: The Psychological Genesis of Violence, Evil and Creativity" by Stephen A. Diamond.

thought of as psychological imprints. They are below the level of normal consciousness and are said to be the root of all impulses, as well as our innate dispositions. They are the root of both our pleasurable and painful experiences."— *Yogapedia*

Yoga, at its essence is a practice that allows us to move beyond our shadow self or samaskaras. Though asana (postures), meditation practices, and breath work can be practiced independently, they are also a foundational aspect of yoga. Together, these practices help us shift the subtle energies and imprints that are latent in our body from our shadow self, from both this life and from others. They help us to not only oxygenate the body, detoxify the system, rejuvenate, and regenerate our vitality, but also help create tranquility and stability in our nervous system, something we absolutely need in order to face our shadow.

Through our yoga practice (asana, breath work, and meditation) we are constantly moving and engaging with these imprints. Have you ever been dropped down to your knees in the middle of a yoga class, inundated by tears of grief, loss, and sorrow by something that happened long ago, yet which was present in your mind today? It was ready to be seen, released, transformed, surrendered to, and now integrated? Samaskaras, or our shadow self, are the imprints of our wounds, of our subconscious and unconscious minds.

Have you ever been camping on a moonless night when your mind *took you for a ride* and you became paralyzed by fear? And when you had a chance to finally turn the flashlight on you found that while some of those fears and projections created by your mind had some sound base in reality, most of it did not? And that bear you were sure was ready to tear into your tent turned out to be a raccoon, or maybe even a mouse?

It is the same with our shadow self. Some of it has indeed a sound base in our experience of reality, but a lot of it is mental projection, an expression of our own unconscious actions from a place of our unhealed wounded-ness.

When you are triggered by an external circumstance or person, or by an emotion rising to the surface, I invite you to remember the value of conflict as an opportunity to grow. I invite you to remember we are all vulnerable, and you and your experience matter. You have the tools to move beyond it, and it is important you take the time and space you need to step into self-inquiry in order to understand the depth of your wound. This will allow you to begin to heal it, transcend it, hurt less in your heart, and cause less hurt in the hearts of others. Not easy, I know. But you got this.

Our triggered states are always in relationship with our wounds, with an unmet need and with the feeling that unmet need is now rising within us. Your process is one of anchoring into a pause in your reaction. This is followed by empathy, the desire to understand your wound, its root, the unmet need, and a deep dive into self-compassion.

The following are a few ***key steps to doing your shadow work.*** Please have writing materials at hand.

- Go to your sacred space or a quiet room. Make sure you will be uninterrupted for at least five minutes.
- Close your eyes and take a few deep breaths.
- Engage in the five-count breath cycle (inhale for five, hold for five, exhale for five) for at least five minutes, and/or meditate for five minutes.
- Pause and feel. Stay within.
- Open your eyes.
- Understand that emotions are not inherently good or bad. They are simply energy in motion.
- Make a list of emotions, self-judgements, and so on that you are currently aware of about yourself. Perhaps just work with one today.
- Then ask yourself these questions…
  - What am I feeling?
  - Why am I feeling this at this time?
  - What unmet need did it trigger in me?
  - What would its root be?
- Breathe deeply. Pause and feel.
- Allow the answers to arise. Sometimes it may take some time. But stay in process. Know that you are guided.
- Become aware of how this feeling truly makes you feel. Are there patterns of feelings, patterns of thought, or patterns of belief systems that get triggered for you? Investigate with self-compassion. Write them down.
- Then draw a big circle, a medicine wheel:

1. At the bottom, or in the south of your medicine wheel, write the following question:

   What needs to be seen at this time?
   Pause and feel … pause and feel …write it down.

2. At the left or in the west of your medicine wheel, write the following question:

    What needs to be released at this time?
    Pause and feel … pause and feel …write it down.

3. At the top or in the north of your medicine wheel, write the following question:

    What needs to be surrendered to at this time?
    Pause and feel … pause and feel …write it down.

4. At the right or in the east of your medicine wheel, write the following question:

    What needs to be transformed at this time?
    Pause and feel … pause and feel …write it down.

5. At the centre of your medicine wheel, write the following question:

    What needs to be integrated at this time?
    Pause and feel … pause and feel …write it down.

Pause and feel. Take a step back and become a witness to your process. Allow the medicine that has just unfolded to infuse your Heart and liberate your Mind. You might just start to feel a little lighter. You might just have an emotional release, and that is a good thing. There is no need to continue carrying a bag full of your shadow self everywhere you go. Real freedom comes from loving every aspect of your self, every aspect of your journey home, even the dark places.

Awareness is at the root of change. Awareness is at the root of exercising our free will and our conscious action into the world to not only better our lives, but also the lives of the seven generations that will come after us, whether biological or not.

The shadow self is an important aspect of our whole self; it will always be there, yet we have the ability to be in relationship with it, rather than it being in ownership of us. We all have the ability to use it as a guide along our journey of healing, use it as a tool to ignite your Mighty inner healer, align with soul, and anchor into your inner source.

Try being in relationship with your shadow self as an opportunity for growth, self-knowledge, and self-awareness. Once you accept its presence, it can serve you as an ally rather than as an enemy we continue to shove deeper into the corners of our being.

TRANSFORM, TRANSMUTE, ILLUMINATE

There is a crack in everything. That's how the light gets in.

—*Leonard Cohen*

Fire is the element of *transformation*. It forces us to get up close and intimate with our shadow self. That is, if we truly want to transform. Honouring our pain from being in this world is a foundational aspect of our healing journey.

In our darkest hour, we often tend to feel alone, the righteous victim of our deep challenges, the righteous victim of our circumstances, and rightly so. In time, as we begin tapping into the power of gratitude, we also have the opportunity to tap into the power of our shadow and our pain, where we greet our greatest teacher of all.

Our shadow, our pain, has been the experience, the process, the trauma of the cracking open of our heart. It contains within it the potential for deep work and soul growth. At its root it is our source of strength and power. We have walked our own dark path; we have battled with our specific demons, limited beliefs, and dis-ease, but can we now bring into our own individual experiences the awareness that it's all a part of our human experience?

Can you forgive yourself for your own humanity?

Can you forgive your self and allow love to come into your heart, and use this expertise to shine your light?

Can you honour your pain by doing the work?

Can we honour the pain of the world by understanding that we are here to learn about love; that we are here to guide and inspire each other?

We cannot know of the light without having first experienced the shadow. We cannot truly appreciate the freedom our heart can feel without having first experienced a broken heart.

As you transform, transmute, shapeshift, and connect with greater clarity to your passions, and to the universal mind of your illumination, you begin to root your own Mighty power at its core.

It is by living in, with, and through your pain and your passions that you begin to awaken to your energetic heartbeat, and truly become the source of your illumination. You become inspired (into spirited) by the world again; you begin to tap into what exactly makes you feel alive, happy and vibrant. Living a vibrant life is about anchoring your Heart, your life through the expression of your passions and the sharing of your illumination.

MINDFULNESS PRACTICES IN STILLNESS AND IN MOVEMENT

You must do the thing you think you can't do.

—*Eleanor Roosevelt*

There are many ***mindfulness practices*** to choose from, and many mindfulness apps to support you along the way. Throughout these pages, I've already shared a few practices with you. But now I want to share a few more that have become a part of my lifestyle, and part of the foundation of my healing and of my being.

The quality of your approach to your own mindfulness practice holds in itself great potential for awareness and awakening. What kind of space will hold you as you begin to mindfully move into stillness?

I encourage you to create a physical sacred space in your home for your mindfulness practice. This will become a quiet space you will always come back to. The more you show up for your practice, the more this space will begin to awaken energetically and become a safe, nourishing expression of who you are. To begin and end the sacred time you will spend in your sacred mindfulness space, create a simple ritual that is meaningful to you. Light a candle or perhaps some incense, or perhaps both. ***The art of creating sacred space*** (page 240) is an opportunity to walk through the portal with grace.

The following are mindfulness practices in stillness and in movement that I will expand on:

1. *Yoga—Union with the universe:* The very word yoga means to *yoke or unite.* Although here in the West we have come to know yoga in mainly a series of stretching exercises (asana), yoga is a mindfulness practice that clears the samaskaras. It creates the right conditions in your body to unite your Mind and Heart through sacred action into the world, as you awaken to the inner space of sacredness within, and the flow of grace or consciousness through you.

2. *Pranayama—Yogic deep breathing exercises: Pranayama* are breath exercises through which you prolong and retain the breath to extend and expand the life-force energy that animates you, your vital energy. Pranayama was created with one intention: to harness a clear mind in a purified body and activate the process of awakening towards your enlightenment, a.k.a. your mightiness. These deep breathing exercises are powerful and should be used respectfully as part of a mindfulness practice to build as solid a foundation, as purified a physical vehicle as possible, for the unfolding of our soul purpose. Traditionally pranayama is taught from teacher to student, only after the student has been practising asana for a few years, and has built a strong enough foundation to be able to handle the intensity of the energetic charge activated through pranayama.

3. *Meditation as self-inquiry:* Meditation is the art of tapping within, of connecting deeply with your true self and creating the sacred space within; a safe, supported vibrational inner space for your soul and heart to find expression, for your mind to anchor, and for your body to deeply heal.

   Meditation is a tool for "processing" your journey through your physical, emotional, mental, and spiritual challenges. It can also serve as a tool for deep nourishment as you tap into deeper levels of awareness of your nature as a human being, and access your own inner nature as an individual.

4. *Shamanism—The alchemy of direct revelation:* Shamanism is an ancient practice of direct revelation, of being in relationship with the inner space of wisdom through engagement with the world of both the seen and the unseen, in sacred reciprocity. Shamanism is an elemental practice, just like the ancient practices of yoga and Ayurveda. They are all practices for a mindful life, through the mindful engagement of the elements in our process of deep healing and creation.

5. ***Forest bathing or Shinrin-yoku forest therapy:*** is the medicine of simply being in a forest (not exercising, hiking, or jogging—but being). Of basking in its atmosphere and healing energy; of taking in the forest through your senses. Shinrin-yoku is like a bridge. By opening your senses, it bridges the gap between you and the natural world.

6. ***Earthing:*** is the art of grounding the human body into the energy field of the earth. The earth is a giant battery with a subtle electrical charge. We are bioelectrical beings. Every process in your body is one of frequency. With the exception of people living in industrialized societies, every living being on this planet is connected to the earth's energy field. Earthing is the technique of "grounding" your body into that energy field to restore coherence to your body's own electrical frequency.

There are many more tools, techniques and practices as unique as each one of us. Try them; explore what you resonate with, and what you don't. Keep what does resonate, then expand and allow the practice to transform you.

Over the next few pages, I expand on each of the above practices, so by the end of this book, you'll be well on your way to establishing mindfulness practices, either to build a more solid foundation, or to expand on the one you already have.

YOGA

Yoga is the intentional stopping of the mind stuff.

—*Joseph Campbell*

Yoga means union, the union of the individual soul with the universal supreme spirit, God, grace, the great originating mystery. It is the union of the seed of the self with the infinite truth, the ultimate reality. Yoga is a mindfulness practice; a pathway to your inner source and a path of remembering your Mighty self. Yet our human sensory experience limits our full understanding of this union. So for most of us, yoga is the path of union of body, mind and soul. Yoga is the intentional stopping of the mind stuff, but that is not the actual goal of yoga.

Yoga developed as a tool for the mind to anchor into the temple of the body as it surrenders to soul. The journey indeed is in and through the body, but originally yoga was intended as a science and a tool for the Mind. Ayurveda, the sister science of yoga, developed as a science and tool for the health of the body.

Your soul is the space of your luminosity and your inner source. The self is the source of infinite wisdom within you. It is not the individual mind, nor is it your body. It is the deep aspect within you that knows the truth, the quiet voice that guides and speaks to you when you look beyond the Ego. Eternal and infinite, it exists within each and every one of us. It is the seed of grace or God we all yearn to come home to.

Here in the West we have a different relationship and approach to yoga. We see it as a power class for the body, a sequence of postures that tone and exercise the body, but that was never the intention or the goal of the science of yoga.

We live in a world of duality, full of polarity and opposites. The pathway to union of that duality is at the heart of the path of yoga. Yoga is not just the practice of asana postures on the mat; it's the practice of transcending the duality, and becoming one with all.

There is only one source, but there are many paths to it. Within yoga, there are four main paths to the one source. As a spiritual seeker, you will most likely walk more than one path to suit where you are at.

Jnana Yoga: The Path of Wisdom

Jnana yoga is the path of the intellect. It is the path of reason, of questioning what is real and what is not, what is the self and what it is not. It is the path of knowledge.

Karma Yoga: The Path of Action (Selfless Service)

Karma yoga is the path of eliminating the Ego and attachments through selfless service to others without attachment to outcome. The goal of this path is the action of being in service. There is no ulterior motive, and the Ego is disengaged. This path creates no karma at all.

Bhakti Yoga: The Path of Devotion

Bhakti yoga is the path of prayer, worship of the divine, and the surrendering the self to a higher power or nature. It is the path of surrendering one's emotions into devotion. Praying, kirtan (devotional singing), chanting, rites, ritual, and temple life are all part of this path.

Raja Yoga: The Path of Mind Control

Raja yoga is the path of concentration and meditation. It starts with the physical body and connects us to the astral body. It is a path controlling the imprints, desires and illusions of the Mind as we come to discover—remember—our relation to the absolute. This path is "in and through" the body as a vehicle for enlightenment.

Hatha Yoga is an aspect of Raja yoga. Hatha yoga is the lineage that informs Iyengar yoga, Shivananda yoga, Ashtanga yoga, Kundalini yoga, Modo yoga, Bikram yoga, Anusara yoga amongst others. The yoga we have come to know here in the West stems from Hatha yoga.

Ha means sun, the sun of our bodies, and **Tha** means moon, our consciousness. Hatha yoga is the mystical union of the sun (our soul) and the moon (consciousness itself). Much like the energy of the sun our soul never fades. We might lose track of it, but it never fades. The energy of the moon fades in and out through its lunar cycle, yet it reminds us, that no matter which "phase we are in," we are always whole.

Your body has an energetic blueprint; an organizing principle that guides your journey of evolution. Time, your environment (space), and your unconscious habits have the power to shift you away from this energetic blueprint; away from your innate state of harmony into dis-ease. Hatha yoga offers a roadmap to realign yourself with your own unique energetic blueprint.

The **asana** aspect or limb of yoga are the postures we hold to become aware of ourselves and to move beyond our samaskaras (impressions of the mind left on the physical body). They are a mindfulness practice in movement. The postures help us to control our bodies, our breath in order to control our Minds. The postures also work in re-establishing the flow of energies and physical processes according to their proper balance, as well as assist the body in its purification processes of cleansing and rebuilding.

Asana facilitates the union of our Minds and bodies through mindful movements, providing stillness to the energy of consciousness that moves through us. As this stillness first extends, we root down in order to rise, then it expands from our core back to the layers of our skin and beyond, and soul begins to fill our entire body. At that very moment, we awaken to our essence, to our truth. At that very moment, *we remember who we are.*

The **pranayama** aspect of yoga, as I already mentioned, is the yogic science of breath control. Prana is our vital energy, and pranayama are deep breathing and breath control, prolongation and retention exercises that powerfully affect and control our Prana. Breath control and awareness of the rhythms of the breath are essential for consciousness to stillness. By controlling the breath we can control consciousness, and by controlling consciousness, we can control the breath.

Meditation practice is another aspect or limb of the science of yoga. It requires our concentration and focused awareness and is the portal through which we can enter samadhi or union with all.

Samadhi is your blissful ecstasy, the mystical union of the seed of grace within us with the absolute cosmic consciousness that created the universe; the divine marriage. Samadhi is beyond time and space, beyond word, beyond our senses, and beyond causality.

Through the path of yoga, union of body, mind and soul with the absolute divine, comes the ultimate freedom—the liberation of one's Mind from the attachments of the body, the ultimate source of our suffering.

Traditionally, yogis engage in asana prior to pranayama as to clear the sacred vessel (body and Mind) for the movement of Prana (intelligent life-force energy) and once the body and Mind have been purified and weaved by Prana, they would engage in deep meditation practices.

So in your personal practice, I invite you to do as the ancient yogis have done before you. First, mindfully move your body. Second, perform a few deep breathing exercises. Third, engage in your meditation practice. You might just find your monkey mind being less of a monkey, and you might just find yourself elated in pure bliss.

As I wrote in the section on shadow work (page 241), through your yoga practice you are constantly moving and engaging with the samaskaras or imprints of the Mind. They need to be consciously detoxified and cleared so as to create a solid foundation for your self; one that is congruent with your current emotional and belief systems.

Though we might begin our healing journey at the physical level, the root of what needs to be healed at this time lies deeper than that. The more you consciously move your body, the more you engage in breathing exercises that charge your body with Prana that bring in coherence and begin to shift the densities that need to be detoxified, the healthier your relationship to self and other will be.

Through your clearing of the samaskaras, you heal your body. You heal the seven generations that came before you, and have the power to affect the seven generations that will come after you, whether biological or not. Through your yoga practice, you begin to anchor your mind into your body as you unite them both with your heart. You begin to engage with the world through sacred action because you awaken to the sacred within you, to the mightiness you have always been and to the flow of grace or consciousness through you.

As you heal yourself, you heal the world.

PRANAYAMA

Breath is the bridge which connects life to consciousness, which unites your body to your thoughts.

—*Thích Nhất Hanh*

As you already know, *breath and consciousness are intimately interconnected.* The power of ***pranayama*** lies in our ability to control consciousness through the breath, and vice versa. Control may not be the right word to describe the depth of the experience. Through the breath you and I are able to know, taste, hear, smell, and feel consciousness. We are able to embody it, we are able to experience it and be moved by it.

Pranayama is a mindfulness practice that uses deep breathing and breath control, prolongation, and retention exercises to purify the body temple, draw the senses within, clear the Mind, amplify our energy field, and bring greater life force energy and, therefore, coherence into our whole-body system. The practice of pranayama requires our concentration and discipline.

If breath is the medium that weaves our bodies and Minds into our Hearts, we can then use our breath as a vehicle for our awakening. You and I can use our breath to align the weaving of our intentions with the expression of our actions. This can further bring into manifestation our potentiality and union with the seed of the divine within us, and the absolute divine without.

Ultimately, pranayama is actually not only about the control of the breath, it's about the control and enhancement of the Prana (life-force energy) in the body. The breath is just the vehicle through which Prana enters the body.

Swami Rama states that "*according to the science of Pranayama, disease is a manifestation of an imbalance in the flow of Prana...*"

So if we can shift, change, and perhaps infuse the force that animates us with life, perhaps we can also bring balance to the body by effectively guiding the breath and the flow of life-force energy that moves through us.

Because of its power, advanced pranayama technique should only be done under the supervision of a qualified teacher.

Breath has three components: inhalation, retention, and exhalation, with retention happening at the end of the inhale and the end of the exhale.

As you inhale, fill the body with Prana, extend through crown of the head, towards the world of spirit.

As you retain the breath after inhalation, allow Prana (divine intelligence) to find and penetrate your divine core.

As you exhale: expand from your core into the world, while holding on to the integrity of the extension and the coherence of the Prana.

As you retain after exhalation, surrender into stillness.

During the inhalation of the breath, we bring in our human potential, inspired by divine cosmic intelligence. During breath retention, our senses, speech, perception, thoughts, and feelings are controlled. We can separate ourselves from our stories, desires, and memories and infuse (charge) the core of our core with Prana.

During exhalation, we expand into the world with a new-found level of coherence and integrity as we also experience emptiness, as B. K. S. Iyengar states in his book, *Light on Life*, *"In exhalation we experience the empty 'I,' the divine void, a nothingness that is complete and perfect, a death that is not the end of life."* As we retain the breath after exhalation, we surrender into stillness.

Pranayama practices involve the control of these three components of the breath to create new rhythms within our system that allow for the separation of oxygen, and the integration of life-force energy contained in the breath.

Pranayama also uses three *locks* designed to draw the masculine and feminine forces within us into the central energy channel, and to raise the Kundalini energy up towards our third eye and crown chakras:

1. Anal lock (moola bandha): contract the anal sphincter muscles. Prevents the escape of Prana from the lower body.

2. Abdominal lock (uddiyana bandha): exhale completely and pull the lower abdomen—belly button—in and up / back towards the spine. This lifts the life-force energy up towards the main energy channel of our bodies.

3. Chin lock (jalandhara bandha): chin presses into chest. It prevents the Prana from escaping from the upper body.

A breath that focuses on the *inhalation* focuses on the upward, warming, invigorating, expanding nature of the inhalation, and will serve to energize and revitalize the body.

A breath that focuses on *retention* serves to clear emotions and the Mind, calm the nervous system, and promote healing and the integration of the life-force energy of the breath into our whole-body systems.

A breath that focuses on the *exhalation* focuses on the downward, cooling forces that are cleansing by nature. The exhalation supports all elimination and detoxification processes of the body, as well as the release of what is no longer needed in the system (emotional and mental densities). It also facilitates a deeper relaxation.

In the classical yogic tradition, there are eight main pranayamas, and many variations of each. Some of the more popular pranayamas are:

Cooling Pranayamas:

*   Ida Nadi Pranayama (Left Nostril Breathing), a variation of Nadi Shodana
*   Sitali Pranayama (Breath of Sweet Nectar)
*   Shitkari Pranayama (Hissing Breath)

Balancing Pranayamas:

*   Surya Bhedana /Nadi Shodhana (Channel of Purification Breathing). Or its variation, Anuloma-Viloma (Alternate Nostril Breathing)
*   Ujjayi Pranayama (Throat Breathing), though considered a balancing breath, it is slightly heating
*   Bhramari Pranayama (Breath of a Humming Bee)

Heating Pranayamas:

- Pingala Nadi Pranayama (Right Nostril Breathing), a variation of Nadi Shodana
- Bhastirka Pranayama (Bellows Breathing) Or its variation, Kapalabhati Pranayama (Fire Breath)

In the Pachakuti Mesa Shamanic tradition of South America, breath is used to cleanse and clear dense energy from the body system, fortify the energy of the system by deliberate intake of Prana and make the healer a better carrier of spirit medicine. *There are five pranayamas or Hampikamayoq breath techniques.*

1. *Breath of Community or Common Unity:* (5-5-5)

- Inhale for 5 seconds, hold for 5 seconds, exhale for 5 seconds
- Inhale again for 5 seconds
- 4-breath cycle per minute
- Repeat for 5–15 minutes

This is actually the first breath technique or pranayama I teach anyone who starts working with me. I find most of us are so stressed out we are not easily able to do this breath pattern to the count of five seconds, which means we are holding so much stress in our body that the breath cannot enter the depths it is intended to enter. This breath should be done without any strain, before moving into any other of the breathing techniques. With this breath, we are starting the process of clearing the body, calming and anchoring the mind into the body.

2. *Wave Breath:* (7-7)

- Inhale and exhale to the count of 7 seconds, with no retention of the breath
- Inhale for 7 seconds, exhale for 7 seconds, inhale again for 7 seconds, and so on
- Create a wave-like pattern with your breath, with no pause in between breaths, and no retention
- 4 breath cycle per minute
- Repeat for 5-15 minutes

This is a cleansing, purifying breath. Imagine inhaling life-force energy into your body, and spreading this energy throughout your body with each exhalation.

3. *Kawsay Energy Breath:* (7-7-7)

- Inhale for 7 seconds, hold for 7 seconds, exhale for 7 seconds
- Inhale again for 7 seconds and so on
- 3-breath cycle per minute
- Repeat for 5–15 minutes

Kawsay is the living essence of all life, the life-force energy. Kawsay energy breath helps connect you to the awareness of energy flow through your body. When using this breath:

- Imagine the energy of the earth entering your body through the soles of your feet as you inhale
- As you hold, the breath spreads through your body
- As you exhale, the breath returns to the earth, carrying with it any densities or impurities along the way

4. *Sami Energy Breath: (10-10-10)*

- Inhale for 10 seconds, hold for 10 seconds, exhale for 10 seconds
- Inhale again for 10 seconds and so on
- 2-breath cycle per minute
- Repeat for 5–15 minutes

Sami refers to a more refined, subtle aspect of life-force energy. This breath activates psi sensitivity, and the capacity for precognition and creative discernment. It allows us as healers to infuse the energetic imprint of the other person. When using this breath:

- Imagine energy coming straight into the back of your heart (the seventh thoracic vertebrae) or your left palm
- As you hold the breath, feel it circulate within you
- As you exhale, feel it pumping through your body
- Feel your heartbeat expand through your whole body and/or imagine/feel the energy travel through your right hand into yourself, or another person

5. *K'anchay Energy Breath:* (20-20-20) Advanced Breath.

- Inhale for 20 seconds, hold for 20 seconds, exhale for 20 seconds
- Inhale again for 20 seconds and so on

- 1-breath cycle per minute
- Repeat for 5–15 minutes

K'anchay refers to the highest form of spiritual energy. This breath induces spiritual illumination, mystical transcendence, and invites us to become the light. When using this breath:

Imagine energy coming into your body through the top of your head, third eye, and nape of the neck or your left hand.

As you hold, feel it circulate within you.

As you exhale, feel it dissolve into the physical outline of your body, or imagine/feel it move through your right hand to the other person and dissolve into the physical outline of their body.

K'anchay is an advanced breath technique, and should only be attempted when one has been practicing long enough, and consistently enough, to have expanded their lung capacity and have created a strong foundation for ourselves to hold the power of the life-force energy we are bringing in and activating within us. If and when you are able to do Sami energy breath comfortably, begin to expand it to the count of 16, then 17, and so on, until you are comfortable at the count of 20. At no point should you be forcing the retention of the breath. Work consistently with discipline and you will get there.

My mighty reader, knowing what you now know about your body and your healing journey, can you begin to use breath practices to facilitate greater healing in your body?

Let me plant some seeds for thought in you. Can you cool you down your body if you are hot or dealing with heat-related inflammatory issues? Can you still and anchor your mind into your body through balancing breaths if you are dealing with anxiety, sleep issues, overwhelmment, or simply want to create more balance in your life? Can you use heating breaths if you are dealing with circulatory issues, constipation, or need to ignite your passions again? Do you see how you can use your own power to ignite your mighty inner healer through your mighty breath? Pst … it's free.

This is just an introduction to the mindfulness practice of pranayama, which can take many years to learn and develop. It is best studied with a teacher, and I do include it in the programs I teach. If you visit www.natyhoward.com, you will find information there about my course programs. If you live in an area where you cannot find a teacher, there are also many books that will provide you with more in depth information and instruction, and you will find them at the back of this book.

MEDITATION

Quiet the mind, and the soul will speak.

— *Ma Jaya Sati Bhagavati*

Meditation is the practice of bearing witness to one's Mind and one's self. The path of mindfulness meditation observes the nature of our experience. It observes awareness and the object of awareness. It observes the nature of a feeling, thought, or sensation. It tries to stay objective, non-reactive—meaning non-attached to the story or to what you become aware of.

Meditation is the process of quieting the Mind in order to transcend it. It is the process through which you and I become intimate with our self as a pathway of liberation from the clutches of the senses, and the subconscious and unconscious mind. It is by transcending our fears, desires, longings, our shit, negative emotions, and ancestral and personal "stories" that we are able to reach a super-conscious state that allows us to identify with the all-blissful higher self. In this state, there is now awareness of both our body and Mind (or duality), and through this state we are able to integrate body and Mind with soul, transcending our duality and therefore *becoming* *one* *with the universe.*

To harness the potential energy of your becoming, you must go within; you must connect, you must create sacred space within. You must tap into your heart and listen. It will speak and, if you allow, it will sing through you. Going within builds an intimate connection with the seat of your intuitive wisdom.

This feeling of intimacy is of key value when in the process of aligning yourself with your true nature. Somewhere along the process of reconnecting and giving your self the sacred space to unfold, your heart opens and you also hear the call of the earth to reclaim your lost intimacy with her.

As you pause and feel, you begin to reclaim the fragmented pieces of your Self, you begin to weave the wisdom of your Heart and the ancestral knowing of your Mind, you being to unfold into the emergence of your true potential, and your life becomes a living sanctuary and a living prayer for peace.

The goal of meditation is to attain an inner state of awareness and activate your personal and spiritual growth process. Through your consistent and dedicated practice, you journey from your Mind into your Heart, from thinking into feeling, from the outer layers of your body to being rooted into source and anchored into your centre.

Our meditation practice is the vehicle through which we create space in between our thoughts, as we notice the nature of our thoughts and witness our thoughts. The longer you stay in the practice, the more you are able to connect with your breath, stay unattached to your thoughts, and the more space between your thoughts begins to occur. You got it! The more you are accessing stillpoint awareness.

Come to your sacred space around the same time every day. Meditation is not just meant to be fit in whenever possible, not another chore, another thing to do … it is your precious time to self-nourish. It is a formal practice, and a tool of deepening that needs its own dedicated time and space, so that your body begins to surrender, to relax and trust you again.

The more you visit your sacred space, the more your cells will instantly relax into a deeper state, and the easier your practice of tuning in to self-inquiry will become. I'm not saying that what will arise will be easy, for sometimes it's not. But because it has risen, now it can be seen and released. This is your time to process the day or the dream state; your time to integrate and to hear your voice, your higher self, and dream yourself alive for the next day.

There are numerous meditation techniques, but they all encourage us to use our concentrated focus on something such as a sound, image, breath, or feeling in order to free one's self from distractions, and then relax into the spaces in between these. If you are new to meditation, start with the simpler techniques here described; choose one practice for a particular set of time. Give each one a week, and feel the deepening in your process. If you already have a meditation practice, then play and invite curiosity to guide your next step.

A note on posture: The posture of your body during your meditation practice is essential. It is the vehicle that will carry you through, so please begin your practice with the correct posture to support your practice. So let's break it down:

- Sit on a meditation cushion on the floor, or on a chair with your back straight
- If using a cushion, sit cross-legged. If sitting in a chair, sit with your feet touching the ground (barefooted would be great), back supported by the back of the chair
- Whether on cushion or chair, scoop your tailbone, draw your belly in and up towards your spine, begin to stack your upper body (shoulder blades move up, then behind you,

and down with the intention of touching each other to lift the heart space). Tuck your chin slightly

- Elongate and extend your spine through the top of your head towards the ceiling
- Hands can be on your lap, palms face up to *receive* energy from the world of heaven, or facing down to "ground and feel supported" by the world of earth
- Take a few deep breaths to ground yourself before you begin any of the meditation practices that follow
- Begin by connecting with your sacred meditation space
- Gently close your eyes

A note on thinking: If you become aware of your thoughts, just acknowledge them and come back to your breath. Don't get caught up in them, or start berating yourself with *here I go again*, but rather acknowledge *oh, there is a thought*, and come back to your breath. So, if you find yourself *thinking*, root into self-compassion, and begin the practice again. Like anything, practice will allow you to dive deeper to the place where counting may not be necessary at all to be present with your breath. If you are able, please practice for at least five minutes, and then expand your practice to twenty or even forty minutes, daily.

Meditation through sound: repetition of a mantra (seed sound), word, specific sound to guide your mind into focus. Some powerful mantras are: Om, Hum, So'ham, Shanti, HU. These sounds are done on an extended out-breath, on any note. Allow the vibration of the drawn-out word to resonate through the cells of your body.

Meditation through gazing: look at an actual object or image with eyes open, yet using a soft gaze. The object can be the flame of a candle, flowers, a crystal, a statue or image of Buddha or Jesus or your spiritual guide, or a picture of an object.

Meditation through visualization: picture an object with your eyes closed, such as a lotus flower, or the energy points in the body (chakras).

Meditation through breath: this meditation is different from the deep breathing exercises I wrote about previously. Our intention is to follow the inner movements of the breath through this technique. Let's try it:

- Focus your awareness on your breath. Do not hold your breath
- Observe and follow the movement of your breath as you inhale and exhale
- As you lengthen the time of your inhalation and exhalation, observe and feel the subtleties of the inner space through which the breath moves through you

Meditation through breathing patterns: through this technique, you follow the pattern of your breath to enter the meditative state, such as inhale for the *Breath of Community* (5-5-5). See page 256 for more complete descriptions of breath work through breath patterns

Meditation through breath counting:

- Follow the *Breath of Community* (page 256) for ten rounds as your first step for this technique. The breath to the pattern of 5-5-5 is a powerful beginning for this meditation practice
- Begin to count your breaths. Perhaps visualize a number in your mind's eye, or use your hearing to count the breaths
- If you become aware of your thinking, let it go, and begin to count again. The action of counting keeps your mind engaged and focused; it actually doesn't matter if you repeat the same number or if you count down from 100. All that matters is that you keep your mind engaged with something other than a thought process
- Practice for at least five minutes
- Gently open your eyes

Meditation through feeling the energy body:

- Follow the *Breath of Community* (page 256) for ten rounds as your first step for this technique. The breath to the pattern of 5-5-5 is a powerful beginning for this meditation practice
- Bring your hands to touch in front of your solar plexus
- Rub the palms of your hands together until you feel heat emanating from your palms.
- Now stop, gently open your palms two inches apart from each other (still facing each other), and focus on the sensation of warmth/heat/magnetism you feel between them
- Focus your attention on the sensation between the palms of your hands. This is your luminous energy body
- As you inhale, slowly move your palms away from each other, palms still facing each other. As you exhale, slowly bring your palms closer together, without touching
- As you inhale, move your palms apart and feel the magnetism or energy field expand. As you exhale, bring your palms closer together but not touching, and feel the magnetism or energy field contract
- Begin to "play" with your energy field. Feel it expand and contract with each deep inhale and exhale
- Continue focusing on your energy body
- If you lose the sensation, start again from the beginning

- If you can't feel it yet, go through the exercise anyway and imagine that you do; soon enough, you will!
- Practice for at least five minutes. Then gently lower your hands to your knees, take a few deep breaths. Bring your palms together in front of your heart, gently tuck your chin to your neck to seal the benefits of this practice
- Gently open your eyes

Heaven and Earth meditation:

- Follow the *Breath of Community* (page 256) for ten rounds as your first step for this technique. The breath to the pattern of 5-5-5 is a powerful beginning for this meditation practice
- Continue to inhale and exhale deeply without breath retention
- Connect with the energy of the earth. Feel (imagine) the energy of the earth coming into your body through your feet, through your sit bone, and moving upwards towards the crown of your head
- Feel (imagine) it leave your body towards the heavens through the top of your head
- Feel the energy of the earth leave its imprint of support, wholesomeness, and being grounded upon your body
- Feel (imagine) this energy creating a silver beam (column) of light from the earth to the heavens
- Now bring your attention to the crown of your head
- Feel (imagine) heavenly cosmic energy come into your body through the crown of your head
- Feel (imagine) it move downward through your body, all the way down to your feet, as if creating a golden beam of light connecting heaven and earth through your body, it being the sacred vehicle for this connection to happen
- Feel (imagine) this heavenly cosmic energy healing your body
- Repeat the whole visualization three times
- Take a few deep breaths. Gently tuck your chin to your neck to seal the benefits of this practice
- Gently open your eyes

SHAMANISM

Shamanism is not a religion. It is a spiritual practice grounded in a reverent awareness that the world is animated, conscious, and energetically interdependent. A Shaman is one who develops a personal and intimate relationship with the Unseen world for the purpose of being of service as a healer. This relationship is cultivated experientially through self-induced altered states of consciousness, ritual, ceremony, and refined energetic awareness.

—*Don Oscar Miro-Quesada*

Shamanism is an ancient practice of *direct revelation*, of being in relationship with the inner space of wisdom through engagement with the world of the seen and the unseen, in sacred reciprocity.

Through shamanism, we awaken to the power of the Elements in sacredness. We awaken to the need for ritual and ceremony in our everyday lives, the need for creating beauty in the world, and the need to be a part of a greater sacred web as we weave the fragmented pieces of ourselves into wholeness. Shamanism offers us the opportunity to live mindfully in sacred relationship. The subtle shifts in energy we experience through that awareness alone can cause miracles.

Within shamanism, we have tools and practices that further our alignment with our self, that mindfully move us into greater awareness of our *story*, our actions, greater alignment with our wisdom and our truth and, potentially, greater integration with the inner space of stillness, the inner space of source. The Hampikamayoq energy breathing techniques (page 256) I described previously are some of those tools, as is shamanic journeying.

A shamanic journey is a guided meditative visualization to the beat of the drum or another binaural sound that focuses on the details of the *story*. As we follow it into the subconscious mind, we bypass the *noise* of our conscious mind and access the seat of our intuitive wisdom. Shamanic journeys allow us to gain further insight or awareness of our present condition, therefore becoming more mindful of our choices and actions at the present moment.

Mindfulness is at the root of shamanism, for one cannot live in sacred reciprocity of the world within, without, seen, and unseen if one is unaware of one's self. Shamanism, the art of direct revelation, is also the art of mindfully living in reverence, anchored in sacredness as we awaken, give shape to and embrace our Mighty inner healer.

FOREST BATHING

Thousands of tired, nerve-shaken, over-civilized people are beginning to find out that going to the mountains is going home. Wilderness is a necessity.

—*John Muir, Our National Parks.*

Forest bathing or Shinrin-yoku therapy is the art of returning to when we knew how to be at one with nature. It is the art of going to a forest, walking slowly, opening your senses, and both breathing in and basking in the healing medicine nature offers. It is the art of taking in the atmosphere of the forest, the beauty, the peace, the magic, and the benefits that await you.

Forest bathing has become a cornerstone of preventative health care and healing in Japanese medicine. A robust body of scientific literature now exists to support and prove the benefits of forest bathing for our healing and well-being.

The key to accessing the gifts of forest bathing lies in allowing nature to enter into your heart through your senses. Listen to the birds sing and the wind rustling the leaves of the trees; feel the sunlight caress your skin; smell the fresh, clear air of the forest. Take a few deep breaths. Inhale wellness. Exhale joy, peace, and happiness. Inhale connectivity to all beings. Exhale separation. Inhale empowerment. Exhale stress. Inhale wholeness. Exhale gratitude. Continue to use your senses and your breath to cross the bridge to happiness and well-being as you activate your cells and your DNA into vibrant health.

Some benefits of Shinrin-yoku therapy are:

- Boosts immune system functioning by increasing in the count of your body's natural killer (NK) cells
- Cleanses and opens your senses
- Reduces blood pressure, stress, and symptoms of depression
- Improves mood, the ability to focus, vitality, and sense of well-being
- Increases flow of energy (Prana/life-force energy) in your body, sense of happiness, and connection to life
- Accelerates your healing processes
- Deepens intuition and brings you back to stillpoint present moment awareness

We all know how good it feels to be in nature. We've always known. The problem is, most of us in North America spend 93% of our time indoors. And though our ancestors lived on the land, in constant communion with the land, the trees, and the forest, we do not.

Imagine yourself walking in a forest. Imagine the scent of the forest, the sound of the leaves rustling in the wind, the fresh clean air, and the sense of being uplifted that you feel deep within. Our imagination is powerful, but even more powerful is to gift yourself the opportunity to experience the benefits of forest bathing first hand. So dear friend, come on. *The forest awaits you. Our DNA awaits to commune with the forces of nature the way our ancestors did.*

EARTHING

Always double up on happiness.

—*My friend, Lee Richmond*

Why would you only bask in the beauty and medicine of the forest when you can also ground into the energy of the earth at the same time, allowing you to double up on the powers that can restore the harmony and coherence of your own energy field?

It just gets better and better.

Earthing is a fast-growing movement based on the discovery that reconnecting to the earth's energy field is foundational for vibrant health. It's now been proven that being indoors and isolated from the earth by non-conductive materials—such as rubber and plastic (our shoes), wood, plastic, laminate and asphalt (flooring surfaces)—leads to fatigue, feelings of isolation and separation, and sometimes depression.

Earthing is also known as grounding for its ability to ground our body's energy field and nervous system as they merge with the energy field of the earth. Remember, you and I are electrical beings always emitting a frequency that must be coherent in order for us to experience well-being. Should disharmony occur, this frequency can be shifted back into coherence through resonance.

Think of your internal "wellness battery" as rechargeable. We have two polarities, and in order to re-charge our battery, we must connect with the greatest charger ever. For us to regain our sense of vitality and well-being, we literally have to plug in into the energy field that supports us. If we don't, our battery will always be running on half-charge.

Just like the sun is an energy source, the earth too is a source of subtle energy that contributes to our optimum health. Earthing can be achieved a number of ways, but *your skin must have direct contact with the ground.* You can stand, sit, lie or walk—but your skin must always be in contact with the ground. So, yes, there is nothing quite like walking barefoot in the forest. Try it. You might just love it as much as I do!

When your body has direct contact with the earth, it's being infused with negative-charged free electrons from the earth's surface. This brings the electric energy levels of the human body into harmony with those of the earth, and this promotes your sense of vitality and well-being, synchronizes hormonal cycles, and balances your physiological rhythms with those of the earth.

I keep having to ask you. Do you remember way back when I wrote about the root cause of the root causes of disease?

I seem to go back to it quite often.

In this modern world, we have largely forgotten our primordial nature. Do you think perhaps earthing might assist you in not only remembering your primordial nature, but also synchronizing your bodily rhythms to those rhythms of nature that are so key to restoring the health of your body system?

I think you are just about to double up on you health and your happiness!

IF YOU HAVE A MIND, YOU HAVE A MISSION

You have to find what sparks a light in you so that you in your own way can illuminate the world.

—*Oprah Winfrey*

I return now to an early inquiry: ***Is your mind full, or is it empty?***

Pause and feel.

Perhaps now inquire deeper into the nature of what your mind is full of, or empty of?

Pause and feel.

If you have a Mind, you have a mission.

You and I were given our mind to help fulfil our mission. When you and I are able to clear our mind of enough of the noise we carry, when we've liberated the mind enough from the hold our subconscious and unconscious mind have on us, when we consciously choose the content of what we will fill our minds and our hearts back with, then and only then, we will have enough clarity of mind to remember our mission.

Clarity of mind comes when you begin to consciously fill your mind back up with that which lifts you up, that which empowers you, that which stems from your true nature, from your intuitive wisdom, from the field of your potentiality.

Mindfulness practices allow you to change the chemistry of your brain, which then changes the body memory of your emotions, and alters the expression of the current conditions your body systems are in. You are, in fact, the master of your body, and the master of your mind. These practices are meant to integrate our fragmentation, providing us a space to pause and feel, a safe space to deeply heal, as we emerge with clear mind and purpose in our heart.

Coherent action can only come when you have access to the space of clear mind. And we can only offer it in sacred reciprocity, once we have rooted into sacredness, into love, and into peace.

The path to remembering your mission has to be sustainable, has to continue to power you up, ignite your transformation, and spark your revolution. So engage your self-care muscle, and bask your body temple with deep nourishment as you continue to create a strong foundation that will allow you to shine. Become the health warrior of peace you have been searching for. Awaken and ignite the mightiness that has always been in you, and remember your mission.

Root down in order to rise. Empty what doesn't serve you. Fill yourself up with the quality of coherent action you seek, which is equally seeking you and that may cause miracles. Allow for your mission to emerge from the space of clear mind. *Own your greatness. Claim your magic.*

ROOT TO RISE

When the roots are deep, there is no reason to fear the wind.

—Chinese Proverb

In yoga, in order to come into the depth of alignment necessary for the fullest expression of a pose, we must root down and create a stable solid foundation with whatever part of the body is touching the ground. This allows you and I to bring our whole body into oneness as we open our hearts to basking in our own medicine. **Root to rise** is an expression, and the best possible way I can end this chapter on the art of mindfulness. Are you ready to root to rise to greatness?

Mindfulness is not about getting out of our body and living in the world of heaven. Although it might sometimes seem nice to escape our reality, it's never really a way that will lead us to happiness. In fact, it's quite the opposite. Mindfulness practices are meant to root you down so deeply into your body, connecting you into your core and the core of the earth and into your present moment, that you embody the fullness of your presence and become one with all that is.

Rooting down creates mindfulness. It allows us space to pause, feel, connect, empower, ignite, and spark our path. Rooting down allows us to consciously choose our intention, and come back into alignment with our actions. Rooting down allows us to move beyond our fears into facing everything and rising beyond them, beyond our wildest dreams. It allows us to integrate our body, heart, mind, and soul with spirit, as a single force greater than the sum of its parts.

We build our foundation always from the ground up. Both the stability and quality of your efforts in solidifying your foundation are vital to building a strong, wise, stable, balanced, harmonious, coherent, and lasting structure on top. What kind of structure are you building right now? What kind of life are you giving expression to right now? *And is it the life you want?*

It's not only important to build a stable and strong foundation, it must be rooted so deeply into the earth that it is unshakeable yet malleable and flexible enough to withstand the winds that may come our way. The winds of fads and change are strong, my friends. The winds of health challenges are even stronger. The universe is demanding that we show up, ignite our Mighty inner healer, and begin to shine as we expand our own grace, our own beauty, our own magic, and gift our own medicine as part of our personal process of evolution. But, equally as important, as part of the evolution of all life on earth.

When you first begin, it may not be easy to *show up*. I get it. But we must, for our health and happiness—indeed, our very survival—are on the line. I believe myself to be an optimist, and as such I must make sure I'm creating with my feet on the ground as I reach out and shine. If not, I run the risk of living in the denial of the past, or the future.

Remember to always create stability over flexibility. Always root to rise. Always ground, as you extend and then expand. Always, in all ways, pause and feel your way through the many ways, tools and practices that can power up your health, ignite your transformation and spark your revolution.

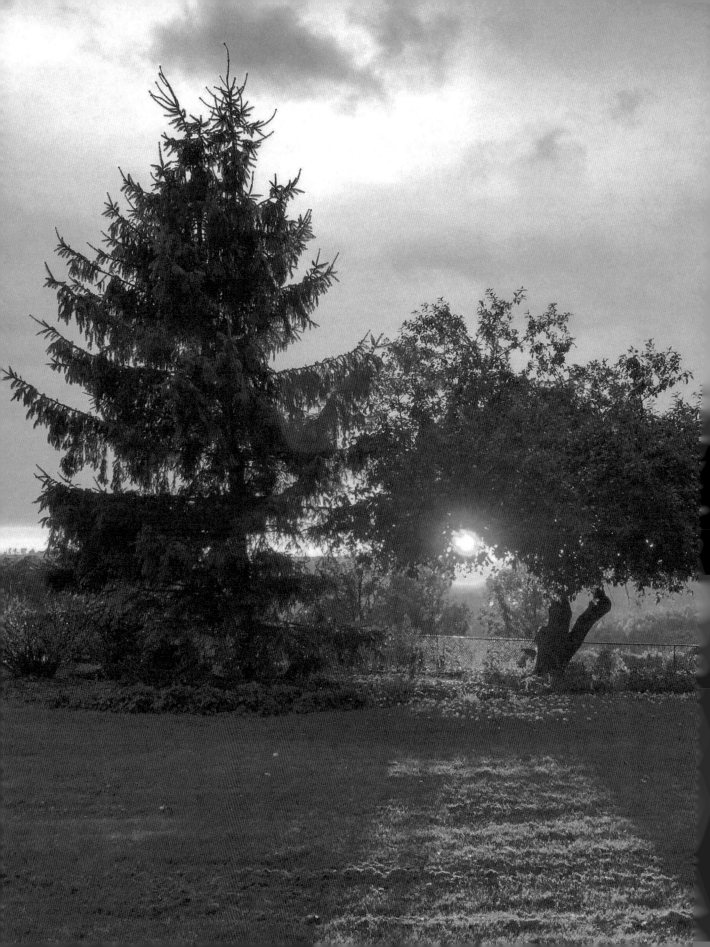

VII

THE ALCHEMY OF
INNER QUESTING

RIGHT ACTION
BORNE OF COMPASSIONATE
SPIRITUAL WISDOM,
UNITES.

—DON OSCAR MIRO-QUESADA

BIOGRAPHY OF OUR LINEAGE

When we learn about our past, we gather strength for the future.

—*Hank Smith*

Our ancestry is written in every fibre of our bodies, from our physical expression to our most intimate emotional landscape. Our history will continue to write us, unless we choose to be the ones to write our stories. *That choice will change everything.*

The ***biography of our lineage*** is an important piece in our own evolution because as we begin and continue to take responsibility over it, *we reclaim our power.* As you and I begin to make peace with it, we can begin to understand and become more aware of our conditioning and of our own stories, and by doing this we begin to reclaim our wholeness. For we can never be whole if we continue to push away, deny, and crucify our ancestry.

When you tap within, are you able to notice some of your ancestral patterns expressing themselves through you? Are you able to see how they affect you, and how they still hold power over you? Are you able to bear witness to how much these ancestral patterns are your own? Can you begin to recognize the great grandmother's thread that weaves itself from your ancestry through your heart?

It's important to recognize the ancestral patterns you carry. It's also important to understand where those patterns came from, and how the seven generations that have come before you really shape, define and run through you. This very realization can be hard to surrender to, I get it. Yet the understanding and compassion that comes can help empower you to change, and then write your own story with awareness of your actions, knowing the power it will have upon the seven generations to come. *It is here, in the power of our actions, and the empowerment our choices can create, that we can find self-liberation and true freedom.*

How can I begin to bring awareness to my true inner voice?

This is the quintessential question. How do we connect with that inner space of truth within our self, our true inner voice that stems from the well of our ancestral wisdom?

The answer: *one breath at a time.* We do this one brief moment of awareness at a time. One realization of our power at a time, one heartbeat, one moment of stillness after another, one felt sense experience of sorrow, one felt experience of bliss, one felt sense experience of the depth of the ancestral wound, and the grace.

The more we begin to show up regularly for ourselves through mindfulness practices such as meditation, yoga, nature awareness, art, or creative expression, the more our true inner voice will begin to communicate through us. The more we will hear our true voice within the boundaries of our own skin. The more we will recognize the space of our true inner voice as our heart compass, and the more we'll develop the ability to access our own true inner voice at will.

Our ancestry carries within it both its wisdom, but also its wound. The shadow aspects of our ancestral lines also become embedded into every cell of who we are. Whether we like it or not, are ready to face it or not, the shadow aspects of our ancestral lines are at the core of our current foundation and current operating system.

Everything affects everything else, and everything is interconnected.

Our tribe often acts as the early onset of our lessons on earth, thus providing our values, understanding, and existence or lack of healthy emotional boundaries. They set the example that we will either accept, reject, or work through for the rest of our lives. Perhaps we can see it as a mad laboratory experiment that sets off the wheels of karma, cause and effect, and our own path of growth and liberation. And that sets the boundaries that will define our Heart and our emotional self, until we become conscious of our power to change and define our Heart and our emotional self on our own terms.

It is important to understand what has set our karmic conditions into play, and fully understand our biological ancestral lineage, in order to gain full access to the depth of our own *story*. We may or may not have a biological bond to our family of origin, but this biological bond gets established even when adopted children come into the family that will raise them and support them, and with whom they will build energetic bonds.

As part of our process, we begin to inquire. What kind of inner landscape does our ancestral self hold within the boundaries of our skin? What kind of hold does it have on our Hearts? What kind of boundaries and limited beliefs does it still anchor us to? We begin to inquire about the positive or negative influences of our ancestral lines on our current emotional inner landscape.

ANCESTRAL WOUND

Sometimes it's the scars that remind you that you survived. Sometimes the scars tell you that you have healed.

—Ashley D. Wallis

The depth of the wound our ancestral lines carry is the depth of the unconscious severing both we and our ancestors have cut away from our wholeness, away from our true inner selves.

Because of the disconnect from the wisdom of our ancestral lineages, we unconsciously negate a core part of our foundation, which also unconsciously negates the wholeness of our true inner self. As a result, we unconsciously stop absorbing the depth of self-nourishment that ancestral wisdom offers, that we desperately need and are seeking.

We negate to give the space of flow to our true inner voices, and, through our body, resentment, anger, and the shadow of our ancestral wound begin to shape our emotional self. But it's by honouring of the shadow of our ***ancestral wound*** that we root further down into reverence, into truth, into sacred conscious action, into rebuilding our lineages in sacredness and deep respect for one another for the seven generations to come.

Complicated, I know. Both our shadow self and the shadow of our ancestral lineage carry with them *density or Hucha* that begins to solidify in our body systems, and that must be addressed for our healing. Until we surrender, truly honour our roots, and arrive anew with the seed of reverence awakened in our hearts, we will not be healing the wound of our ancestral lineages to the depth that we seek healing in our lives. We cannot change our history, but we can honour our roots so as not to repeat it.

As we more consciously choose to heal, to reclaim our wholeness, and to address what hasn't been addressed before, and as we more consciously choose to create healthier boundaries by following our inner voice and tapping into the essence of who we truly are, then we'll be able to move through the emotions that have always limited our healing, and allow the harmful emotional energy to finally be released.

We've become very adept at hiding the harmful energy from this emotional discordance deep into our cellular anatomy in order to create the illusion of being safe. Yet by doing so, we have only further harmed ourselves. We have held onto this poison, and now it's time to release it in order to become whole and truly find the liberation our heart needs.

The current feelings of anger and resentment, of blame and shame are not new to us, but now the universe conspires for us to take a deeper look within. Are we going to hold on to them? Are we going to let them continue to define our emotional landscape? Or, are we ready to get out of our own way and surrender into flow?

We have the ability to know now (and feel it in our bones) that we have created a *safe* space within our Heart where we can self-support ourselves, even when life brings us situations that cause those feelings to rise again within us. Through word and density / Hucha burning ceremony, we consciously have the power to release them (page 307). We have the ability to create the space of safety within our each and every cell. And so, in the name of love, we must gift ourselves that which we are willing to gift to others.

Whether you believe it or not, we live in sacred reciprocity, in relationship with all life in both the seen and the unseen worlds. And while we may think we are individuals living in an individualistic world, our world, in fact, is a universal one. In order to open our heart to the vastness, richness, abundance, love, and compassion of the universe, we must first make peace with our ancestral lineage. Their wisdom creates our bridge into the universe, a gateway into universal consciousness, and to living from a place of expression of our highest potential.

So as we begin to connect with our ancestral lineage—with both their wounds and their wisdom, we begin to connect with the names, stories, characters, constellations, and patterns that make us who we are, and with the life that has been lived before us. We begin to connect with all of life. We begin to access the awareness that we are all interconnected. Actually *all is interconnected with the all.*

We perhaps will begin to surrender to the awareness that our interconnectedness *exists in sacred reciprocity to all.*

PEACE WITH OUR ANCESTRY AND OUR EMOTIONS

Courage is the price that life exacts for granting peace.

—*Amelia Earhart*

So what can we do with all that emotional weight we feel? Put it on paper! It's time to give it a space outside your body, and remember this is a process that may need to be done more than once. Perform the *Hucha (density) ceremony* monthly (page 307), use *mindfulness practices*, become aware of what you carry, so you can release, transform, surrender, and integrate the teachings into your core. Connect with the world of spirit, and through your reconnection begin to witness the small miracles.

You are here, tapping deeper into your quest for personal liberation. Take some time to connect deeply with what you are grateful for. Revisit the strengths that have come out of your own story. We are a product of the seven generations that have come before us, but what beauty, what gifts, what strength, and what growth have these seven generations given you? *Because they have also given you that.*

What awakenings have you had in your own personal life because of the choices and actions those generations consciously and unconsciously choose? Can you stand barefoot upon the earth and feel the pulse of love beating through your own heart, even at the hardest of times? Can you now tap into her support and feel the grace that comes as we take ownership of our lives, and of our karma?

Making peace with our ancestral lineage means making peace with our family. Making peace with our origins and with the portal that has made us who we are, in all of our expression. Making peace with our ancestral lineage also begins the process of shifting our awareness from the individual self to the universal self, a process that may take the rest of our lives to journey through.

As we come to terms with our ancestral lineage, we also begin to make peace with our emotions, with the patterns that have moved through us and continue to shape who we are today. Making peace with our emotions is a process. Understanding where our strengths and weaknesses, negative behaviours, and emotional patterns come from takes work. But it's a very big step in empowering ourselves to find the tools and processes we need to manage them, and a big step in becoming aware that our emotions and behaviours are not who we are.

The process of making peace with our ancestral lineage and our emotions allows us to *feel* and flow with the depth of the feeling, without storing the emotional residue at a cellular level. Making peace with our ancestral lineage brings us the gift of accessing stillpoint awareness. We no longer need to carry our emotional baggage, nor the baggage of those who have walked before us, for we begin to find spaces outside our selves where we can gently place our emotions. Knowing we are safe to feel allows us to feel rather than freeze; knowing we can trust ourselves and our own evolution allows us the gift of the present.

SPIRAL INTO AWAKENING

Energy moves in cycles, circles, spirals, vortexes, whirls, pulsations, waves, and rhythms—rarely if ever in simple straight lines.

—Starhawk, The Earth Path: Grounding Your Spirit in the Rhythms of Nature.

Our movement along the ***spiritual path is a spiral;*** moving from the outer rims of our perceptions, through the innermost sacred chambers of our Heart, into the core of our core—the spaces in between that hold us together. It's a fine balance between matter (mass) and spirit (energy). Its elemental or subtle energy sources are always being converted into cellular material and body tissue, and vice-versa.

The spiral gathers the mass of our outer expression into the world, and converts it into the more subtle aspects of our relationship with spirit, consciousness itself, the sacred vessel that contains our experience. At the same time, it gathers together our own core beliefs about ourselves and the world, and converts them into our physical reality.

This movement happens simultaneously, and is interdependent. Thus, it is extremely important to become aware of our subtle energies, or the ways in which we are feeling the world energetically, the ways in which we interpret our experiences, as well as our core beliefs about ourselves and others. As you see, our biography becomes our biology, and our biology further reinforces our biography.

Our spiritual path to becoming our mightiness is all about moving from our human potential towards higher consciousness. The more we purify our living sanctuaries (whole-body system), the more we bring awareness to our path, the more we become conscious of our thoughts, our beliefs, and our actions into the world, the more we will have access to higher levels of consciousness and the more these higher levels of consciousness will begin to shape shift our whole-body systems and change our lives.

Our journey along the spiritual path is to awaken our understanding that we are soul having a human experience. To understand that our purpose is to learn about *love* and our mission is to *share it.* To become aware that our path is one to be lived in sacred reciprocity with ***all life,*** with both seen and unseen forces, Mother Earth, and all beings. This reciprocal living requires us to live in balance with our visionary knowledge, compassionate love, and right action.

Although our journey requires us to engage with spiritual and metaphysical realities to get to know ourselves more intimately and understand our source, it's the very act of anchoring into the physical world that allows us to evolve. We must grow roots deep into Mother Earth in order to reach for the stars.

The process of awakening into your mightiness follows the ***spiral-like*** force of awakening that begins in and through our physical reality (body, challenges, pain) and moves into our heart (emotions, trauma), challenges our beliefs and our relationship with spirit, and opens our mind to the greater universal mind and to our higher self, away from ego, as it anchors us deeply into the space of soul.

Each direction of the spiral is in relationship to an element (are you surprised?), and in relationship with one of the five bodies (are you now going whhhhhaaaatttt?)—I know. I did that too when I first found out.

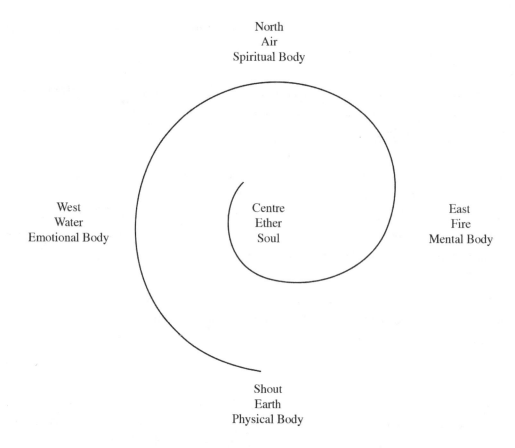

North
Air
Spiritual Body

West
Water
Emotional Body

Centre
Ether
Soul

East
Fire
Mental Body

Shout
Earth
Physical Body

Spiral of Awakening. Pachakuti Mesa Tradition of Cross-Cultural Shamanism.

It turns out we have been walking the spiral of awakening all along. We were just sleepwalking through it, that's all. But the *spiral of awakening is only part of the journey, for as we begin to anchor into soul, we begin to reverse our walk through the spiral into one of embodying our mightiness.* It's through activating our own revolution that we get to live in greater harmony. Through refining our actions, we get to bring congruency into the world. By becoming our own master, we get to fulfil our destinies, fill our Heart with love, and radiate peace into the world.

We need to connect with spirit daily to fill our sacred vessel and access our soul purpose. We need to fully embody our physical reality in order to live our Dharma (soul purpose— always benevolent by nature) and gift it back into the world. Simply knowing our purpose is not enough; we must act upon it. If we have a mind, we have a mission.

So, our journey is never just our own; it is infused by soul and needed by the world. Many a gift will be received by opening our Heart to the journey, and many a lesson will be learned.

Along the way, we will re-wild our whole being and begin to live from the space of our personal truths. These are not just for our own benefit, but always for the benefit of all. Along the way, we will awaken to what it means to be in sacred relationship with our self and the world; awaken to remembering the inner space of sacredness that exists within the back chambers of our heart, for it is here where soul resides. Soul is the portal into our sacredness, the core of the spiral, and the anchor of our journey.

B.S. | BELIEF SYSTEMS

I'm not interested in your limiting beliefs, I'm interested in what makes you limitless.

—Brendon Burchard

Our belief systems become our life patterns. Our psychology becomes our biology. Our life patterns not only give shape to our bodies, but they also give shape to the expression of health or disease in our body. That is why my dearest friend, ***our belief systems, are also our BS.***

Part of reclaiming your sacredness is establishing a new relationship with your self. Creating a more peaceful inner dialogue will allow you to connect deeper within, but also allow you to shift the perception of your reality, the way you treat yourself, and the way you act and *react* to the world around you.

When you look back at your life, can you identify a place in time where you lost connection to your sacredness?

Perhaps you weren't even aware that you were a sacred being?

Perhaps you violated yourself somehow in your quest for approval and external love?

Perhaps you were violated by others?

Perhaps you put your magical world to sleep, for no one else believed in it, and you felt you just didn't belong when you so desperately wanted to belong?

Perhaps you just don't remember? Perhaps you do remember, but carry too much trauma, sadness, grief, anger, fear, shame, and guilt within to acknowledge it?

How do we even begin making peace inside while still carrying that heavy burden? How can we ever reconnect with our sacredness when we still feel/carry the effects of our trauma in each and every one of our cells? How can we embrace-in-order-to-heal that which we have put away, hoping to never have to face it?

By now we've gotten pretty good at fooling ourselves, at denying. We've created walls and fortresses that keep our heart safe. We've created a big long list of beliefs that define who we are, and which give boundary and a sense of safety to our lives. But are our limiting beliefs really true? Are they the source of our liberation, or the source of our suffering? Are they our bridge to our essential nature, or the gate that prevents access to our essential nature? Are they the bond that connects us to our sacredness, or are they the Ego that pulls us away from our true self as soul?

In the exercise the follows, I invite you to take a look at your BS. Get intimate and really honest; inquire about and examine the way in which your beliefs have kept you bound, and perhaps been the source of, or a part of your current disharmony.

Brew yourself your favourite elixir or tea. Sit at your sacred space. Take a few deepening breaths and connect with the truth or perceived truth that lives within you.

This exercise is just for you. Nobody is watching, and if you need to you can burn it afterwards. What matters is that you release onto paper the weight of your heart, and begin to see some of the ways in which your beliefs limit you. This is an opportunity to begin to rewire your belief structure into one that will serve your current evolution.

For the sake of keeping it short, I am going to ask you to identify at least three limiting beliefs you feel are currently holding you back, or affecting you in a negative way. And then I want you to dive into them. Know that you can come back at any time to identify other limiting beliefs or to deepen your process.

I invite you to take a look at any limiting beliefs you can identify in any or all of the following areas:

- *Your self.* For example: I can only write a book about healing once I have healed myself completely. If I had stayed believing my own BS, this book would never have come into being. That would have been such a missed opportunity for me to heal deeply, and for you to have tools and practices to also heal deeply, and climb your own mountain!

- *Your habits.* For example: I'm a procrastinator. Or, I can do it myself, I don't need anyone's help. Or, I don't have enough discipline to do that.

- *Your body.* For example: I can't exercise or do yoga. My body is always stiff. Or, I'm too far gone now to start taking care of my body.

- *Your mind.* For example: I just can't meditate. My mind is always racing.

- *Your age.* For example: I am too old to learn how to do a somersault. Or, I'm too young to be thinking about my health.

- *Your role at this time.* For example: life is so busy, as an engaged mother I have no time to write, or do yoga practice, or take care of myself, or learn about my challenge. The dishes await!

- *Your partner or limiting belief about not having one.* For example: you have to work hard at a relationship for it to work. Or, I'm just not "relationship material."

- *Parenthood or limiting beliefs about not being a biological parent.* For example: I am a terrible parent for yelling at my kids when they misbehave. Or, I can never have meaningful relationships with children because I'm not a parent.

- *Your family unit.* For example: I can't pursue my dreams because my family needs me now. I need to make their meals, take them places, oh gosh! never mind the laundry!

- *Your family of origin.* For example: I can't because I wasn't born into the right kind of family. Or, my family will abandon me if I change. Or, there is no way anyone else in my family can do meals, laundry and the dishes if I don't. (you get my drift).

- *Your ancestral lineage.* For example: as _____ (name your faith), we are always being _____ .

- Work with one limiting belief at a time, but do the exercise with three different limiting beliefs. There is a reason why limiting beliefs are ... limiting. You will soon start to see a pattern that weaves between all your limiting beliefs. This might just be time to upgrade your operating system. It's a good thing!

I now invite you to write down your limiting belief. Explain it in detail. Dig deeper.

I will use my own as an example:

> **Limiting Belief:** *I can only write a book about healing, once I have healed myself completely.*

First of all, who am I to write a book? English is my second language. I haven't completely healed. I am not an expert. I have so many things that have helped me heal, it is so diverse! No one will ever read it!

Plus, I have three boys in hockey (which makes me a hockey mom), and I barely have time to go to the washroom, never mind write a frickin' book! My husband is always traveling for work, I feel like a married single parent when he is away, and who is going to make their meals, do laundry and the dishes and take the garbage out?

Ha! Who am I kidding? I suck at writing. I barely passed ESL (English as a Second Language). I'm just not a writer. I am an artist, a photographer and painter, a yoga teacher and shamanic practitioner! Yes, a total ***Renaissance artist!*** Words? Na … words ain't my thing.

And healing? Well, it seems like I'm always in "healing mode." Though I must say I'm so much better than before. My right side is no longer numb. Heavy metal levels are way down, almost normal. My mind is definitely more centered. My yoga practice has deepened and I love, just love teaching. Juicing is my bliss and makes my brain tickle. But I am still healing. I am still addressing deep layers of my journey. I am not a doctor, I am just me. I simply decided I wouldn't numb my numbing pain, and I gave my mind one task only—learn, heal, repeat. Okay, maybe three.

And so, dear reader, you are holding the book that resulted from letting go of my BS (limiting beliefs) about myself. And you can do the same. You can see how ridiculous I can be about some of it, and how when we finally put on paper we can create the space we need to make a conscious action to not believe and feed our BS anymore.

Now, find the feeling in your body associated with it (shame, anger, guilt, fear, sorrow, etc.).

For example:

I feel shame and fear about writing this book. And sometimes I feel anger at feeling shame and fear.

I feel shame because I haven't healed completely. I mean, I'm not the poster child of healing, so how can I write about it? I feel shame when my face breaks out due to the liver detox I've been doing. I feel fear that I may not heal to the depth my heart desperately seeks. I feel anger at the fact that I know I know my s##t, yet I still get challenged by layers of my issues, and by the constant questioning … *Oh do you really know what you are doing? You're not a doctor, you know. Did you know that wheatgrass is not good for you after all? I just saw it in the news! See, I've told you so for years."*

Arggghhhhhhhhhhhh!!! Read the bloody research! Get educated! Yes! I do know I've been on this path for quite some time, and I'm still at it. And no, you will not always hear the whole story on the news. If you would like to read the almost fifty books I have on the subject, perhaps you will come to your own conclusion!!

I used to feel sorrow deep within, for it has been a lonely journey. I am better now, for I have found the fullness in the empty spaces, and I've found a soul tribe full of heart.

Ask yourself, where in your body do you feel it?

For example:

I feel shame in my face. I feel shame when my face breaks out. No, it's not hormonal.

I feel fear in my chest. My breath gets shallow. My throat tightens. I can hardly breathe.

I feel sorrow deep behind my throat. Deep behind my heart weeping down my belly into my sacrum. I feel my breath go shallow and my belly fear my breath. I feel like crying but I can't.

I feel unsafe. I feel unsupported. I feel like either the world has gone mad, or I have gone mad. I feel like claiming my own island in the middle of the ocean far away from it all.

It's okay to get raw and personal. We can only release what we can see. *We can only let go off what we give space to arise.* So go deep, allow yourself to feel, and give your feelings space outside your cells.

Breathe. Pause and feel.

Breathe. Pause and feel.

Once you have worked through three limiting beliefs, sit in meditation. Do a few deep breathing exercises. Give yourself space from what has now been seen.

Can you begin to see a pattern? If so, write it down.

For example:

My pattern, through many a limited belief is shame and fear. They seem to be the anchors to a lot of my BS.

Can you begin to see a pattern whose seed is ancestral? If so, write it down.

For example:

My ancestral pattern is also shame and fear, with a wedge of anger. Safety, or rather, the lack of safety has been at the root cause of the shame, fear, and anger.

But I have only arrived at this place after understanding my family's story, and the story of my lineage. And that, dear friend, is a whole other book. But for now, imagine that you are a narrator telling your ancestral story from an outsider's perspective. Write it down in the third person. Go into the feelings, the emotions behind the story. Sometimes they seem to jump straight at you, and sometimes they are harder to see. But I invite you to first ground yourself with the tools and practices you have already learned, then dive into the unknown. Trust that any emotion you see or identify is revealing itself to be set free.

By working in and through the layers of your BS, you will come to recognize your patterns, the loop on auto-play that drives your unconscious mind and gives shape to so much of your reality. The good news is that by choosing to show up and face your BS, you will move beyond it, to the point where it will no longer be the software that runs your current operating system. Are you ready to unleash your mightiness?

ARE YOU STILL LISTENING TO THAT OLD TAPE? ON AUTOPLAY?

And the day came when the risk to remain tight in a bud was more painful than the risk it took to blossom.

—Anaïs Nin

As we begin to tap deeper within we may begin to recognize the ***loop of our BS on autoplay.*** I know I have, and I also know that sometimes I fall back into this inner pattern of shame and fear. This is an old, toxic inner emotional pattern for me, as it is for most people.

But along the journey, we begin to recognize these old patterns running on autopilot. We also begin to take action towards building a new inner landscape for our emotional self to feel safe in, and for it to develop a new language to engage our heart in healthier boundaries, first with our self, and then with those around us.

We cannot create healthier boundaries with those around us unless we can first create and sustain them with our self. We cannot demand healthier boundaries from others, until we can show up for our self in the very same way we demand of them. Though our mind and our awareness may not know this yet, our heart does, and there is no fooling it!

So, whose old cassette tape are you playing? How toxic is it? Is it running on autoplay? How can you begin to slow it down, stop the autoplay, and finally remove it altogether?

We begin by bearing witness to our mind, to the voice within, to the self-shame and blame and emotional toxicity that voice creates within us. We become aware of the coping mechanisms that show up uninvited when we fall into our autopilot emotional reactions and resulting behaviour patterns. So, just like on our old tape player, and now on our phones, we can hit the PAUSE button, we must now create a CANCEL button within our own habitual emotional self.

Any time you find yourself in the emotional self autopilot inner conversation, say to yourself, "Cancel, Cancel, Cancel." Then replace the negative thought with an updated affirmation you have prepared and ready, which will begin to change your inner dialogue and landscape.

For a lot of us the inner landscape of the ancestral self is quite dense and filled with negativity. Yet we have the power to redefine our ancestral self with the positive examples and influences of those who have guided our lives in a positive direction, and have organically become our positive ancestral self. We can begin to remember the ancestral wisdom, benevolent by nature, that is the seed of truth of our ancestral lineages and that has been awaiting our awakening.

Pause that tape. Feel. Breathe.

Pause. Feel.	Witness.	Pause. Feel. Breathe.	Release. Pause. Feel.	Create Space.
Pause. Feel.	Breathe.	Choose. Pause. Feel.	Reset. Pause. Feel.	Breathe. Root.
Pause. Feel.	Anchor.	Pause. Feel. Breathe.	Choose. Pause. Feel.	Transform.
Pause. Feel.	Breathe.	Surrender. Pause. Feel.	Integrate. Pause. Feel.	Breathe. Rise.
Pause. Feel.	Shine.	Pause. Feel. Breathe.		

FLIP THE VIBE

Whether you think you can, or think you can't, you're probably right.

—Henry Ford

Infuse your BS with a whole lot of love! Self-love.

When we are on an airplane and it is going down, I mean really going down, the first instruction we receive is to *place the oxygen mask on yourself, before helping your child, or any other loved ones.* As you begin to work with your BS, the same rule applies.

You must get yourself out of your own BS, as no one else can do the work for you. You've gotta become your own cheerleader, and *flip the vibe!*

Flip the vibe is a five-step process:

1. ***Acknowledge your BS.*** It is important that you see it, name it, and give it space on paper outside of your body. You have done this through the previous exercise.

2. *Trust.* You continue to develop trust in your self and your process through your mindfulness practices, through self-compassion, through engaging with your subconscious mind, and by showing up for yourself in all the new ways you now know how.

3. *Replacement through affirmations.* You've cleared out some junk. Now you need to fill the empty spaces with a new and more positive tape to play on autoplay—and an affirmation works great. When working with affirmations, I first like to release the old BS I'm working with, and then replace it with a more positive affirmation. Find a new, empowering belief to replace the old one for your subconscious mind to use. It's so important to choose carefully what thoughts and self-talk we fill ourselves up with.

4. *Tap into the new core feeling* of your affirmation to activate and ignite its power and effect at a cellular level.

5. *Anchor into the inner space you have just created.* Root your new core feeling into this space. This is your new sacred foundation.

For example: knowing all you now know about me, there are a few limiting beliefs I have to address. The first was around the writing of this very book, which, thankfully, by now I've let go of.

Limiting Belief: I can only write a book about healing once I have healed myself completely.

Flip the Vibe: I have the wisdom to write a book about healing because I've been through it. I have healed, I have walked the path and gathered many tools that can help others deepen their healing. I got this.

New Core Feeling: I am grateful for the opportunity to heal deeply, to write, to guide, to create, to inspire, to be of service, and to help others.

My new inner space is a sweet expansive space. My new sacred foundation feels deeply nourishing to me.

But why stop at that when I know deeply that my vibe is being affected by the core feelings of shame and fear, with a wedge of anger?

Let's *flip the vibe* on those, too.

Shame: Flip the Vibe. "I clear and release all my conscious or unconscious thoughts and feelings of shame. With every breath I take, I am sending love, gratitude, and healing to every single cell in my body. I am enough."

Pause and feel. Tap into the expansive feeling of being enough this affirmation creates within you. Bring that feeling into your heart space. Integrate it into your core.

Fear: Flip the Vibe. "I clear and release all my conscious or unconscious thoughts and feelings of fear. With every breath I take I am sending love, gratitude and healing to every single cell in my body. I am courageous. I can face everything and rise."

Pause and feel. Tap into the expansive feeling of courage this affirmation creates within you. Bring that feeling into your heart space. Integrate it into your core. Feel into gratitude for the opportunity to anchor into courage.

Anger: Flip the Vibe. "I clear and release all conscious or unconscious thoughts and feelings of anger. With every breath I take, I am sending love, gratitude, and healing to every single cell in my body. I am peace. I live my life joyfully."

Pause and feel. Tap into the expansive feeling of peace and joy this affirmation creates within you. Bring that feeling into your heart space. Integrate it into your core. Feel into gratitude for the opportunity to align with peace and joy.

Feeling Unsafe: Flip the Vibe. "I am now free to release all ideas, thoughts, feelings, and past experiences that I need to in order to stay safe. I am now safe to be myself in the world."

Pause and feel. Tap into the expansive feeling of safety this affirmation creates within you. Bring that feeling into your heart space. Integrate it into your core. Feel into gratitude for the opportunity to feel safe in your body and as you shine your mightiness into the world.

Whenever you find yourself doubting your mighty power or limiting yourself, I invite you to look closely into your BS. I invite you to press PAUSE or CANCEL and re-wire yourself with a more positive affirmation.

SHAME ON WHOM?

Shame is a focus on self, guilt is a focus on behaviour… Guilt: I'm sorry. I made a mistake. Shame: I am sorry. I am a mistake.

—Brené Brown

We often disconnect from our self because we feel deep **shame** at our core. Either consciously or unconsciously, we feel it. Maybe we cannot easily identify it as shame, but if we dig deep, it will be there. Shame.

Did we bring our self to shame, or were we brought to shame by our circumstances and or early traumas? Probably both. But shame on whom?

For most of our lives, we have more consciously been holding onto projecting onto those around us the old saying, *Shame on you. How could you? How could you have done that? Shame on you.*

But deep inside, our inner younger self feels more like *How could I? How could I have let this happen? How could I have? Shame on me.* The shame of the small child who, before the age of five, was neglected, abandoned, abused, ignored, criticized, or invalidated in some way, has distilled down into the core shame that when you dig down deep, is some version of *I'm not good enough. I'll never be good enough. There is something wrong with me. I'm bad.*

The burden of this shame eats away at our sacredness and at our heart. It eats away at our self-esteem, at our happiness, and at the possibility of becoming the expression of our highest potential. It is Ego at its best, for it keeps us away from our true nature and our compassion. It is the harsh blaming voice of the adult, with the finger pointing right at the heart of that still-young child within.

Shame is a strong wall in our fortress of self-limiting beliefs. Is it possible to inquire into our shame and see it for what it is? Is it possible to go back in time to when that wounded child stored that shame within her cells, and re-write that story?

Perhaps allow your adult eyes to become the guide for that wounded child to see how the challenge has shaped you, and how it became a core part of the light of which you are today, and the life you have created for yourself. Gently, softly, with great compassion, you can begin to shift away from shame, and into self-forgiveness, self-acceptance, and then self-love.

Softly, gently, with great compassion, you can begin to flow out of the rigid walls of your fortress into the arms of trust and into the awareness that everything that has happened in your life has been key to your own evolutionary development of soul.

AUTHORSHIP VS. VICTIMHOOD

If you want something you've never had, you must be willing to do something you've never done.

—*Thomas Jefferson*

Authorship or victimhood. Two sides of the same coin. Which one do we choose? Which one do we slide into 'cause you know, we all do? *It's part of our humanity.*

As we journey from childhood to adulthood, we can sometimes begin to shift from the feelings/consciousness of *victimhood into authorship.* We may begin to question what is serving us and what is not. We may be challenged by new circumstances, but you and I now know we can be guided to act from a different place within our self. But sometimes it takes more than that. Sometimes our traumas have anchored so deeply into our body and our Ego that the journey from *victimhood into authorship* is not such an easy one.

Traumas can keep us bound. Depending on the trauma, it can keep us stuck in the cycle of violence, abuse, abandonment, fear, betrayal, invalidation, and/or self-sabotage (to name just a few), for it's all we know. This is all great food for the Ego, which prefers the self-righteous indignation of victimhood, so the Ego wants nothing to do with even the thought of authorship. To the Ego, authorship is its enemy. But to the soul, authorship is everything.

So how do we begin the process? For it is a process and it likes to dance. The better we get at rewiring our brains and anchoring into authorship, the less often we will slip back into victimhood. And if (and when) we do (because we probably will), we will now be equipped with the tools and resources to recognize it quickly, and shapeshift our way back into authorship with less hardship.

You and I begin by creating inner space, and start taking inventory of our patterns, our thoughts, and our indications of self-sabotage. We begin by bearing witness to our self, to our mind, and to our body. We begin by choosing to do things differently, and make different choices than we've done before, for this is the only way to obtain a different result. We begin with one step, with one choice. For some of us, we begin by grabbing the lifejacket that has always been by our side and stating to our self and to the universe: **_enough._**

We begin to take one step forward and two steps back. Get ready to dance the salsa!

One step forward, two steps back. Or at least that's how it feels some days. But there is only one thing that those who have walked the path to the Heart and have gotten there have done: **_blisscipline._** Show up, show up, and continue to show up. Through blisscipline, you will be able to access the unimaginable. What once was a big effort will become effortless. What felt like a duty will become a passion. You create new habits and rid yourself of what no longer serves you. You can bring your practice with you when you leave your cushion or your mat as you anchor with boldness into the life you want to live. You get a chance to discover your self, the depth of your existence, and the depth you are willing to travel to reclaim your self alive.

So play the music loud, Babe, and let it rip.

OUR ISSUES ARE IN OUR TISSUES

The cure for the pain is in the pain.

—_Rumi_

It is said that our **_issues are in our tissues,_** and our body is always speaking to us, but often we don't know what it is saying. It is not because we don't want to know, although that may be true for some, but I'd like to believe that for most us, we do want to know, but we simply have forgotten how to understand our body's code.

Every issue in our tissue can be traced back to an emotion that got _stuck_ in a belief system that is now being triggered into expression. I invite you to look at your tissues both through the lens of your dis-ease or dis-harmony, and also through the lens of symbolism and emotion. By decoding your body's message, you will move through that which has been limiting you, that which has kept you bound and become a source of suffering.

Symbolically, issues in the following tissues or parts of our body are related to issues with:

"*Arm:* represents the capacity and ability to hold the experiences of life.

Back Issues: Represents the support of life. *Back Problems:* – *Rounded shoulders:* Carrying the burdens of life. Helpless and hopeless. – *Lower Back Pain:* Fear of money or lack of financial support. – *Mid-Back Pain:* Guilt. Stuck in all that stuff back there. "Get off my back!" – *Upper Back Pain:* Lack of emotional support. Feeling unloved. Holding back love. – *Back Curvature:* The inability to flow with the support of life. Fear and trying to hold on to old ideas. Not trusting life.

Breast: represents mothering and nurturing and nourishment.

Breast cysts, lumps: a refusal to nourish the self. Putting everyone else first. Over mothering. Overprotection.

Colitis: insecurity. Represents the ease of letting go of that which is over.

Ear: Represents the capacity to hear. – *Ache:* Anger. Not wanting to hear. Too much turmoil.

Eye: Represents the capacity to see clearly past, present, future.

Face: represents what we show to the world.

Galllstones: bitterness. Hard thoughts. Condemning. Pride.

Headaches: invalidating the self. Self-criticism. Fear.

Heart: Represents the center of love and security. – *Heart Attack:* Squeezing all the joy out of the heart in favor of money or position. Feeling alone and scared. "I'm not good enough. I don't do enough. I'll never make it." – *Heart Problems:* Longstanding emotional problems. Lack of joy.

Hip: carries the body in perfect balance. Major thrust in moving forward. Fear of going forward in major decisions. Nothing to move forward to.

Intestines: represent assimilation and absorption.

Jaw: anger issues.

Kidney Problems: Criticism, disappointment, failure. Shame.

Knee: represents pride and ego. Stubborn ego and pride. Inability to bend. Fear. Inflexibility. Won't give in.

Left Side of Body: represents receptivity, taking in, feminine energy, women. Mother.

Leg: carry us forward in life.

Liver: seat of anger and primitive emotions. Chronic complaining. Justifying fault-finding to deceive yourself. Feeling bad.

Lung: the ability to take in life. Grief. Depression. Not feeling worthy of living life fully.

Neck: represents flexibility. The ability to see what's back there. Refusing to see other sides of a question. Stubbornness, inflexibility. Unbending stubbornness.

Ovaries: represent points of creation. Creativity.

Pancreas: represents the sweetness of life.

Prostate: represents the masculine principle. Mental fears weaken the masculinity. Giving up.

Right Side of Body: giving out, letting go, masculine energy, men. Father.

Shin: Represents the standards of life. Breaking down ideals.

Shoulders: trust issues, hopeless, helpless, feel burdened, responsibility issues.

Shoulders (rounded): carrying the burdens of life. Helpless and hopeless.

Skin: protects our individuality. Anxiety, fear. Old buried things. I am being threatened.

Spleen: obsessions. Being obsessed about things.

Stomach: holds nourishment. Digests ideas. Dread. Fear of the new or inability to assimilate the new.

Throat: avenue of expression. Channel of creativity. *Throat problems:* inability to speak up for one's self. Swallowed anger. Stifled creativity. Refusal to change. *Throat (sore):* holding in angry words. Feeling unable to express the self.

Uterus: represents the home of creativity."[21]

Through the previous exercise (writing out your limiting beliefs), you have begun connecting your current belief system to your current expression of health. In beginning to understand the relationship between your beliefs, your emotions, and where they live in your body, you will have new revelation and insight into your body's code. If you find this process overwhelming, remember to *pause and feel.* Use the Mighty powers of your breath to anchor you into the safety of your body.

We will now take that exercise one step further.

Is there a part of your body that came up a lot for you in the previous exercise, or that has come up for you while reading the list above? Is there a part of your body you would like to understand or be in communication with? Grab a sheet of paper. Write that down in the middle of the page. Draw a circle around it.

Now, in free-flow style, begin to write words, emotions, feelings, attitudes, and beliefs that you associate with and around that part of your body, from the obvious to the symbolic, from the centre of the page out towards the edges. And then write more free-word associations about those. Write down what seems obvious to you; write down the emotions you now know to be associated with that part of your body; write also any symbolic meanings that might arise within you and what, through free-flow writing, might just pour out of you. It might just be the right word that unlocks your puzzle.

There might be two parts of your body that are related, or where you might be experiencing your disharmony. Write them both down. Gift yourself the opportunity to play with this exercise. Stay curious. See where it takes you.

---

21   Louise Hay, You Can Heal Your Life (Carlsbad, CA; Hay House, 1999).

Once you have done the exercise, allow whatever other words need to flow out of you to flow. Give them space on paper. You might be surprised with a little gift of body/soul wisdom. Now, go back and highlight what is most true to your current situation, condition, or state.

Pause and feel. Breathe. Pause and feel.

What did you learn about yourself? What did you learn about your body?

What is your body trying to tell you? In what direction is it pointing?

What are the emotions related to your specific part of the body?

What feelings have come up for you?

What beliefs have come up for you in doing this exercise?

Were you aware of them prior to doing this exercise?

Pause and feel. Breathe. Pause and feel.

I recommend you do this exercise whenever you feel your body is trying to tell you something, whenever you feel stuck, or in need of greater insight, understanding, or awareness about your current situation. Your Mighty inner healer may be trying to tell you something. The more we know, the more we can do about it. Now you also know that living in today's world, has also led to the accumulation of toxicity in your body and that you now have the tools to address both the symbolic meaning of the issues in your tissues and the underlaying reality of the toxicity in your system. Right? Right.

THE POWER OF CHOICE

Discovering who we are is a choice and knowing that we have power over our thoughts, feelings and responses helps us take personal responsibility. This frees us to consciously shape our lives and create a world reflecting deeper dreams and values.

—*Llyn Roberts and Robert Levy*

As you become more intimate with your self, you will begin to recognize that while you cannot control your external circumstances, you have a **choice** in how you react/respond to those circumstances, how they affect you and make you feel, either by further creating an unconscious biology, or by choosing to become conscious of your play and the choices you make.

As you become more conscious of your role and your part in your process all along, and more conscious of the power ***you*** have to choose something different, you will tap into your own potential. If you are not happy about XYZ, *you have the power to change it.*

You may not be able to change what is happening in *your story,* but you can absolutely change your relationship to it and the emotion it brings up in you. You may not be able to change what happens *to* you, or what is happening *around* you, but you can change your relationship with your self, knowing you now have the voice, strength, and support system to manage and deal with life. You can choose to no longer be the victim of your circumstances.

Recognizing you and I have the power of choice brings us great liberation and freedom. In knowing we are no longer bound to our family of origin's story, we can reclaim our personal power, a key step along our evolutionary healing. Once you can connect with your personal power, you will also better able to decode the messages your body is trying to tell you.

The power of choice awakens the ***hope activist within,*** for what you and I do matters, and how we go about creating our dreams on earth matters. It activates your whole being to living in the present moment, aware that what you choose and how you choose to act have consequences. Once this fact is real for us, we are now in charge of determining which consequences we can live with, and which we no longer choose to live with.

When you choose to do the work, you activate your personal power, and then you begin to align with a deeper space of truth and love more in synch with your current value system. You can choose to leave behind that which no longer fits you, and create clear boundaries for your physical and emotional body.

Having made peace with your inner child for what you were unable to do/cope with before, you can now choose to live from a different place of authenticity. You know you now have the ability to fully support your self. You are here to learn to support your self, and to learn about love. Learning to love your mighty self, just as you are, is one of the most important choices you and I will ever make.

I choose to honour and deeply support my self through love. Read that aloud to yourself three times.

SHAMANIC CALLING

Two roads diverged in a wood, and I - I took the one less travelled by, and it made all the difference.

—*Robert Frost*

There are many ways to awaken to the spiritual path. Some people are born awakened. Some surrender easily to their awakening. For some of us, though, we've had to kiss the ground running a few times, and learn to surrender to big challenges and traumas before we were ready to come back to living in alignment with soul and source.

The *shamanic calling* is the process of awakening towards the spiritual path, and it can take make forms: personal trauma, self-doubt and inner confusion, identity crisis, family or environmental chaos, severe illness or health problems, acting out through bizarre behaviour, UFO encounters or other phenomena, near-death experiences, life-transforming dreams and/or spontaneous visions.

It's important to understand that *all your challenges have a purpose; they bring you back into alignment with your path to mightiness.* They remind us of our wholeness, of where we forgot our essence and our soul purpose. Our challenges and traumas build our character. They deconstruct the false facades we have built, tear down the walls to our heart, and bring us back to our path. Our challenges help shape us into who we are, and gift us the sensitivity to feel the depth of the world in more subtle ways.

Often the shamanic call is heard in the midst of your deepest challenge. It is only through the cracking of your heart that the light can shine into your deepest, darkest aspects, and remind you of your wholeness. Remind you of your essential nature as soul having a human experience. Remind you that true harmony is a state of living in sacred reciprocity with all of life.

It is through your greatest wounds that you are able to emerge whole. It is through your greatest wounds that you will hear your calling.

The shamanic calling is one that can take many shapes, but all involve the death of the old. As you release old beliefs and reclaim the fragmented pieces of your self; like the phoenix, you will rise from the ashes, and be reborn. This death can be physical or symbolic, but it awakens in us the more subtle elements of our sensory perceptions, our psychic abilities, and a yearning to be of service to the world.

ANSWERING THE CALL OF SOUL

Practice listening to your intuition, your inner voice; ask questions; be curious; see what you see; hear what you hear; and then act upon what you know to be true. These intuitive powers were given to your soul at birth.

— *Clarissa Pinkola Estés, Women Who Run With the Wolves: Myths and Stories of the Wild Woman Archetype*

Soul has always been within you, guiding your each and every breath. Your awareness of your self as soul may not always have been there, or perhaps it drifted in and out of your consciousness over the years. Here on this human journey we often forget we are the embodiment of soul, rather than just a body. Your body is not you, it is yours. Your mind is not you, it is yours. They are aspects of your true nature as soul—expressing its dream in form.

Some people arrive early at the core/felt sense/understanding of living from that place of your authentic self/true nature/soul, but for most of us this is a quest, a journey of re-embodiment. A journey of recalibrating your heart compass to guide you back home to wholeness, and to the reclaiming of your divine identity.

For many of us, this journey starts through trauma, through the cracking of our heart, through facing dis-ease and dis-harmony. Ultimately, it leads us to the dark night of the soul. Here, we are forced to face our self, our limited beliefs, our ancestral wound and the wisdom of our ancestral lineage, the densities we have gathered, the karmic conditions we have brought forth, and the understanding of our generational karma. As we pass through this dark night of soul, we move into a new place of deep intimate relationship with our self, and with soul.

*When we consciously choose to answer the **call of soul**, everything changes.* Up until that moment, our challenges were our struggles, and brought tears and fears and **why me?** to our life. Yet when we consciously choose to answer the call of soul, our challenges become our teachers, and we begin to understand that we're on a quest.

Our quest is what you and I came here to do, to unravel the heart and anchor knee-deep into earth's rhythms and consciousness. You begin to understand there is more to life than what you'd been doing up until this point, that life is asking you to show up from a deeper place, not only for your self but in service to humanity, the world and as part of the shift towards Peace.

Answering the call of soul is not easy. It takes great courage to delve into our darkness, to peel back the layers and expose the generational patterns of trauma and addictions and the ancestral wound. But only by seeing, acknowledging, and facing them can you and I begin to release them. And only by releasing them can you begin to write your own chapter in your generational book in a new direction: towards the weaving of peace, healing your traumas, creating peace in your relations, and your life being a force of peace towards next generations.

So dear beating heart, you heard her call. We are here together opening the door. *As within, so without. As above, so below. As in heaven, so on earth. As in spirit, so in soul.* Know I've got your heart as I know you have mine. Go on—make the change you seek to make in the universe.

SHAMANIC TOOLS

The mystical traditions that speak to the ability to transform and transmute poisons are a valuable resource. Their stories of how certain gifted people harmonized with nature to restore health to the environment have much to teach us.

—*Sandra Ingerman*

Within the spiritual practice of shamanism we have tools, rituals and ceremonies that facilitate the awakening of our ancestral wisdom and deepen the healing of our ancestral wounds. These tools allow us to connect with the consciousness and the spirit that animates all matter.

These rituals require that we honour our processes with great transparency and utmost impeccable intention to heal and awaken in service to the world and the seven generations forward.

Becoming Hollow Bone

I first came across the concept of becoming hollow bone through my work as a photojournalist. In 1997, I was working on a photo documentary about deafblind individuals in Canada and abroad. Kay Clarke was a deafblind ham radio (Morse code) operator and, she was, above all, one of the finest ladies I have ever come across.

Kay, in her eighties, always wore red lipstick and dressed to the nines in red high heels. In order to use her ham radio, she had devised and adjusted a small car speaker to fit her set so when she put her hand on it, she could actually feel the vibrational patterns of the Morse code signal and was able to translate the message. She called this "bone conduction," an innovation that allowed her, using Morse code, to communicate with the whole wide world. It was one of her portals to living in freedom and independence.

Years later, as I studied shamanism, I encountered again the idea of bone conduction, in a slightly different way. We have the ability to feel the subtle vibrations of sound and life-force energy through our bones, to become a bone conductor, ourselves. We have the ability to translate and share it, to allow the healing life-force energy of the cosmos to pass through us, and be in healing service to our self and others.

This is the art of becoming hollow bone. *The ability to quiet ourselves so deeply as to become a vessel of transference of healing energy into ourselves or others.* It is not us doing the healing; rather, we are the vehicle through which the healing energy of the cosmos is able to flow into others. Becoming hollow bone is a shamanic tool for deep healing, one we can use for ourselves, and one we can gift to others.

The Hucha Ceremony

The word Hucha means density. The Hucha ceremony is the practice of giving the densities that reside within us, whether inherited, self-created, picked up from those around us, or acquired from the space outside our bodies. The Hucha ceremony allows you to give space to your *ancestral wounds outside yourself, as you continue to heal and integrate their teachings and the gifts of their medicine.*

It is a simple ritual that can have a profound effect, for the impact of your emotions and their densities exists in the timeless spaces in between your cells. This ritual works best when done in alignment with the new moon. The darkness of the moonless sky allows us to see with clarity into the world within. It is a quiet time of inner revelation.

Ingredients & supplies you will need:

- paper & pen
- ceramic bowl, matches
- glass mason jar with lid
- water
- baking soda
- quiet time

Step 1:

- Come to your sacred space.
- Centre yourself, pause and feel.
- Use any of the deep breathing exercises/pranayamas to quiet and anchor the mind.
- Write your Hucha letter. Allow yourself to write down onto paper the densities that have been weighing you down. These densities can be an emotion (sadness, grief, anger, fear, shame, guilt), a thought, a relationship, or whatever you can identify.

Note: This Hucha letter is just for you. It is not meant to be read by anyone else, so go for it; be as raw and truthful as you can. Allow yourself to use all the words you need (even the not so nice ones—yes, it's okay!) in order to release the emotional charge responsible for creating incoherence at a cellular level.

Step 2:

- Burn the letter. Yes, you read it right. Burn it to fully release the density those words still hold. You will need to keep the ashes, so whether you choose to burn it inside or outside, use a ceramic bowl to burn your Hucha letter.
- Place the ashes of your letter in a glass Mason jar. To whatever amount of ash you have, add equal amounts of baking soda and water to it. Mix it well. The baking soda will begin to neutralize the energetic density of the ashes. Place it in the freezer until the Full Moon.

Step 3:

- The day before the coming Full Moon, remove the jar from the freezer and allow it to thaw.
- On the day of the Full Moon, release it into a moving body of water. Let it flow, let it flow. Offer a prayer of gratitude to the Great Spirit for the opportunity to release these densities, and for the opportunity for them to be recycled into healing cosmic energy.

Remember the first law of thermodynamics? Energy can neither be created nor destroyed; it can only be transformed.

Energetically, the portal of energy that becomes heightened during the New and Full moons lasts for three days. Both the day before and the day after the new and full moons are also days of heightened energy, offering the best opportunity to perform this Hucha ceremony.

May this ritual serve you to release density from within your body, mind, heart and soul, and bring you into greater harmony with the magic and the sacred medicine of the Moon.

Hampikamayoq Breath Techniques or Shamanic Breathing

As you already know, our breath simultaneously weaves its power to both awaken our ancestral wisdom and heal our ancestral wound. Deep breathing exercises bring coherence into our body systems, and through resonance shift them into more coherent patterns of expression.

I wrote about the Hampikamayoq breath techniques on page 256 . I hope by now you've had the opportunity to explore them, and begin to feel the benefits of your practice.

Alignment with the Five Elements, the Five Directions, and Their Medicine

Alignment is key. *Alignment with your Elemental nature is the only path to wellness that will address the root causes of your discordance.* Awakening *your* ancestral wisdom is, in part, awakening *your* awareness of *your* Elemental nature. The five Elements: Ether, Air, Fire, Water, and Earth are also in relationship with the five directions and the five bodies.

Through the ritual and practices of toning, evoking (chanting) the five directions, we invoke the opening of their medicines within us. Through toning, evoking, and honouring their power, we invoke their animated essence into our own, activating their ability to serve as portals for awareness, deep healing, and communion with the all.

According to the universal cross-cultural Pachakuti Mesa Andean shamanic tradition, the five Elements and the five directions are in interrelationship, as follows; their expression is the journey of the spiral of awakening (page 282).

South is the seat of the Element of Earth, and situated at the beginning of the spiral. We are spiritual, energetic beings having a physical, human experience. Our awakening will always begin in the body, through our physical form, through the element of Earth. South is the portal for healing the physical body.

West is the seat of the Element of Water. As we further our awakening and our healing, we must learn to flow with the waters of our emotional bodies. West is the portal for healing the emotional body.

North is the seat of the Element of Air. As we learn to flow, we surrender to the great originating mystery, Spirit—which moves through the Element of Air, breath, Prana, into our spiritual bodies. North is the portal for healing the spiritual body.

East is the seat of the Element of Fire. What needs to be released, what needs to be transformed. Fire, the great transformer, the great alchemist of the Mind, which sparks the heart into passion and action. East is the portal for healing the mental body.

Centre is the seat of the Element of *Ether,* and is situated at the core of the spiral where all movement leads to and emerges from. Ether is the sacred vessel that holds the All. Centre is the portal for healing soul.

Connecting with Your Power Animals

Every tradition of shamanism has grown in direct communication with their immediate environment. This leads them to form stronger bonds with certain animals over others. Yet, there is a universality to the power and message of the animal kingdom we can all integrate into our own path of healing and awakening.

Power animals or animal allies serve in shamanism as guides, as great alchemists, as archetypes and portals of consciousness. They serve as both messages and messengers of the truth and wisdom that reside beyond our conscious mind that we can access through the guidance and wisdom of our power animals or animal allies.

Power animals carry meaning, power, and great wisdom. They are embedded in symbolism and they reveal their guidance to us, as we deepen our relationship with them. Power animals can relate to aspects of our personality; they can relate to skills that we have cultivated or have yet to develop, a situation that has recently come into form, or simply offer us insight into understanding our selves, others and our environment that much better.

The following are a few power animals and their meaning:

Bat: rebirth and renewal.

Bear: strength, confidence, healing, grounding.

Butterflies: personal transformation, metamorphosis, moving through different life cycles.

Cougar: strength, courage, instincts, leadership, and sensual mystique.

Crow: reminder that magic is everywhere, what has not taken form yet, carries the energy of life mysteries, power for deep inner transformation. Insight, fearlessness, determination.

Deer: gentleness, innocence, grace, wisdom. Connection with the innocence of the inner child.

Dragonfly: change, transformation, adaptability, joy, lightness of being.

Eagle: rise above and soar to new heights, new perspectives, widen your vision.

Fox: discernment, responsive, agility, intelligence.

Frog: cleansing, detoxification of emotional densities, release old belief systems, rebirth, transformation, associated with life mysteries and the unknown.

Hawk: focus, clear vision, perspective, spirit messenger.

Horse: driving force, passionate desires, strong emotions, what your thrive for or what carries you in life.

Hummingbird: love, lightness of being, playfulness, beauty, enjoyment of life, wisdom to accomplish great feats, strong sensibility.

Lion: strength, assertiveness, personal power, courage.

Owl: access to intuition and wisdom, seer.

Peacock: self-love, beauty with a delicate balance of humility and confidence.

Racoon: disguise, secrecy, curiosity, intelligence, illusion, adventurous.

Raven: ignites the energy of magic, keeper of secrets, messenger between heaven and earth, introspection, self-knowledge, healing, shape shifter, mystic, change in consciousness.

Spider: weaver of the web of creation, feminine energy, patience, weaver of destiny. Shadow self, darker aspects of life or personality.

Turkey: connection with the spirit of the land, with Mother Earth, abundance, honouring community and the sharing of the fruits of our labours.

Turtle: symbol of the world, earth. Walking one's path, slowing down, pacing yourself, determination, ancient wisdom of the earth, determination.

Wolf: intelligence, instincts, social.

This is a very brief and general approach, but if you want to go into greater detail about the meaning of each power animal, and deepen your relationship with the wisdom of the animal kingdom, please check the book resources at the back of this book for suggested reading.

Shamanic Journeying

Shamanic journeying was developed as a tool to transcend the mind, or at least, transcend the illusion of the conscious mind. It was developed as a tool for shamans to travel in between worlds to gain wisdom, guidance, and healing for a person or for their community.

Today, shamanic journeying can be used as a tool for self-discovery and deep healing; to deepen your path of awakening, to gain insight about *your story*, to seek guidance and healing from the power animals that guide you on your journeys, and as a tool for remembering.

Vision Questing

Vision questing is the alchemy of deep self-inquiry. In Indigenous traditions, a person coming of age would be sent on a vision quest as a rite of passage to "find themselves" as they come into adulthood. The purpose of a vision quest is to awaken the participant to his/her own personal medicine and personal power, as well as facilitate a *remembering* of their soul purpose for coming into the world.

Vision questing is also done to deepen the healing of the body system as we awaken to our divine nature. A vision quest always strengthens the relationship between the participant, the great originating mystery and nature.

Indigenous traditions believe the vision quest is crucial to the destiny of the individual, and the dream visitors who come during a vision quest are believed to remain as guides for that person for rest of their life.

A vision quest is one of the most powerful tools we can use to awaken our ancestral wisdom and our ecological consciousness. It is one of the most powerful tools we have to heal our ancestral wound as we reclaim not only our physical body, but also begin to reclaim our larger ecological body: Mother Earth.

A vision quest is the vessel that holds our quest to the innermost chambers of our being.

THE SHAMANIC JOURNEY

The creative is the place where no one else has ever been. You have to leave the city of your comfort and go into the wilderness of your intuition. What you'll discover will be wonderful. What you'll discover is yourself.

—*Alan Alda*

Shamanic journeying is a guided meditation following the beat of the drum or rattle and it is one of the most common practices used in shamanism today. It is a practice of direct revelation, and its experiential nature allows us to make contact with our helping spirit guides and/or power animals to access empowerment, guidance and healing.

The shamanic journey is the journey to the realms beyond the veil, to the world of things hidden, where helping spirit guides and power animals reside, eager to be of assistance along our path of healing and awakening.

Traditionally, shamans used journeys make contact with their helping spirits to access empowerment, personal guidance, and healing help for the individual or community. You can personally use shamanic journeying to gather insight from your subconscious and unconscious mind, as well as insight from your intuitive wisdom, to which you may not have access in your everyday reality.

The beat of the drum or rattle creates a binaural sound, which allows both hemispheres of your brain to synch. It also facilitates your brain entering theta brain waves, the dreamlike state between wakefulness and sleep through which you enter a meditative or visionary state of consciousness. It is here where you find that numinous[22] state between worlds. It is here that we follow "the story" deep into our subconscious mind, transcending the limits of our ego-based mind, and simply allow that which needs to be seen, experienced and heard—to happen.

Theta rhythms increase creativity, enhance learning, reduce stress, and awaken intuition. They weave and reconnect your mind and your heart. Theta rhythms allow you to leap forward in your own process of evolution, as you are able to have access into the inner space of wisdom and deep healing, where you can ignite your self alive, and therefore ignite your Mighty inner healer.

---

22   Numinous is defined as "supernatural, mysterious; filled with a sense of the presence of divinity, holy." Merriam Webster.

In shamanism, there are three worlds through which the shaman journeys to gather wisdom, knowing, and healing.

The upper world is the ethereal world of gods and goddesses, the ancestors, the ascended masters, and the compassionate angelic forces that are willing to be of service in our healing and gaining spiritual wisdom.

The middle world is the world of hidden reality, the dream aspect of the everyday world we live in. It has ordinary and non-ordinary aspects to it, both seen and unseen.

The lower world is the subconscious inner or lower world. The archetypical realm of the shadows.

Traditionally, monotonous drumming and/or rattling are used to serve as the portal to enter the shamanic state of consciousness, as well as guide our own awareness through the journey.

In my practice, I find people are sometimes hesitant of journeying, not because of fear, but rather because of they are not sure of what to do, or how.

Steps of the Shamanic Journey:

1. Be in a quiet space. Make sure you will not be disturbed for at least thirty minutes.

2. Relax your physical body through mindful movement or mindful breathing. Do a couple of deep breathing exercises to anchor soul in your body, connect with the inner space of sacredness to shift into a heart space.

3. Set an intention. If journeying on your own, this step is crucial as it serves both as the compass and the anchor of your journey. Which world will you visit? Which portal will you use? In addition, the intent for your journeying should be very clear.

4. Sit or lie down.

5. Listen to monotonous drumming or rattle music, or drum for yourself (but this is harder to do if you want to journey at the same time).

6. Enter your journey, and allow the process to guide you.

7. After returning from your journey, spend a few minutes in your quiet healing space. Allow yourself to integrate what you have witnessed.

8. *With as little movement as possible,* record your journey in detail. Remember you've had access to a higher state of consciousness in your journey, and as you begin to return to your normal state of consciousness, you will not likely remember your journey the way you do now. So now is the best time to write it down, and record it.

There is no right or wrong way to journey. Everything you witness in your journey will have a personal symbolic meaning that you may or may not understand at this time. Explore different worlds, levels in between worlds, different music. Explore sitting or lying down. Explore!

Keeping a *journey journal* is a great way to begin linking the symbolism you are shown during your practice of shamanic journeying. Always write down your journeys. For, just like a dream, while they may seem very alive at the moment, in time they will fade. But their essence will remain. Sometimes we just have to sit with our journeys, and clarity will come in time.

To best interpret a journey, ask open-ended questions about it and, as you sit with your journal, let yourself speak or write in a flowing manner, recording whatever comes to mind. Sometimes the answers will just flow straight to your pen, bypassing the mind.

Shamanic journeying is a practice that can greatly inform your life. The key is to establish a long-term relationship with your helping spirit guides and power animals with whom you can develop trust and good communication, over time. Remember, your journey is your own. And though we might be inclined to ask for feedback from others on our journeys, it is important to understand the way in which spirit is speaking to you is just as important as the journey. The stories, myths, impressions, archetypes, symbols, and metaphors are given to you to awaken the mystical within you; to awaken to your own mystery of self creation. So listen to your own intuition and your own wisdom first, which is, in itself, a big lesson.

THE VISION QUEST

I have learned that the point of life's walk is not where or how far I move my feet but how I am moved in my heart.

—*Anasazi Foundation, The Seven Paths: Changing One's Way of Walking in the World.*

The *vision quest* is a rite of passage, similar to an initiation, used by the Indigenous traditions of our world. Throughout time and across the spectrum of faiths, vision questing has been used as a tool to create a stronger connection with the divine, and every faith and culture has their own way of doing it. Vision questing is the ancient practice of opening the mind into our inner vision. A vision quest is a journey into the innermost aspects of your being, through your demons, through your grace, and into the heart of soul.

Traditionally, the vision quest is done out in nature. It begins with several days of preparation and teachings prior to the actual quest, which may involve three to four days and nights of dry fasting (no food, no water) alone in a place of wilderness. This is then followed by a few days of reintegration. Through the alchemy of the teachings, the preparation of the body for the intention of the soul through prayers, and the act of spiritual fasting and being in nature with no other distractions, we enter into an altered state of consciousness that leads us through visions into a powerful state of healing.

When approached in this way, a dry fast becomes a spiritual fast and is used to enhance your communion with the world of the unseen, to purify your mind and heart, and gift you with great clarity of vision. Spending time alone in nature, with no distractions, awakens us to our sense of belonging in the world, our sense of interconnectedness and of living in sacred reciprocity with all of life. Being in nature has been used as a tool to reconnect us to our inner nature, and brings us back into alignment with the rhythm of nature. Vision questing is a tool for self-realization.

A vision quest is a turning point in one's life, and its intention is to awaken in your consciousness a deeper understanding of your purpose and life direction, a deeper connection to the ancestral wisdom that resides within, a deeper connection to all life as well as the transformation of your demons and your wounds, both personal and ancestral, through the cracks that allow the light to come into your heart.

A vision quest is a ritual and a tool for tapping into your own medicine and anchoring into your body. It provides the tools for anchoring into the power of your intentions, for hearing the call of the soul and answering the door; for connecting into the power of your actions and of your deepest yearning to be whole. We often look for the answers to our challenges outside our self. We have forgotten that we have, and we are, the answers we seek. A vision quest cuts through the veils of our illusion and disharmony, and shows us the path back to wholeness, our own power, and the vision of our truth.

Through vision questing we remember deep in our cells the art of being. The experience brings you-us into stillpoint awareness and takes you into the wisdom of your ancestral lineage. Through vision questing, we come to better understand the biography of our lineage and awaken to the depth of the ancestral wisdom within. You also awaken to the ancestral wound and your BS. As you begin your process of cutting through them, you awaken to your shame (or other deep seated feelings) and begin to move from victimhood into authorship.

Through vision questing, we get to know who we truly are, both our demons and our grace. We get to make peace with our ancestry, our family, and our emotional self. We are able to tap into the world of the beyond for healing and for guidance. We are able to answer the call of soul, as we re-member the fragmented pieces of our selves into wholeness.

It is important to be *held* and supported during a vision quest. By this, I mean it's important to be energetically held by a teacher or an elder, by the wisdom of their teachings and the medicine of the lodge; by the sacred songs and the sound of the sacred drum, brought by the winds at our most challenging times, protected by prayer as the cedar burns in the sacred fire, and awakened by the soft fragrant scent of sweetgrass. I do not recommend that you go out into the bush for four days and four nights on a dry fast without being properly initiated and guided into the power and ritual of this process.

A vision quest is a tool to move beyond the veils of our own illusion into a place that is deeply anchored in universal truth. We remember who we are, we embody the ancestral wisdom within and, as we carve sacred space within, and we also begin to carve an outward expression of who we are here and now. We become more conscious of our journey, of the process, and of the subtle elements that make up our whole existence.

A vision quest allows you (and me) to rebuild our sacred vessel, our body temple, into a living sanctuary as it anchors us deeply into sacredness. Vision questing is the vessel that holds our inner quest towards wholeness.

THE ALCHEMY OF INNER QUESTING

Your vision will become clear only when you look into your heart. He who looks outside, dreams. He who looks inside, awakens.

—Carl Jung

Our quest towards wholeness is an inner process and, as such, it demands that you ask your self questions that bring you back into alignment with your higher self, your mightiness, your values, and your pathway towards your inner space of sacredness and source. What does it actually mean to come into alignment with yourself and your values? What does it feel like? Many questions arise when we are confronted with the task of self-inquiry.

While for some of us the path of a vision quest is part of our pathway in and through, the alchemy of self-inquiry in everyday living can also be a powerful ally in our journey.

Inner questing allows us to consciously tap within, ask those hard questions we've been avoiding and facing your self with the answers; it re-wires your belief system and upgrades your current operating system. Inner questing inherently uses mindfulness practices, through which we can recalibrate our heart compass deep into the core of the earth with great accuracy.

It's time to pause and reconnect. Grab a pen and paper, and spend a few minutes to recalibrate and check in with yourself.

Ask yourself:

- What is my soul's desire?
- What is my heart compass showing me?
- Can I lead the way?
- Can I trust that I am guided?
- Can I honestly take a look at my life and surrender to my heart?

If you struggle with getting started, ask to be guided. Before you go to bed tonight, ask to be shown: What does your heart desire the most? How can I pursue it? Hint, hint ... it is something you're already talented at that makes you happiest! We've all been given our talents and gifts for a reason; follow the giant arrow that points straight to your heart.

The *alchemy of inner questing* lies in using all your tools to ignite your heart into greater action. Your personal revolution awaits! You are powerful beyond measure, and have within you everything you need to be the source of your own medicine and the spark of your own magic. You are Mighty and the time has come to unleash your mightiness!

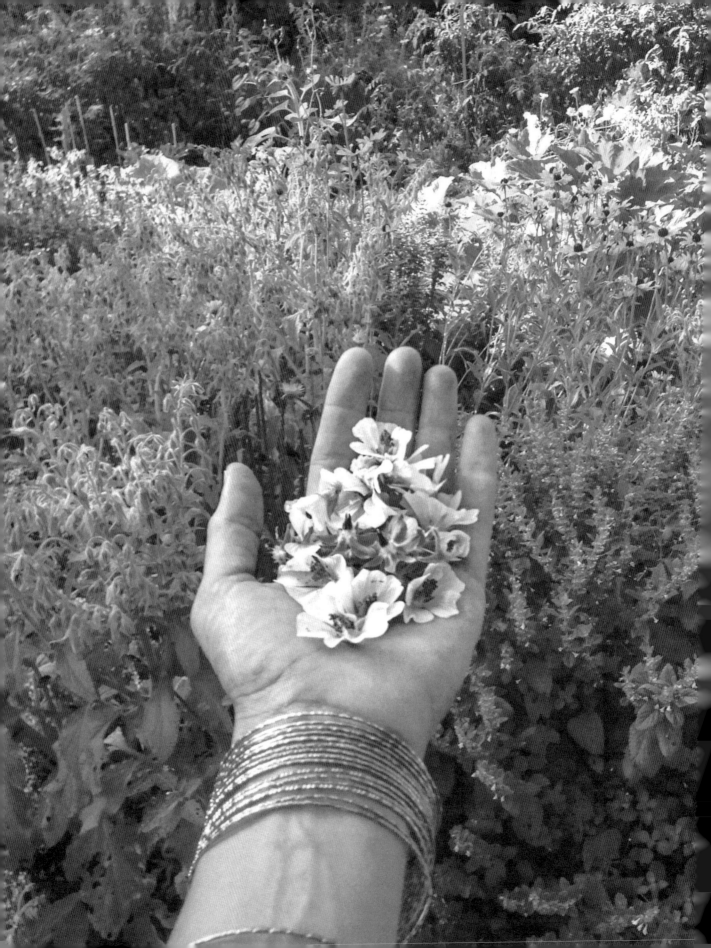

VIII

BE YOUR OWN REVOLUTION

TELL ME, WHAT IS IT YOU PLAN TO DO WITH YOUR ONE
WILD AND PRECIOUS LIFE?

—MARY OLIVER

12 THINGS I LEARNED FROM MY 40-DAY JUICE FAST

Fasting is the first principle of medicine; fast, and behold the strength of the Spirit.

—Rumi

January 15, 2012. My First 40-Day Juice Fast.

I had already been raw vegan for two and a half years, but something in me wanted a deeper experience, a deeper healing, a deeper cellular understanding, a deeper connection within, and a deeper experience of radiant health all throughout.

I decided to do the 40-day juice fast along with a 40-day deepening of both my meditation practice (40 minutes a day for 40 days) and my yoga practice. Rain or shine. I also decided to write publicly about it to create a deeper commitment within myself. At the time, 40 days seemed like a long time, and writing so openly allowed me to document my journey; my experience, my progress, my challenges, and my inspirations, and inspire others as I was inspiring myself. It was also a process of accountability.

My combo #3—a.k.a. 40-day juice fast / 40-day deeper meditation commitment / 40-day deeper yoga practice—changed my healing journey. I witnessed my body change from the inside out, and every blood test reassured me I was headed in the right direction.

Looking back on my 40-Day juice/meditation/yoga feast, there's a lot that I learned that I would like to share with you. I hope these tips, that I continue to use, serve you well as you build your own self-supported toolbox:

1. Fasting, or any combination of practices that support the inner journey, will inevitably allow your emotions, energy, thoughts, and attachments to move through you instead of getting stuck, and to feel it all is a good thing.

2. Become your own health expert; you know your self best. Today we have access to wonderful, insightful information about our health—at every level. All the answers are out there, if you are willing to seek them and make the effort to take advantage of them.

3. Commit, show up, seek support. Commit, show up, establish support from within. Making a commitment to stay on your healing journey with an open heart is a big step in showing up. When you dig in and commit, it's easier to seek support because you know where you're standing.

4. Set your intention(s) and continue to refer to them as they lead your way. Clearly stating your intentions—in writing—makes them more real, and allows you to navigate a clear path forward on your journey.

5. Slow down. In this hyper-fast-moving world in which we live, any practice that invites you to slow down is an incredible gift to your body, and to your higher self or soul.

6. Create the space for the witness to unfold. Connect with stillness. Set the boundaries you need to journey within, and ahead, to connect with your intentions and desires.

7. *Move your body with the intention of awareness, through the lens of mindfulness. Connect with your breath. Move and shift the impressions of your experiences still living in your bones and in your soul. Just let it go!*

8. Purify and sharpen your senses. Ignite your intuition. Through my journey, I began noticing how sharp and keen my senses were becoming. Notice how your senses sharpen as you proceed on yours.

9. Alkalize your what? Alkalize your that! Fresh, raw, organic, homemade vegetable juices provide the high-octane nutrition you need to heal, rest, reconnect, and rebuild. Juicing, meditating, and conscious movement practices are all great alkalizers!

10. Root into peace. Tap into gratitude. Shine your light. Making a conscious effort to root your choice in peace and gratitude can be difficult, but recognizing the power you have to move from victim consciousness to authorship is both empowering and liberating.

11. TRUST. Trust that life is inherently benevolent and will hold your heart. We often tend to trust in the doctors and specialists more than we trust ourselves. Once you engage your intention and effort, then you need to trust that you are being guided, even if your healing journey has not been linear.

12. Nope, there are no magic tricks or fancy curtains, just a lot of digging in.

DRIVE STRAIGHT THROUGH

In order to write about life, first you must live it.

—Hemingway

In this fast-times-at-fast-speed world we live in, your health can no longer afford the drive-thru as you know it. From now on the only drive-thru you will enter is the new and improved ***drive-straight-through;*** you know, the one with the giant arrow that points straight to your heart. Your new mantra: if it doesn't support, power up, or ignite your health, then, *drive straight through* and do not pick up the junk.

If it is wholeness and wellness that you seek, it is time to leave the fast food revolution behind and embrace the whole food revolution. But I must warn you. Once you go *in and through*, you might just find the healing you seek, the one that has been equally seeking you.

Nothing will happen without you, period. And *everything will happen the second you choose to take action.* That one single choice to take massive, imperfect, sustainable action will be the driving force along your roadmap to wellness.

Your drive straight through will not only transform your health, it will transform our current food system that is broken, and it will transform your relationship to food and your relationship with your self. It will awaken your desire to heal the fragmented aspects of your heart and your mind, and it will inspire you to claim your part in the healing of the Earth.

Know the journey will have ups and downs, but also know that you got this. Know that your actions and conscious non-actions, your power, your force to move mountains will ignite your Mighty inner healer as you power up your health, transform, and spark your own revolution into Mighty wellness.

Today, you and I are blessed with the opportunity of having ancient wisdom hold each and every step and breath we take. We have available to us tools and practices for deep healing at the root cause of our dis-ease or dis-harmony. Remember, we don't have to reinvent the wheel. We just have to be willing to get the wheel moving again.

Combining liquid nutrition (inclusive of the ritual of detox) and mindfulness practices with inner questing activates the spiral of awakening, allowing you to leap through your process at the *speed of light*. (Okay, maybe just with Mighty speed, but still…) In this way, you'll be able to bring about greater stability and create a strong foundation for you to root into as you rise.

Your roadmap to wellness allows you to bask your body in the deepest of medicines. It allows you to become conscious of your unconscious patterns and habits as you reclaim your power, create space for freedom, and softly remember and embody your authentic self.

MAKING PEACE WITH YOUR BODY

Plant kindness and gather love.

—Proverb

Each of us has our own story—the one about how we got to where we are. Along the way, we may have experienced trauma, sadness, grief, pain, anger, fear, rage, shame, guilt, self-hatred, negative self-talk, and all our heart's despair as we try to make sense of the injustices we've experienced and that we see in the world. Along the way, some of us got a chance to stare into the abyss, which brought a chance to make a clear choice: to continue on doing things as we were, numbing ourselves, perhaps without awareness, so as not to feel our pain. Or, we could choose to stop the negative cycles of pain and violence that have afflicted us, that we've been carrying for generations.

You and I have the choice to do things differently now and begin to take ownership of, and responsibility for, our body again; take ownership of our heart, our pain, our suffering, and our despair, allowing them to move through us and release them, creating new space for love.

Making peace with your body *is a journey.* The path for glowing health is right here, right now. Treat your body as a ***living sanctuary.*** Nourish yourself through whole and wholesome food, love, and plenty of time spent in nature, mindfulness, and self-inquiry practices. As you know by now, these are all tools that align us with our path towards wholeness.

What you eat, drink, assimilate, and think today will be at the cellular core of who you are tomorrow, and a core belief in how you act the day after that. We are not just our cells, not just our bodies, not just our emotions, not just our thoughts nor the mind that holds those thoughts, and not just our Soul. We are all of these and more. We are the space and the sacredness that holds us and weaves us together. Beyond a sacred temple, you are a living sanctuary.

Yes, repeat out loud with me: *I am a living sanctuary.*

Doesn't that sound and feel beautiful? Read it again. Read it again quietly and then out loud.

I am a living sanctuary, a place and an inner space of peace, love, radiant vibrant health, sacredness and refuge, through grace.

How would you treat this living sanctuary? How would you allow others to treat your living sanctuary? What would you do and not do within this sacred space? It is through tools and practices that bring awareness, consciousness, radiant, and vibrant health into your life that you begin to tap into the awareness of being a living sanctuary.

Perhaps, at the core of our awakening, we will come to accept our selves and our lives as we are. Perhaps, at the root of our awakening into sacredness, we will come to accept our selves and our lives as we are, in love. As above, so below. The space of love.

NON-NEGOTIABLE

Non·ne·go·ti·a·ble /ˌnä(n)nə ˈgōSHəbəl/[23]

adjective:

1. *not open to discussion or modification.*

As you anchor into the awakening of your Mighty Inner Healer, I invite you to choose one or perhaps three non-negotiable actions towards yourself that will allow you to build yourself up and begin to rise.

A non-negotiable action is one stemming from deep self-compassion; one that will allow you to power up and spark your personal revolution beyond your habitual actions, habitual thought patterns, self-sabotage, and any of your circumstances that conspire against you—because they

---

23   "Non-negotiable", Oxford English Dictionary.

will. A non-negotiable action is a personal choice - meant to be one of your greatest allies in your pursuit towards wellness, radiant health and happiness.

Changing your habits may not be easy at first, but with the aid of the non-negotiable you will begin to get out of your own way. Have you ever turned your alarm to snooze, knowing full well that if you simply got up the way you intended to and did your meditation practice, your day would most likely turn into the best day ever? Yet still your mind starts to chatter and convince you that those extra twenty minutes in bed are worth hitting the snooze button? Then, when you finally get up you are groggy and slow, and you really, really wish you had overcome your mind and simply gotten up, because now you are so totally not ready for the day, never mind for it to be the best day ever? I know I have.

Until I began to use my "non-negotiable" as a tool to not allow my mind and my process of Evolution-Going-On (Ego) to interfere with my mission to heal deeply, I was an expert at hitting the snooze button. I hit the snooze when it was time to eat healthier meals; I hit the snooze when it was time to juice daily; I hit the snooze when it was time to exercise. Yes, I hit the snooze plenty of times until life came knocking at my door and I had to make a decision. Because yes, it is simply a decision.

Stop hitting the snooze button. Identify your own non-negotiables, and make a decision. Once you do, you'll begin to climb out of your self-sabotage and unclaimed personal power, and own your story as you begin to live in your truth. Deep healing happens just as we make that decision, and choose to do that single action.

A non-negotiable can be choosing to have one cup of coffee a day instead of five. It can be choosing to start your day with a jar of liquid nutrition, or claiming some time and space for yourself each day to simply be present to your Self, or to breathe deep with eyes closed while you place your hand on your heart. We are all different, and there are as many possible non-negotiable actions as there are humans on this Earth. We all need something different and out of that need, your own non-negotiables will arise.

You may know what your first non-negotiable is already, or you may not. Either way, spend some time in the inquiry.

What boundary or non-negotiable do I need to set up for myself to deepen my healing? To ignite the change that I seek within myself?

Start with one – and make a decision.
Commit to it.
Show up.
Be present.
Teach love by the way you live.
Repeat.

REWILDING

Rewild, v; to foster and maintain a sustainable way of life through hunter-gatherer-gardener social and economical systems; including, but not limited to, the encouragement of social, physical, spiritual, mental and environmental biodiversity and the prevention and undoing of social, physical, spiritual, mental and environmental domestication and enslavement.

—Peter Michael Bauer

Rewilding is a progressive approach to conservation through the process of creating the right conditions for a place, ecosystem, or species to be able to take care of itself. Rewilding allows wildlife's natural rhythms to create wilder, more thriving, biodiverse habitats. When we get out of nature's way, nature knows how to survive, how to heal itself, how to self-govern and self-regulate. Nature finds a way to thrive and evolve, and always come back to the space of love.

As humans, we too are in a process of rewilding, of learning how to best create the right inner conditions for the life within to begin to thrive again. You and I are learning how to best get out of our own ways, so as to allow the body to heal and self-regulate. We are learning how to rewild as we align our body's elemental rhythms with those of nature, and how to reconnect with our inner source, our inner space of grace and love.

As humans, we used to live in intimate relationship with the land and the elements around us. Our survival depended upon our ability to be present to the land, and deeply connected to our bodies. As the domesticated animals we have come to be, we've lost our connection to the land

and to our bodies, for we believe our survival does not depend on that connection. Perhaps it is time to re-evaluate.

Rewilding is a movement of awakening into the mightiness of your heart, and the rewilding of your senses to live a more authentic life, aligned with your true nature. We ignite our inner fires as we remember the only way to survive is to come back into connection and relationship with the land and with our bodies.

The goal of rewilding is to *restore your own ecosystem so it can come to look after itself.* The process requires awareness and accountability, and demands that we claim responsibility for our actions towards ourselves and others. Your true nature away from being rigid is rather a fluid state of communion. Your journey home to your wild true nature demands that you become independent thinkers and doers, that you engage with a new-found depth of care for one another, and that you cultivate healthy, authentic, deep interactions with both humans and the "more-than-human" realms of our existence.

INNER OUTER

Everything relies on everything else in order to manifest.

—Thich Nhat Hanh

Your body is a community of human cells in relationship with/to countless other tiny organisms without whom you wouldn't be able to think, move, speak or be who you are in this very moment. Yet most of the time we fail to recognize that just like your body is a giant living community working together in symbiosis, so is our Earth a living, breathing, giant ecosystem of which we are a part. We forget that whatever happens in our inner realms is also happening in our outer reality. We forget that the microcosm is in constant relationship with the macrocosm, and that whatever happens in one, will affect the other and vice versa.

So as you power up, ignite, transform and reclaim yourself, I invite you to extend your process beyond the boundaries of your skin, and step into ever more congruent, sacred relationship with all living beings inclusive of Gaia, Mother Earth.

As we heal ourselves, we heal the Earth. As we restore our own ecosystem into a sustainable, healthy source of life-giving radiance and wellness, we begin to also understand the need to care deeply for our outer ecosystem. The way in which we engage in relationship with ourself is the way we engage with each other, and with Mother Earth. We must come to understand that the ability of our own bodies to truly thrive is interdependent and interrelated to the ability of our greater ecosystem to thrive, inclusive of the ecological and cultural diversity of all natural systems. The human species has come to live in the erroneous belief that we are owners of this Earth, as if the Earth was simply a mechanical instrument for us to exploit for our so called well-being. We have forgotten the Earth is indeed a living system, with whom we live in relationship with rather than ownership of.

As you expand your conceptual and perceptual awareness of yourself beyond the boundary of your skin you will come to experience, understand and awaken to yourself as a relational self, or ecological self.

Vietnamese Buddhist monk Thich Nhat Hanh coined the term inter-being to best describe the true nature of our existence. We cannot exist alone; we can only exist in relation to one another. Our relational self or ecological self, recognizes that we are all a part of the greater web of existence. It invites us to define ourself, not only through the relationships we have with other human beings, but through the relationship we have with the larger community of all living beings, inclusive of our beautiful Earth.

This awareness of our ecological self is at the root of the environmental philosophy and social movement known as Deep Ecology. "Deep Ecology is based in the belief that humans must radically change their relationship to nature from one that values nature solely for its usefulness to human beings, to one that recognizes that nature has an inherent value." [24]

Through our personal journeys we come to realize we've always been dancing the inner outer dance of healing ourselves through healing the Earth, and through answering the call to heal the Earth, healing ourselves. Your ability to be self reflective allows you to transform your own wounding through sacred congruent action with the Earth. It allows you to root into what-has-cracked-your-heart-open, and establish a path of action as you embrace your Self with compassion, acceptance, receptivity and an openness to be present.

Inner outer are reflections of one another, in inter-existence.

---

24   "Deep Ecology", Encyclopaedia Britannica

THE POWER OF ALIGNMENT

The source of all creation is pure consciousness... pure potentiality seeking expression from the unmanifest to the manifest. And when we realize that our true Self is one of pure potentiality, we align with the power that manifests everything in the universe.

—Deepak Chopra, *The Law of Pure Potentiality.*

Alignment can be defined as: *"an arrangement of objects in a way that makes a line or row; or as parts of something that are in the proper position relative to each other."*[25]

For me, the power of alignment resides in the feeling of being one with the universe, the power of living your purpose, and the power of living consciously.

To me, alignment is the process of merging the fires in my belly, mind, and heart in sacred relationship and the unleashing of my potential, my mightiness, into the world through sacred action.

Alignment is the process of living a conscious, ethically, and ecologically responsible life, rooted in the values of self (and global) respect, honesty, interconnectedness, and the pursuit of peace within, with our self and the world at large.

Alignment, to me, is stacking the odds *for* me not *against* me. It is stacking my actions towards greater health and wellness of body, heart, and mind, with soul. It is layering the three pillars for wellness along with the many tools and practices that continue to build me up every single day.

What does alignment mean to you?

Know that the depth of alignment you seek is possible. *It's all possible.* Our commitment to ourselves will lead the way to the journey to our true self, and to the freedom that comes when living with an open heart, to the depth of healing your Mighty inner healer will unlock, and its power to ignite and transform you.

Seek your truth.

Remember it, align with it, embrace it, surrender to it, walk it. Be it.

---

25   "Alignment", YourDictionary.com

THE PURPOSE OF DEDICATION

I've learned that people will forget what you said, people will forget what you did,
but people will never forget how you made them feel.

—Maya Angelou

As we begin to consciously become part of the whole, we realize the power our life has to be a force for change and good. We realize that each and every action has the power to shift our whole experience of life, and therefore the experience others have of us in our life together. We are all interconnected. The one affects the whole and the whole affects the one.

As our heart unfolds, surrenders, and merges into the world, we begin to dedicate our life to others with a sense of deep respect for all sentient beings. We begin opening our self up to the nourishment and beauty of life; to the gifts, the mystical, the magic, and the miracles happening constantly around us. **We realize we can only truly rise when we elevate others.**

So, as you rise, (because you will), think about who you are elevating. Who are you dedicating your journey to? Who are you dedicating your mightiness to, besides your self? For, you know, the ride is sweeter when we share it. And together we are stronger.

As you dedicate your self forward, what kind of choices will you make? What kind of choices won't you make?

Can your individual acts be a resource, and a part of the solution? Can the sum of our single actions change the world?

As we dedicate our life to the greater *life*, a deeper sense of responsibility of self, other, and All emerges from within. As we elevate others, we embody our wholeness, our interconnectedness. Our sense of self widens into an empowered state, and there is a new-found depth of alignment that brings even greater coherent action into our lives.

Take a few minutes now and think about who you would like to dedicate your emergence to.

PRAY IT FORWARD

prayer /prer/[26]

noun

1. *a solemn request for help or expression of thanks addressed to God or an object of worship.*
2. *an earnest hope or wish.*

Is prayer the act of asking to receive, or is it the act of giving forward?

What does prayer mean to you?

As you heal, ignite your mightiness, dig in and through, can the dedication of your journey or perhaps the gratitude for your journey become a prayer?

Can you feel into the gratitude for your journey, for the teachings, for the magic, and for the medicine?

Can you expand into the feeling of gratitude, from deep in your core, as a prayer for peace?

Can the dedication of your movements, your actions, your healing, become an active prayer to make both your body and this earth a better place?

Can you perhaps commit to sending ripples of prayers forward as you become your mighty health warrior, or even just because?

Prayer is a powerful force that activates the universe into conspiring action. It is a Mighty force that changes our body chemistry, our thoughts, our emotions, and the mindfulness in our actions.

Connecting with something greater than yourself, through prayer, continues to align your mind with the universal mind, continues to inspire you into action, continues to ignite your heart into a leap of faith so Mighty that it too will become your ally.

So go ahead. Connect in with something greater than yourself, even if your prayer is just for your self—your wish or hope to get better. Go ahead. Ask to receive. Feel into it. Then feel into

---

26 "Prayer", Oxford English Dictionary.

the feeling of having received your heartfelt prayer. Allow that feeling to expand. Anchor deeply into it.

Thank you. Thank you. Then, pray it forward.

AWAKENING OF DEVOTION

What is important is not the specific manner in which God is worshiped but the degree to which the devotee is filled with love.

—Prem Prakash, The Yoga of Spiritual Devotion A Modern Translation of the Narada Bhakti Sutras.

Devotion or bhakti is one of the four main yogic paths to enlightenment; its only requirement is an open loving heart. *Some of us surrender into devotion through our challenges; most of us awaken into devotion through our practices.*

Devotion is the art of falling in love. Its ultimate goal is to awaken to our higher self, and to the feeling of pure bliss attained through the devotional surrender to the divine. This time, it is in and through our heart that we surrender into devotional love. It's in and through the cultivation of our practice that our heart unites our soul with the object of our devotion.

The path of devotion ultimately leads to our outer life becoming an ever-increasing expression of our higher self, as it begins more and more to manifest and express itself into the world. Our life itself then becomes a dance, a form of worship, of being in a state of constant sacred reciprocity. The path of devotion is many-layered indeed. It requires an inner offering of selfless love towards our very own heart, and an outer offering of ayni (sacred reciprocity) to feed the world around us with our love.

And though we have techniques, tools, and practices to facilitate our awakening into love, our own awakening is beyond them; it stems from the intuitive experience perceived by the heart of the world of the within, where time and space cease to exist.

How do we cultivate devotion? I have shared many tools and techniques with you already, but here I will name a few within the context of devotion:

- Allow yourself to fall into love with your self, and all the life that surrounds you
- Set your heart intention before your mindfulness practice
- Engage in ritual/ceremony to stay connected with the space of sacredness within and live in sacred reciprocity
- Create a heart-full outer living sanctuary to remind you of the fullness of your inner heart
- Continue to bring your heart back into your mindfulness practice. In your practice, use devotional chanting (or its music), mantra meditation, and use the Sanskrit names of the yoga poses to reconnect you to the subtle energy each pose is meant to awaken within you
- Use pranayama (deep breathing exercises) to calm and centre your being
- Wear your heart on your sleeve and speak it out loud
- Keep showing up; keep coming back to the space of the heart, keep reconnecting with stillpoint awareness as your core
- Offer a prayer into the world

LIVING IN REVERENCE

If you want the secrets to the universe, think in terms of energy, frequency and vibration.

—Nikola Tesla

As we awaken into devotion, we surrender into living in ***reverence.***

Living in reverence is the art of living in sacred reciprocity, the art of engaging in sacred action through life-affirming practices, rituals, and ceremonies of remembering. It's the harmonious act of a mutual respectful exchange, in alignment with both your personal truth and the consciousness that created you. It's the alchemy of claiming your magic and gifting your medicine for the benefit of another, for the benefit of our planet.

The three pillars that make your roadmap to wellness will engage you to also live in reverence as you ignite your own alchemy of wellness. Living in reverence is a core principle of the shamanic path, also known as ayni (sacred reciprocity in the Quechua language of the Incas), as the three ethics in permaculture (page 31), and as Dharma in the Vedic (Yoga and Ayurveda) traditions.

Through sacred reciprocity, we re-establish the sacred web that once held us. By tapping into the inner space of sacredness within, we heal through remembering our primordial nature (the root cause of the root causes of disease), we strengthen the sacred ground upon which we stand, and through love we begin to weave the sacred fabric of all our relationships, to self, other and Mother Earth.

The practices that ignite your mightiness also purify your five bodies, open your heart and ground your mind into it, align you with both spirit and the core of your core, and anchor you into soul. These practices bring you into greater alignment with the rhythms of your inner nature and the cosmic nature. They serve you to reclaim your health, your personal power, and the ancient that speaks through you. They awaken you to your duty and responsibility as an Earth citizen. They infuse you with your sense of belonging, and your power to be your best self going forward, in reverence to all of life.

DAILY PRACTICE

The important point of spiritual practice is not to try and escape your life, but to face it—exactly and completely.

—Dainin Katagiri

As you continue the process of anchoring knee deep into the earth and embodying your sacred temple again, creating and maintaining a ***daily practice—Sadhana*** is crucial to your journey of becoming mighty.

Having a daily practice begins with carving out sacred space, and connecting with your self on a daily basis. It becomes the time and space where you connect first with your breath, and then connect in with your higher self or soul. It allows you to stay connected with your heart, and provides you with a safe place to process whatever is going on for you right now. It allows quiet time and inner space for processing new insights, understanding and perspective. It is also the time where you connect with the source within where you can feel supported and feel grace. It is a practice that leads to self-realization.

Making this daily commitment to your self is vital to becoming your own revolution. As you take ownership of your life, you begin to anchor back into your body, building a stronger foundation, releasing what you no longer need, and keeping only that which serves you. Although your daily spiritual practice is an external practice, its purpose is to anchor you into the internal landscape of sacredness, peace, and grace. It is a felt sense experience and, in the daily doing of it, you begin to access ever deeper layers of yourself, most of which you didn't even know existed.

The *daily* aspect of your practice is crucial because today we live in such a fast-paced world of distraction. Our world, in general, functions because most of us are spending all our time outside ourselves, outside our bodies, disconnected from our hearts, disconnected from our minds, and disconnected from our purpose. In other words, in total *dysfunction*.

The rat race in all its craziness is simply getting faster and faster because we're not stopping / anchoring / feeling the generational consequences of our actions. The mind is the first to go out of balance, and the nervous system follows. We are now bearing witness to the global effects of our disharmony—and it has a price tag.

One of the best ways to calm your unbalanced nervous system is through some kind of daily practice. This might include meditation, yoga, chanting, toning, spending time in nature, conscious movement practices, slowing down, breathing exercises, awareness-based practices, or creative expression practices.

Your daily practices will change over time, but the commitment to creating the sacred time and space for your self remains unchanged. The gifts that come from going within include the expansion of your consciousness, the activating or awakening of the kundalini energy, remembering and igniting your Mighty inner healer and ultimately your own enlightenment or self-liberation—*a.k.a. **unleashing your mightiness!** Remember, the practice is the practice.*

AWAKENING KUNDALINI ENERGY

Kundalini is the higher evolutionary force hidden within you that has the ability to unfold your spiritual potential.

—David Frawley

Kundalini is a higher evolutionary psycho-spiritual force, the energy of the consciousness that lies dormant within you until it is activated spontaneously or by your spiritual practices. It is your creative soul potential, and has the ability to bring new states of consciousness, including mystical illumination and transcendence of self. The word *kundalini* comes from the Sanskrit language and means snake or serpent power. It is believed that once the kundalini energy awakens, it moves from the base of your spine (root chakra), in the form of a snake, up towards the top of your head (seventh chakra).

> *"The word 'Kundalini' generally refers to that dimension of energy that is yet to realize its potential. There is a huge volume of energy within you that is yet to find its potential. It is just there waiting, because what you call a human being is still in the making. You are not yet a human being, you are a 'human becoming.' You are not an absolute entity of being human. There is constant scope to make yourself into a better human being."—Sadhguru.*

The awakening of kundalini energy is enhanced by tools of self-realization, such as mindfulness practices, yoga, meditation, being of service, eating a diet high in raw foods, juicing protocols, fasting, water fasting, liquid feasting, detox, sacred practices, vision quests, inner questing, and the daily observance of a spiritual discipline or practice.

I find that for most people, it's a process of tuning in to the world of the subtle. Tuning in to that part of yourself, to root into that place where your authentic, essential self (soul) lives, and making a commitment to live from that place, wearing your heart on your sleeve. Throughout this book, I speak often of aligning your forces in synergy. When you combine several tools for igniting your mightiness, you speed up your own process of awakening. It's a beautiful thing to awaken to your potential, to heal into the deeper layers of your tissues, to arrive at a place of trusting your soul, and to remember who you are.

As you purify your body, align your whole-body system with your soul, quiet your mind, and tap into your heart, you will bring great coherence and vitality to your life.

Awakening kundalini energy can be experienced as the awakening of the treasure within. It is your most creative potential waiting to be discovered by your heart. It is the source of your truth and energy, and the universal consciousness within you.

The awakening of kundalini energy is the process of your own awakening and liberation, which happens in and through the awakening and rebalancing of the five bodies (physical, emotional, mental, soul, and spirit bodies) and the seven key energy centres in your body—your seven chakras—whose reclaiming is needed for you to align with the wholeness and the mightiness that you are.

BECOMING YOUR OWN MASTER ALCHEMIST

The real alchemy is transforming the base self into gold or into spiritual awareness. That's really what new alchemy's all about.

—*Fred Alan Wolf, Mind into Matter, and Matter into Feeling.*

Alchemists are the masters of transformation. They hold the key to the portal of wellness, for they shapeshift and transmute mercury into gold, toxicity into radiance, a broken heart into a well of love. Alchemists know there is great power in the sacred subtle dimensions of our existence, and know our bodies are but vehicles for spiritual transcendence.

Alchemists may choose to reside in the far away caves of the Himalayas, away from the busyness of the world. But today, more and more, you and I are becoming our own master alchemists, for we know our bodies best. Today, this brave new world is demanding that we step up, seek the support and stability the ancient rituals offer, and awaken to the truth that our very own mightiness is needed.

Alchemists know the secrets to longevity are not actually secrets after all. Synergy always plays a wild card and, if we stack the cards right, longevity, radiance and radiant health are a few steps away. Our challenges become our greatest teachers. They crack our hearts open and we are reborn with new insights, new perspectives, new tools, and new practices that build our sacred container for the abundant, thriving life to step forward.

As you and I remember we are the alchemists of our own lives, it is up to us to turn ourselves into gold. We have available to us ancient tools for deep healing, which lead to radiance. But can we step away from the old habits that no longer serve us? Can we try new practices that build us up? Can we tap into new beliefs that move us forward, and release old ones that keep us trapped? Can we empower ourselves to seek our own medicine? And can this medicine be, most of all, the deep nourishment we choose to gift to ourselves?

You and I both have the power, the ability, and the responsibility to become our own master alchemist. The journey ahead may not be linear, but it will bring to us the greatest gifts. And the thing is, we need each other. We need each other to be our best potential, to live our soul's purpose, to radiate not only radiance but also happiness, joy, peace, and freedom. For when we do this, we elevate all those around us with our presence, we make the world a better place, and we live more fulfilled lives that change everything and everyone around us.

Deeply nurture and nourish yourself. You are a living sanctuary, and as such need to self-care. It doesn't have to take a long time; it just must be soul food.

So go ahead, *become your own mighty master alchemist.* You are worth it. I believe you have the power to change, to transform, to shape shift, to break away from the old boundaries holding you back, both inherited and self-created, and to live in freedom.

18 TOOLS TO UNLEASH YOUR MIGHTINESS

might·y /ˈmīdē/[27]

Adjective: ***Mighty;*** *comparative adjective:* ***mightier;*** *superlative adjective:* ***mightiest***

1. *possessing great and impressive power or strength, especially on account of size.*

By now, I hope you believe me when I tell you, **you are mighty beyond measure.** And **you've** got what it takes. You are powerful; you have the strength to move in and through your journey. And the size of your intention to heal? Well, it will move mountains.

---

27   "Mighty", Oxford English Dictionary.

As you now know, liquid nutrition (inclusive of the ritual of detox), mindfulness, and inner questing are three important pillars in your foundation, along your roadmap to wellness. To ignite your mightiness, it is important to examine that foundation on a regular basis.

Here are eighteen tools and attitudes to unleash your mightiness.

1. *Connect within to your higher self.* Even if you are not currently challenged, are you including any or all of these vital tools to create better health, to detoxify, to rebuild, and to heal yourself? To discover and get in touch with your authentic self, and be the best possible version of yourself? All of the above? *Every day, every breath, and every action are an opportunity to transform. An invitation to be reborn.*

2. *Decide: What or how do you want to feel? What is it you want to receive? What is it you want to give?* Write this feeling down. Write down some goals that will allow you to feel this way today. Start your day with this inquiry, and bear witness to your mightiness in action.

   Gaining clarity on what and how you want to feel today is crucial in helping redefine your goals and your intentions, and will save you a lot of unwanted turns along your healing journey.

   Having clear goals that are anchored in feeling well daily will help you shift old habits, attitudes, and behaviours and adapt new ones with less resistance.

3. *Ignite and balance your inner fire.* Ignite and balance the fire in your belly, the fire in your heart, your passions, your joy, your love, the fire in your mind, and your inspiration. Get in-spirited as you ignite and balance your ancestral sacred fire!

4. *Identify attachment to old habits, attitudes, and behaviours, and flip the vibe.* Are your attachments a source of your suffering? If so, which ones? Are the foods you eat and the drinks you drink currently contributing to your health goals? Are your attitudes, BS, current emotions, and fears building you up? Or are they contributing to your challenges? Are you facing resistance to change? Fear of change, fear of letting go, fear of stepping into authorship, fear of being responsible? Fear of being well?

   Pause and feel. You have the ability to flip the vibe. You have the ability to witness your self in action, and witness the actions that are no longer serving you, your healing or your health. Go back to the feeling you wrote about in point #2, and to the goals that support that feeling. Is the attachment you have to XYZ supporting the way you want to feel? If not, it's time to reassess. Time to create some space between you, and that thing you're attached to.

Silencing the negative inner voice. We all have a little voice in our head that's often negative. Listen to it as you set your goals and go about trying to implement new habits. What is it saying? (*This won't work, you can't do this, this is too much work, this is a waste of time, it's too expensive, nothing I do ever works … and on and on and on.*) Sound familiar? Listen for it—and when you hear it talking—write it down so you will recognize it quickly when it shows up. There's a wealth of information there to help you see how you may be holding yourself back! Once you identify it, it's important to silence it quickly. It's not in charge. You are. Have a positive affirming statement ready to replace it. "*This will work. I can do this. I've got this. This is the best investment I've ever made. I AM worth it.*" Be ready, because at some point you will need these words.

5. ***Drink your greens, mindfully move, be still, and connect with Nature to get to know yourself better.*** Green is the colour of the heart chakra. It is the colour that abounds in nature, the colour that soothes a hot mind, and the colour that grounds an anxious scattered mind. When we drink our greens, it brings mineral density back into our lives. Your health revolution is also a mighty green revolution, in more ways than one.

6. ***Care for the earth. Care for people. Fair share.*** These are the three ethics of permaculture. They are also three ethics to keep in mind when tuning into and unleashing your mightiness.

In a world where we have lost sight of personal responsibilities, it is important, actually, key to our healing and survival that we anchor deeply into ethics and begin to take responsibility for our actions.

> *Permaculture is a holistic design system for creating sustainable human settlements and food production systems. It is a movement concerned with sustainable, environmentally sound land use and the building of stable communities, through the harmonious interrelationship of humans, plants, animals and the Earth.*
>
> *By this very definition, this system necessitates that our conduct is focused on the good of the planet, Nature and the people. It cannot work otherwise.*— *deepgreenpermaculture.com*

Just like in permaculture, once we ignite our mightiness, it's important that we keep it focused on the good of the planet, nature, and the people. It cannot work otherwise. Strive to create and support sustainable systems that extend beyond your self into the care of the earth, care for people, and fair share.

Our own healing, actions, and relationship to self are interdependent and interconnected with our relationship with *the environment,* Mother Earth, Gaia. So as we care for the earth, as we care for people, as we continue to share our gifts and our purpose along with the sharing of resources to create healthier, striving communities, we engage in life-affirming actions that awaken us to living in reverence, even as we deepen our own healing.

As you heal your self, you heal the world. And we can only truly rise when we elevate others.

7. ***Commit to taking massive, imperfect, sustainable action.*** Sometimes our challenges require us to change fast. Sometimes we have the luxury of time. Focus on creating sustainable actions that will continue to build you up beyond the end of today. Sustainable actions will support your mind, emotions, and nervous system, bring more coherence into your life, and weave support systems into your journey.

Mightiness develops like a muscle. How are you developing your mightiness? What can you do next that is sustainable for you … *right now*?

Perhaps is it adding some liquid nutrition power once a day, or even just once a week—*right now*. Perhaps it's ending your day with five minutes of mindfulness deep breathing practice—*right now*. Perhaps it's spending ten minutes a week in quiet contemplation or self-inquiry. You can implement very simple practices immediately. *Right now.*

Don't add more stress to your life. You don't need it, nobody does. Keep it simple, ***but commit to taking action.***

Mindfulness of your process will take you a long way; it is one of your greatest gifts.

8. ***Ignite the law of addition.*** *Add on,* and what you wish to let go of will simply fall away! When you embark on changing your habits and lifestyle, it can be quite overwhelming to take things away (foods and habits) and replace them with the new foods, habits, and the lifestyle you desire. It can be more than overwhelming, and will require a transition time. You bet your body just might freak out.

Adding on will leave you in a state of abundance; taking away can easily leave you in a negative state, feeling deprived. So why take away when all you need to do is add? The patterns and habits you were so attached to—that you thought were oh-so-important in your life—will simply slowly vanish. Once we start to feel good, we want to continue feeling good. Right?

For example, start your day with a juice, smoothie, or elixir *before* you have your morning coffee. Then you might just have one cup of coffee instead of three, and be fully satisfied, or might have just a small cup, before you lose interest in it all together.

Having said that, sometimes we are challenged in a way that requires us to change quickly, to rapidly shift, and to adapt to this brave new world fast and furiously. So honour where you are, and if this is needed—then you go for it.

9. *Plan for your success.* The food you eat and the lifestyle you enjoy play a big role in your feeling of well-being. Get involved in preparing and making your food and your liquid gold. Pause and feel, and reset your lifestyle to nurture you.

    When you plan for success, you feel more nourished, more supported, and believe you can successfully transition into a healthier lifestyle. Some of your goals might include enjoying liquid nutrition once a day, beginning your day with mindfulness practice, and/or doing a Mighty detox once or twice a year. Planning will not only save you time, but it also will save you stress and money, and add strength and resolution to your journey.

    Food and lifestyle choices can build us up or tear us down. Connect deeply. Build yourself up. Make one change, pause and feel, evolve. Then make another. One step at a time. You've got this.

10. *Explore. Stay curious. Variety and spice give happiness to life.* Staying curious about your process will allow you to perhaps investigate, and open doors you never would have considered. So, keep the flame of curiosity alive, ignite your inner fire, and rewild your self alive!

    When using liquid nutrition to build a stronger foundation, focus on variety to keep your Mighty self engaged, inspired, sparkly, and alive. Spices are key to staying balanced, especially in the north, where we must adjust to the seasons.

    Rotating the vegetables and greens you juice and include in your smoothies will ensure you get a wide variety of nutrient density into your system. Including a variety of flavours, from sweet to savoury and everything in between, will keep you going and inspired. Being playful with your exploration regarding colours, textures, aromas, and coolness/warmth will add other dimensions to your experience of liquid nutrition.

When approaching mindfulness practices, I invite you to experiment with the various practices I have offered, until you find what resonates deeply within you. Then stick with that one. Commit to your practice, rain or shine. Allow it to become a portal to your evolution.

When engaging with the alchemy of inner questing ask a variety of questions. Ask for what needs to be seen, ask-ask-ask … for it's in the asking that we stop hiding.

11. *Be gentle with your self.* It is easier to be compassionate and gentle towards those around us, even towards strangers passing by, than to our self. And it's always so much easier to have awareness and insight into the healing journeys of others, than of our own.

We can be quite blinded by our habits, by our deeply rooted beliefs. So, when we get challenged (because we will), it is so important to turn that open heart towards ourselves. We are multidimensional beings, and your journey is unique to you. Embrace your own heart and your own journey with compassion, with inquiry, with tenderness and a gentle caress.

12. *Create a support system. Reach out to your community, or create your own soul tribe!* We humans are social beings. Most of us don't live in isolation. Most of us thrive and do best when surrounded by people and systems that build us up; that keep us safe, and allow us to explore yet hold the space for us to succeed. So, as you transition into new habits and routines, it's key to seek out people already on the journey on which you are embarking. It's so important to feel deeply that you are not alone, and you have all the support you need to succeed.

13. *Claim your magic! Commit to your journey. Strive to be limitless.* Know it will have ups and downs and sometimes even plateau. But know also—*that you've got this.* This ride is yours for the taking. It's yours for the claiming. Strive to move beyond the limits that currently define you. You are worth it.

14. *Blisscipline.* Yes. Discipline yourself for bliss. We have to. Create the sacred space in which your great unfolding will happen. You have to create that new non-negotiable routine, establish that new non-negotiable habit that will allow you to transform your current state of affairs into the one you dream of. One juice at a time, one smoothie at a time, one elixir at a time. One breath, one thought, one action at a time. Are you ready to revolution your self alive?

15. ***Add some G power to your attitude!*** Choose an attitude of gratitude as the source of your new-found vision, as your lifejacket to dive deeper into your self. Fill yourself with gratitude for all the good things already in your life, gratitude for the experiences that have led you to this place as you begin to recognize them as your teacher, as you are guided into this journey of reclaiming your sacred self and your Mighty sacred heart.

    Connecting with gratitude allows us to see the light at the end of the tunnel. We begin to know we can do this, and we're not alone. The helplessness of our victim consciousness begins to shift into the empowerment of authorship. We begin to detach slightly from our story, and this allows us to create room within to implement all those tools for deep alignment we've been yearning for. The very ones we (falsely) believed we could not do.

    In order to leap to the next version of our self, we must jump from the cliff of old habits and old patterns; re-examine our attitudes, beliefs and feelings, and let go of what no longer serves us. Make space for trust. Make space for gratitude. Make space for magic. Make space for Grace. Make space for the universe to conspire in and through you, as you dear one, have always been a mighty healer.

16. ***Celebrate your AWESOMENESS!! Celebrate your steps; they will make your journey that much sweeter!*** We often want to get from point A to point B as quickly and easily as possible, and then move quickly on to the next. Sounds familiar? But what if you stopped for a moment, and celebrated the little steps that are getting you to point B; the new habits, the new thoughts, the new moments of discovery, the new wisdom, the new a-ha moments? If we can just take a moment to notice our successes and then celebrate them with gratitude, we might just skip point B all together and find ourselves living a life that is beyond our wildest dreams. *Gratitude, celebration, love, and self-healing like to hang out together.*

17. ***Trust in the bigger picture. Awaken the hope activist within.*** It is so easy to get lost in the world of "I". We get lost in our very personal story, in only the aspects we can physically sense of our story, the depth of our shadow, and the pain and despair we may feel. The current expression of dis-ease and dis-harmony. But our physical/mental/emotional story is also our soul's story, and there is much we don't know yet.

    There is so much for us to discover in this brave new world, and so much power behind the actions towards wellness that you will now take. Gather your breath and your resilience, and anchor into the hope activist within as you trust in your power to make Mighty things happen.

Last, but not least ...

18. ***Bookend your day. Start the day with a homemade green juice, end your day with a mindfulness practice—every day!*** If there is one concept you can take away from this book, one tool to build a stronger foundation for your self—it's to bookend your day.

    The days go by fast, and how we start our day sets the tone for the rest of it. How we end our day allows us to savour it. So, begin your day with a glass of homemade green juice or a smoothie. Think of it as your multivitamin. It will cleanse you, build you, tickle your brain, and promote your health and the bounce in your step to the next level.

    End your day with a mindfulness practice that allows you to process and savour the day, to honour where you're at, a practice that keeps you in self-inquiry and brings you into stillpoint awareness. It will change what you choose to keep from the day to inform your tomorrow.

Unleashing your mightiness is a process. There truly are no magic pills, but this one comes pretty close to it.

REMEMBER ... There is a revolution going on!

BE YOUR OWN REVOLUTION

Revolution might sound a little dramatic, but in this world, choosing authenticity and worthiness is an absolute act of resistance. Choosing to live and love with our whole hearts is an act of defiance.

— Brenéé Brown, *The Gifts of Imperfection.*

You are the Medicine.

Gather your tools. Know they are a map into your sacred heart. They are not you, nor are they your heart. But make these tools your own; add a dash of your own spice and blend them into your core.

Remember your truth is your own. Yet collectively we hold one purpose, and that is to love, and one mission, to share that **love**.

Gather your tools, and along the way others on their own journey will greet you. Gather your tools, and revolution yourself alive!

Trust your body. Trust your heart.

Be your own revolution. Leap into wellness in sacred balance. Live in the now.

Take the time to know your self, away from your Ego. Take the time to become your self, follow your heart. Take the time to shine your very best light forward. Take the time to become a shining radiant one.

Take the time to pause and feel. For if not now, when? For if not you, then who will?

Seek the ways in which your soul's purpose and your radiance allow you to love bigger, allow you to engage in sacred reciprocity …

Seek what has always been seeking you. Seek it, remember it, embrace it, surrender to it, and walk it.

Let your life be a prayer. Let your medicine be ours, in service to the seven generations to come.

Let your process be your revolution; let it inspire me into loving you more deeply.

DARLING, YOU GOT THIS

I am not what happened to me,
I am what I choose to become.

—*Carl G. Jung*

As you journey on your quest of alignment with your Mighty inner healer and with radiant health, darling, know you are unique. Darling, know that you, and only you, know yourself best, deep within the boundaries of your skin. And darling, know you've got this.

Liquid nutrition (inclusive of the ritual of detox), mindfulness practices, and inner questing are a magical realm. Explore them. Stay curious. Gift your self the time to get to know them, and through them get to know your self. Revolution yourself from the inside out.

As a yogi and shamanic practitioner, my teachings are informed by my practice in as much as by my teachers of both traditions. They are informed by my own healing journey and all the tools I have used, and continue to use to heal and transform. So, what I have offered you, throughout the pages of this book, has been informed by own my path—an integrated universal path to access the inner space of deep healing and source available to all who seek their own inner space of truth.

One path that contains many roads, many universal truths and laws, yet it has one purpose: to anchor into love and living in sacred relationship, and to share it. I invite you to join me along this very precious earth walk to your inner path of sacredness, interrelationship, mightiness, love, truth, deep healing, and deep nourishment; for the more we nourish the world, the more we are nourished by the world.

Now, as we begin to part, I invite you to seek and implement the practices that build you up, that power up your health and ignite your becoming. I invite you to actively witness that which nourishes you and brings vitality, and that which leaves you drained and not feeling well. I have offered many tools, practices, and rituals for you to try, test, and feel into. Now you get to decide for yourself what works for you, and what does not. You decide what you will keep and what you will let go of. Above all, I invite you to pursue your own tipping point: that moment when the expression of health and harmony will be stronger than the expression of disease and disharmony, and you will step into the vibrant, radiant good health you have been seeking.

I urge you to seek, to become, to be your best self forward, for the entire universe is calling. May our journeys cross again. May you revolution yourself alive as you rewild your heart and anchor your mind into it. May the depth of what you seek inform your path of remembering.

There is only one path: yours, uniquely yours, always informed by the path of many who have walked this Earth before you.

Reclaim your one path. Awaken into your mightiness. ***Darling, you've got this.***

IS YOUR HEART FOLLOWING ITS CREED?

Awaken to the power of your truth. Surrender to the power of your heart.

Reclaim your sacredness for you are already whole. Journey through the seven generations of your ancestral being, because they are a part of your foundation.

Plant the seed of care in each other. Feel the love of the seven generations that will come after your time on Earth has passed.

Recalibrate your heart compass. Eat raw food. Reconnect the hope activist within.

Make each day better. Believe in your power. Align with your purpose.

Get your hands into the earth. Grow. Grow your own food.

Express yourself alive. Create. Create yourself alive. Be love. Lovely be.

Wear your sacred heart on your sleeve.

Travel the longest journey of all: the 17 inches that separate your mind from your heart.

Be your own revolution.

Juice every damn day. Power up your health. Drink your medicine. Rawck it all!

Become a living sanctuary. You, yes, you. Embody yourself alive.

Let your breath fill every inch of your body from the inside out. Move. Link movement to breath. Shake it all down. Be still.

Anchor your breath in your heart. Bear witness. Get outside. Connect with nature.

Find your blisscipline and stick with it.

Walk barefoot. Ground knee deep into the Earth as you touch the sky. Bask in the moonlight.

Journey on … become soul. Soul is calling … do you feel her pull?

*May your heart be sparked like a **wildfire!***

In sacred awareness,

XOXO,

Naty Howard

PROGRAMS BY NATY HOWARD

Your Mighty Inner Healer

- An eight-week virtual course based on the content of this transformational book, this course will help you root into the teachings I have shared, as you create a stronger foundation for healing, health, and well-being. Through each practice, you will consistently shift into radiance, anchor into your centre, and align with your truth.

Unleash Your Mightiness MasterClass

- This eight-month online program is an in-depth course to dive deep into unleashing your own mightiness! In alignment with this book, each month is an opportunity to awaken, align, and ignite your self through wisdom, tools, and practices to shift you into thriving.

3 or 7 Day Mighty Detox

- This detox is an online guided juice/smoothie feast to cleanse and detoxify as you deeply nourish yourself to radiance, using the three pillars of your roadmap to wellness: juice/smoothie feasting, mindfulness practices, and inner questing.

Mighty Juice- transform your health with the power of liquid nutrition

- This is a nine-module online program into the art and the power of liquid nutrition: juices, smoothies, teas, broths, and elixirs as a tool for reclaiming your health and deepening your healing.

Moon Magic

- A six-week online journey into the heart of soul that uses yoga, breath work, ritual, ceremony, crystal activation, and shamanic journeying in alignment with the magic of the moon.

Detox Yoga Flow

- An online yoga class to awaken, align, and anchor as you release and detoxify your body temple. Includes Detox Yoga Flow Video Class (80 min) and the Ritual of Detox Worksheet.

New and Full Moon Yoga Spirit Medicine Circles

- Bi-monthly in-person circles to gather and anchor into sacredness in alignment with the moon through ritual, ceremony, vinyasa yoga flow, shamanic journeying, and sharing circles. Filled with magic, these evenings are a complete recalibration of your heart.

Spirit Speaks

- In-Person Shamanic Apprenticeship Level 1 and Level 2. Refine your skills as a healer and make this ancient practice a part of your toolkit. Learn about the principles and the five Elements of shamanism. Build your own shamanic sacred altar. Transform your relationship with yourself, your soul as you anchor into your true nature. Align your mind, heart, and soul into congruent action.

In-Person Workshops and Retreats.

- These programs are always being adjusted and updated. For more and up-to-date information, please visit: www.natyhoward.com

SUGGESTED READINGS

The following books have inspired and informed my healing journey. You will find an expanded updated list online at https://www.natyhoward.com/inspiring-wisdom

Raw foods, Whole Foods and Liquid Nutrition

- *Conscious Eating*, Gabriel Cousens, MD
- *Spiritual Nutrition*, Gabriel Cousens, MD
- *The Hippocrates Diet and Health Program*, Ann Wigmore
- *Enlightened Eating*, Caroline Dupont
- *Going Raw*, Judith Wignall

Ayurveda

- *Ayurvedic Tongue Diagnosis*, Walter "Shantree" Kacera
- *A Life of Balance*, Maya Tiwari
- *The Idiot's Guide to Ayurveda*, Sahara Rose
- *The Ayurvedic Cookbook*, Amadea Morningstar

Mindfulness and Meditation

- *Meditation and Mantras*, Swami Vishnu-Devananda
- *The Power of Now*, Eckart Tolle
- *The Miracle of Mindfulness: An Introduction to the Practice of Meditation*; Thich Nhat Hanh
- *How to See Yourself As You Really Are*, His Holiness The Dalai Lama

Quantum Healing

- *You Can Heal Your Life*, Louise Hay
- *Perfect Health*, Deepak Chopra
- *Quantum Healing*, Deepak Chopra
- *Ordering From the Cosmic Kitchen*, Patricia J. Crane

Yoga

- *Yoga and the Sacred Fire*, David Frawley
- *Light on Life*, B. K. S. Iyengar
- *Light on Yoga*, B. K. S. Iyengar
- *Anatomy of the Spirit*, Caroline Myss, PhD
- *Eastern Body, Western Mind*, Anodea Judith

Shamanism

- *Shapeshifting into Higher Consciousness*, Llyn Roberts
- *Awakening to the Spirit World*, Sandra Ingerman and Hank Wesselman
- *Letters of Courage*, Don Oscar Miro-Quesada
- *Peruvian Shamanism: The Pachakuti Mesa*, Matthew Magee
- *Animal Spirit Guides*, Steven D. Farmer, PhD
- *Medicine Cards: The Discovery of Power Through the Ways of Animals*, Jamie Sams & David Carson

Spirituality

- *In Search of the Medicine Buddha, A Himalayan Journey*, David Crow
- *The Ringing Cedars Series*, Vladimir Megre
- *The Alchemist*, Paulo Cohelo
- *Autobiography of a Yogi*, Paramahansa Yogananda

ACKNOWLEDGEMENTS

There are many people to acknowledge, for the creation of a book is never a solo effort. First, I want to thank my teachers, and the people who helped shape my healing journey beyond the writing of this book. Some of them have become great friends and I still bask in the medicine of their teachings. Some I have heard speak at lectures or I have read their books, but have never met in person. Still, their influence has still been key along my path of emergence.

Angela Nickle and Happy Farms, Angie Di Orio and Andrew Blake, Brian Clement and Hippocrates Institute, Brian Gangel, Caroline Dupont, Chong Wu, Cindy Miro-Quesada, Cindy Sellers and the Angel Farms Team, Crystal Veenstra, David Schonfeld, Don Oscar Miro-Quesada, Emily Wolff, Felicia Weinstein, Karen Pfister, Kelly Parker, Kohav Howard, Lizbeth Schonfeld, Michael Siddall, Schonfeld Fam Jam, Sean Corn, Shaman Bolivar, Shantree Kacera and The Living Centre, Thomas Mock, Rabbi Gabriel Cousens, MD, MD(H), ND(hc), DD, and Tree of Life Center.

To the five grandmothers named Dian(ne)/a whose medicine I deeply carry within:
Diana Atherton Davies, Dianne Bourbonies, Grandmother Dianne Ottereyes-Reed, Diana Syverston, Diana Zweygardt.

To my muse, who distills the words from the Above into my heart.

To my editor *Janet Matthews and my publisher FriesenPress:* In the vast ocean of editors and publishing houses, you are both truly one of a kind.

Last but not least, to my husband Noah and my children Louie, Theo, and Ezra, you are my greatest gifts. What an honour it is, to get to fall in love with you over and over again.

DRINK THE LIGHT
EAT THE LIGHT
THINK THE LIGHT
LIVE IN THE LIGHT
BE THE LIGHT

Printed in Canada